JUN 21

ALSO BY LAWRENCE WRIGHT

The End of October
God Save Texas
The Terror Years
Thirteen Days in September
Going Clear
The Looming Tower
God's Favorite
Twins
Remembering Satan
Saints and Sinners
In the New World
City Children, Country Summer

THE
PLAGUE
YEAR

THE
PLAGUE
YEAR

America in the Time of Covid

Lawrence Wright

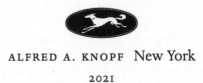

ALFRED A. KNOPF New York

2021

THIS IS A BORZOI BOOK
PUBLISHED BY ALFRED A. KNOPF

Copyright © 2021 by Lawrence Wright

All rights reserved. Published in the United States by Alfred A. Knopf,
a division of Penguin Random House LLC, New York, and distributed
in Canada by Penguin Random House Canada Limited, Toronto.
This is an expanded version of "The Plague Year" which originally
appeared in *The New Yorker* on December 8, 2020.

www.aaknopf.com

Knopf, Borzoi Books, and the colophon are registered
trademarks of Penguin Random House LLC.

ISBN: 9780593320723
LCCN: 2021932374

Jacket photograph by Callaghan O'Hare / Reuters / Alamy
Jacket design by Chip Kidd

Manufactured in Canada
First Edition

In memory of those no longer with us

Contents

THE
PLAGUE
YEAR

Prologue

HISTORY HAS PAID a call on Wuhan before. In 1966, Mao Zedong, the seventy-two-year-old chairman of the Communist Party, visited the city. He already had the death of tens of millions of people on his hands: the forced industrialization campaign of the Great Leap Forward led to the greatest famine in human history. Mao inaugurated that catastrophe by swimming in the Yangtze, the largest river in China, at one of its widest points, in Wuhan. Now he worried that his grasp on power was weakening. There were rumors that he was in ill health or near death. He needed to prove them wrong. He had just announced the latest stage of his plan for China, the Cultural Revolution. He would swim the river again.

A legend was concocted in the party press about how far and how quickly the old man swam that day—more than nine miles in sixty-five minutes, according to the state newspaper, which would have been a world record. Video of the event shows him doing a leisurely side stroke, surrounded by bodyguards and thousands of enthusiastic supporters who plunged in after him. The swim was a turning point in Mao's chaotic rule, amplifying a personality cult among young people who now saw him as their champion. They became the Red Guards, the vanguard of the reign of terror that lasted until Mao's death ten years later.

Mao visited Wuhan again the following year, but this time he was greeted by insurrection. Demonstrators, some carrying iron bars, others with machine guns, surrounded Mao's villa, shouting slogans through loudspeakers and actually breaking into the compound. Mao was spirited away, but it was the most perilous moment in his nearly two decades of rule. Wuhan was purged; 184,000 citizens and soldiers were reported killed or injured in Hubei Province.

Present-day Wuhan is a city of eleven million people in the heartland of the country. Like Chicago, Wuhan is a major transportation center, a crossroads of railways and expressways; the Wuhan Tianhe International Airport is a hub of the Chinese airline system, with direct flights to major cities all over the world. It is an intensely modern city, but like all of China, it sits atop a mountain of trauma.

On December 26, 2019, at Hubei Provincial Hospital of Integrated Chinese and Western Medicine, Dr. Zhang Jixian examined an elderly couple complaining of fever and a cough—flulike symptoms—but a CT scan showed a form of pneumonia the doctor hadn't seen before. She summoned the couple's son and found that he, too, was suffering from an unknown pneumonia. She observed, "It is unlikely that all three members of a family caught the same disease at the same time unless it is an infectious disease." At about the same time, healthcare workers were falling ill with similar symptoms, indicating human-to-human transmissions of the new pathogen was taking place. That fact was not acknowledged by government officials until nearly a month later; instead, authorities instructed the medical staff not to wear masks or gowns because they might give rise to panic.

On December 30, 2019, Ai Fen, the director of the emergency department of Wuhan Central Hospital, received a lab report of an atypical pneumonia. Like other doctors, Ai had noticed a stream of patients with unfamiliar pneumonias. A novel disease probably had been circulating in Hubei Province since November or possibly mid-October. Some of the cases seemed to be connected to the Huanan Seafood Wholesale Market not far from Dr. Ai's hospital. Ten of its 653 stalls offered exotic animals—including badgers, snakes, crocodiles, and pangolins—which were sold live and slaughtered in front of the customers. It was called a "wet market" because it was covered with scales and blood and water that splashed out of the fish tanks. Often, animal cages were stacked on top of each other, so that a palm civet nursing a virus might pass it to a hedgehog in the cage below. People also get infections from animals, but they are not considered human diseases unless they are shown to be transmitted from one person to another.

The lab report diagnosed Dr. Ai's patient as suffering from SARS coronavirus. That report would prove inaccurate; it was actually a previously unknown SARS coronavirus that causes a disease that would come to be called Covid-19.

Dr. Ai was used to dealing with crises—anyone who works in an emergency department has to have a steady temperament—but the lab report left her shaken. She circled the diagnosis in red and shared it with a few colleagues, reminding them to "pay attention to protecting themselves."

There was good reason for Dr. Ai's concern. Severe acute respiratory syndrome, or SARS, a coronavirus that erupted in China in November 2002, had thrown the country into its worst political crisis since the 1989 Tiananmen Square uprising. The initial response of the Chinese government and the ruling Communist Party had been to hide the outbreak, even from its own public health officers. Under the cloak of the news blackout, SARS spread through the country, reaching Beijing the following March. Doctors in charge of the treatment had no idea what was going on, so closely held was the information, but frightened rumors spread by text messages. Pharmacies sold out of antibiotics and flu medicines. The new disease killed nearly 10 percent of the people it infected, becoming the first epidemic since HIV/AIDS dangerous enough to threaten the entire world. SARS is thought to have passed from horseshoe bats into masked palm civets and presumably into its first human hosts in the wet markets of Guangdong.

When World Health Organization (WHO) authorities were finally allowed into the country to inspect Beijing hospitals, in mid-April of 2003, patients suffering from the disease were smuggled into ambulances and driven around the city or checked into hotels until the inspectors finished their tour. By that time the contagion had already skipped from China to Hong Kong, Hanoi, Singapore, Taiwan, Ulaanbaatar, Toronto, and San Francisco. That outbreak eventually reached thirty-two countries, but through heroic efforts on the part of public health officials around the world, and simple luck, the disease was contained in July 2003, nine months after it first appeared.

Another coronavirus, MERS-CoV, which causes Middle East respiratory syndrome, or MERS, was first reported in Saudi Arabia in 2012. It proved to be less contagious than SARS but much deadlier, killing about 35 percent of the people it infected. Public health officials everywhere were on edge about the potential danger of coronaviruses, but fortunately MERS spread rather poorly.

The SARS contagion allowed the entire world to peer into Chinese society through the lens of a mortal disease. The international scorn directed at the Chinese government shattered the country's confidence and sidelined its ambition to take its place at the head of the table of nations. There were reasons for the cover-up of SARS, including the fear, typical of repressive systems, of passing bad news up the ranks; a tangled bureaucracy; and the singular priority of economic growth over all other considerations; but the naked fact stood that the Chinese government was willing to sacrifice its own people and place the entire world in jeopardy, risking millions of lives, simply to avoid accountability for the outbreak.

In 2005, because of SARS, new global health regulations were instituted, requiring greater transparency. The Chinese government seemed to be entering an era of openness, but in the seventeen years since the humiliation of the SARS epidemic, that intention had not been seriously tested.

News of the novel virus circulated quickly, frustrating the government's attempts to block it. One of the doctors who received Dr. Ai's message was Li Wenliang, an ophthalmologist at the same hospital, who reposted it to former medical school classmates on a private WeChat group, warning them to tell their families and friends to take precautions but also to keep the news confidential. He suspected there was human-to-human transmission because patients were being quarantined. That same day, the Wuhan Municipal Health Commission ordered hospitals to treat patients suffering from an unknown pneumonia, apparently because victims had been turned away. It's unclear how much the central government knew until that point, but almost immediately scanned copies of the official messages were leaked onto social media.

The Taiwan Centers for Disease Control, having noticed the posts, contacted health authorities in mainland China and were told that the cluster existed but that it had turned out not to be SARS, an assertion that the Taiwanese had reason to doubt. Taiwan pressed the WHO for more information and shared its suspicion that the new disease was likely to be communicable among humans.

Mainland China refuses to allow Taiwan to participate in international organizations, including the United Nations and the WHO, insisting it is not an actual nation but a province of the People's Republic. The WHO did send a message to its country office in mainland China to follow up on the Taiwanese request, but China wouldn't admit that the pathogen was transmissible between humans for another three weeks, which contributed to the fatal delay of so many countries to prepare for the onslaught. Left to draw their own conclusions, the Taiwanese began early screening and quarantines, which would result in a strikingly low rate of infection on the island.

On December 31, the morning after Dr. Ai posted her note, Chinese technology companies began censoring phrases on social media, such as "unknown Wuhan pneumonia" and "Wuhan Seafood Market." But that same day, an official report from Hubei Province said that there were twenty-seven patients with similar respiratory symptoms in the city's hospitals, seven of whom were critically ill. The news was out.

Dr. Ai's superiors at the hospital reprimanded her for spreading rumors that might cause panic and "damage stability." When she suggested that the virus could be contagious, she was told not to discuss it with anyone. She was ashamed and terrified. When she went home, she told her husband, "If something happens to me, you will have to take good care of the children." She was haunted by the blank face of a man receiving the death certificate for his thirty-two-year-old son. Another man had arrived at the hospital too sick to get out of his car. By the time Dr. Ai went to fetch him, he was dead. "If I had known what was to happen, I would not have cared about the reprimand," she recalled. "I would have fucking talked about it to whomever, wherever I could."

Dr. Li Wenliang, the ophthalmologist who had reposted Dr. Ai's note, was charged with rumor mongering that "severely disturbed the social order." He was forced to sign a confession. His punishment, and that of seven other doctors who had publicly discussed the outbreak, was broadcast on China Central Television, a clear message to others who might attempt to undermine the government's narrative. Humble and compassionate, Li had a quiet charisma that made his punishment seem notably unfair. A few days after Li returned to the hospital, he caught the virus from a patient. "How can the bulletins still be saying there is no human-to-human transmission, and no medical worker infections?" he wondered.

Chinese authorities continued to scour web pages and social media posts concerning the outbreak and forced reporters into detention disguised as quarantine. On January 11, an ER nurse at Dr. Ai's hospital became infected with the virus, but hospital authorities again denied that human-to-human transmission was occurring.

When Dr. Ai gave an interview to the Chinese magazine *Renwu* (People) in March, it was immediately removed from the internet. Some highly inventive dissidents rewrote the interview to get around the censors, using emojis, Morse code, braille, and even Sindarin, the fictional language spoken by elves in J. R. R. Tolkien's Hobbit books. By that time, however, the Chinese government had shut down Wuhan and regained control of the narrative.

FACED ONCE MORE with a new virus that had the potential to become a catastrophic pandemic, the Chinese government again failed to warn the WHO or even its own people about the dangers of the new disease until the news was already out. Several Chinese labs quickly sequenced the new virus. The genomic sequence is the first step toward understanding the virus and serves as a starting gun for the creation of a vaccine. But Chinese authorities ordered unauthorized labs to stop testing samples from Wuhan and to destroy existing stock. These steps slowed the flow of information about the virus, and they also impeded the science required to develop a reliable test in countries that were not given samples to work with. On January 5, a group of scientists, led by Professor Yong-zhen Zhang, at Fudan University, in Shanghai, defiantly submitted the genome to the U.S. National Institutes of Health GenBank. Thereupon, Shanghai authorities shut down Professor Zhang's laboratory for "rectification." The Chinese Centers for Disease Control did not officially release the sequence until January 10.

American intelligence would later surmise that the central government had been caught by surprise because of the duplicity of local officials, but it is also true that Chinese authorities continued to downplay the threat once they knew about it. They demanded that researchers stop publishing about the virus without government authorization and cease warning about the danger of the outbreak. They continued to deny that there was evidence of human transmission. The government refused to share virus samples with the U.S., which set back the production of the tests needed to detect the disease by a couple of weeks. The WHO field office in China was finally allowed a brief visit to Wuhan on January 20, followed by a carefully managed delegation of WHO officials, led by the director-general, Dr. Tedros Adhanom Ghebreyesus, to Beijing one week later, a month after the first case surfaced.

The government likely disguised the true mortality figures; for instance, the official death toll in Wuhan was 2,579 (later revised to 3,869), but there were social media reports that the city's eight crematoriums were operating around the clock, and photos showing long lines of citizens waiting to pick up the urns containing the ashes of their loved ones—perhaps as many as 3,500 urns per day. One preliminary study estimated that the true death toll in Wuhan was around 36,000, nearly ten times the official figure.

Dr. Li died on February 6, the first known of the thousands of healthcare workers around the world who would perish in the contagion, including four other doctors from his own hospital. He left behind a five-year-old child and a pregnant wife. The mass mourning that greeted his death was an expression of the anguish expressed by great numbers of Chinese people. They saw Li as a whistleblower and a martyr for free speech. They laid flowers in front of the Wuhan hospital and blew whistles in his honor all over China. It was a telling indicator of the provisional nature of Communist Party rule. Before he died, Dr. Li told Caixin magazine, "A healthy society shouldn't have only one voice."

The coronavirus revealed China as a country struggling in the grip of one-party control, at once fearful and defiant, ambitious and proud of its rise in the world but also seething with popular resentment at the political calculations that valued the party's image over human life. The reluctance to disclose the scope of the outbreak and to share the science that was necessary to stop its spread displayed an indifference to life that is the enduring legacy of Maoism.

In Wuhan, on January 18, the traditional Chinese New Year potluck banquet took place around the city with 40,000 households participating and no authorities standing in the way. On January 20, with the number of deaths rising, Zhong Nanshan, the best-known face of China's public health community, finally confirmed that the new virus was a communicable disease. Not until then was protective gear provided to the medical teams. Two days later, China announced a total quarantine of Wuhan. Eventually about 650 million people, nearly half the population of China, were placed in quarantine. Nothing in history compared with the scale of it. The contagion was smothered, along with dissent.

By that time nearly half the population of Wuhan had already left the city for Chinese New Year, the most important holiday on the calendar, when people return to their hometowns, visit relatives and friends, and travel for vacation. Chinese authorities estimated nearly three billion trips would be taken during the forty-day festival. An immense portion of the travelers would pass through Wuhan along their way. International students went home for the holidays. It is the world's largest annual migration.

Covid-19 was on the move.

1

"It's Going to Be Just Fine"

ONE MINUTE BEFORE midnight on December 30, 2019, ProMED, a closely watched online publication of the International Society for Infectious Diseases, posted an article translated from Chinese media stating that twenty-seven cases of what was termed a "pneumonia of unknown cause" had been found in Wuhan. The Centers for Disease Control and Prevention (CDC) and the World Health Organization learned of it almost immediately.

Robert Redfield, the sixty-eight-year-old director of the CDC, was vacationing with his family in Deep Creek, Maryland, when he read the ProMED notice on New Year's Eve. Several alarming details jumped out. The pneumonia appeared to be associated with a seafood market in Wuhan. Patients suffering from the pneumonia were placed in isolation, which was prudent, but suggestive that the health authorities were concerned about human-to-human transmission. "Whether or not it is SARS has not yet been clarified," the document said, "and citizens need not panic."

On January 3, 2020, Redfield spoke with his counterpart in China, George Fu Gao. Like many similarly named organizations around the world, the Chinese Center for Disease Control and Prevention was modeled on the American original. Redfield had heard that the first twenty-seven reported cases included three family clusters. It was unlikely that each of them had been simultaneously infected by a caged civet cat in a wet market. When pressed, Gao assured Redfield that there was no evidence of human-to-human transmission. It seemed to Redfield that Gao was only just learning of the outbreak himself. Redfield offered to send a team of CDC disease detectives from the U.S to investigate, but Gao said he was not authorized to invite them. He told Redfield to make a formal request to the Chinese government. Redfield did so, and immediately assembled a team of two dozen epidemiologists and disease specialists, but no invitation ever arrived.

The specter of SARS hung over both men. Gao was teaching at Oxford during the 2003 outbreak. He returned to China the following year to head the Institute of Microbiology at the Chinese Academy of Sciences, and in 2017 he was appointed director of the Chinese CDC. A widely published and world-renowned virologist and immunologist, Gao was hired as part of the intense investment that China made in medical science after the SARS debacle, establishing almost from scratch the world's largest reporting system for health emergencies and infectious disease outbreaks, building clinics and specialty hospitals, expanding research budgets, and providing free universal healthcare for its citizens. In short order, China appeared poised to become a leader in global health. The Chinese CDC was a critical part of that design, and its main mission was to detect emerging diseases, including anything that looked like SARS. But in the face of the new disease, the Chinese public health system had once again totally failed. There was no way of really knowing how many people were infected.

When Redfield first spoke to Gao, the "unknown pneumonia" was presumed to be confined to China, not yet posing an imminent threat to the rest of the world. In fact, the virus was already present in California, Oregon, and Washington State, and within the next two weeks would be spreading in Massachusetts, Wisconsin, Iowa, Connecticut, Michigan, and Rhode Island—well before America's first official case was detected.

In another conversation that first week of the new year, Dr. Gao started to cry. "I think we're too late," he told Redfield. "We're too late."

MATTHEW POTTINGER WAS getting nervous. As the Trump administration was entering its final year, he was one of few who had been there from the start. Perhaps his durability stemmed from being so hard to categorize. Fluent in Mandarin, he had spent seven years in China, reporting for Reuters and the *Wall Street Journal*. He left journalism at the age of thirty-two and joined the Marines, a career switch that confounded everyone who knew him. In Afghanistan, he co-authored an influential paper with Lieutenant General Michael Flynn on improving military intelligence. When Trump picked Flynn to be his national security adviser, Flynn lured Pottinger to be his Asia director. Scandal evicted Flynn from his job almost overnight, but Pottinger stayed, serving five subsequent national security chiefs. In September 2019, Trump appointed Pottinger deputy national security adviser. In a very noisy administration, he had quietly become one of the most influential people shaping American foreign policy.

Pottinger is of medium height, with blue eyes, his dark blond hair still cropped in a military cut. His eyebrows are a brighter blond, lending him the quality of appearing extra awake. In 2003, he was in China reporting on the SARS cover-up for the *Wall Street Journal*. Now, when Chinese authorities were assuring the U.S. that there was little evidence of human-to-human transmission, that the virus was fragile and would not stand up to warmer weather, and that the situation was under control, familiar alarms were ringing in Pottinger's mind.

He was struck by the disparity between official accounts of the novel coronavirus in China, which scarcely mentioned the disease, and Chinese social media, which was aflame with rumors and anecdotes. Someone posted a photograph of a sign on the door of a Wuhan hospital saying that the emergency room was closed because staff were infected. Meantime, the WHO—relying on Chinese assurances—tweeted that there was no clear evidence of human-to-human transmission, countering a statement made the same day in a press briefing by a WHO scientist who said the opposite.

The National Security Council (NSC) addresses global developments and offers the president options to consider. On January 14, Pottinger authorized a briefing for the NSC staff by the State Department and the Department of Health and Human Services, along with CDC director Redfield. That first interagency meeting to discuss the situation in Wuhan wasn't prompted by official intelligence; in fact, there was practically none of that.

The next day, two hundred guests assembled in the East Room of the White House to witness the signing of the first phase of the U.S.-China trade deal. Cabinet members and corporate leaders mingled with members of Congress, governors, Fox News stars, and the Chinese delegation. "Together we are righting the wrongs of the past and delivering a future of economic justice and security for American workers, farmers, and families," the president said, in front of a bank of American and Chinese flags. He called Chinese president Xi Jinping "a very, very good friend."

On January 20, the coronavirus officially arrived in America. "This is a thirty-five-year-old young man who works here in the United States, who visited Wuhan," Dr. Anthony Fauci, director of the National Institute of Allergy and Infectious Diseases (NIAID), said on a Voice of America broadcast. "There was no doubt that sooner or later we were going to see a case. And we have." President Trump took note of the event at the World Economic Forum in Davos. "It's one person coming in from China, and we have it under control," he remarked. "It's going to be just fine."

COVID-19 ARRIVED in America at a vulnerable moment in the nation's history. The country was undergoing a wrenching political realignment, brought to a head by the 2016 election of Donald Trump, whose policies on trade, deficit, alliances, and immigration were at odds with traditional Republican conservativism. His election pulled the country further into a cataclysm of identity politics, shrinking the GOP into a pool of aging white voters who felt disparaged, resentful, and left behind. The #MeToo movement had ignited an edgy dialogue between the sexes. As the stock market soared, long-delayed questions of income disparity and racial justice were pressing forward. Every dissonant chord among the parties, the races, and the genders was amplified within the echo chambers the fractured communities had made of themselves.

Into this turbulent, deeply troubled, but prideful society, the coronavirus would act as a hurricane of change, flattening the most powerful economy in the world, leveling not the physical cities but the idea of cities, strewing misfortune and blame and regrets along with the tens, the hundreds, the thousands, the hundreds of thousands of obituaries.

No country would escape the destruction the virus inflicted, but none had as much to lose as America. Wealth and power breed hubris, and perhaps Covid-19 was the force that America needed—to be humbled, to reckon with itself, to once again attempt to create the democracy it had always intended to be.

On the other hand, America's moment at the forefront of history might have passed, and Covid-19 was a blow it was no longer strong enough to fend off. Rival powers—with China at the top—were competing for control of the new millennium. This was a challenge to democracy, which was America's cause in the world. The alternative to American preeminence was not a globe full of mini-Americas but a world dominated by tyrants. Freedom was at stake, as it always is, but America had tied itself into a political knot. The cyclonic forces of fascism and nihilism gained in power as the center weakened. The only thing that kept democracy from winding up in a suicidal brawl of self-interest was a sense of common purpose, but the pandemic exposed that the United States no longer had one.

In those early days, when politics mattered most, few paid attention when nature entered the ring. It had been a century since the last great pandemic, which was nursed in the trenches and troop ships of the First World War and spread even into tropical jungles and Eskimo villages. That flu lasted two years and killed between forty and a hundred million people. Back then, scientists scarcely knew what a virus was, so how could they fight it? By the twenty-first century, however, infectious disease was considered a nuisance, not a mortal threat to civilization—at least, this was a common assumption among the elected officials who were charged with protecting the country. This lack of concern was reflected in the diminished budgets that nourished the great institutions that had led the world in countering disease and keeping Americans healthy. Hospitals closed; stockpiles of emergency equipment were not replenished. The specter of an unknown respiratory virus arising in China gave nightmares to public health officials, but it was not on the agenda of most American policymakers. In January 2017, days before Donald Trump was inaugurated, Dr. Fauci had warned there was "no doubt" that the incoming president would be dealing with an infectious disease outbreak. "We will definitely get surprised in the next few years," he predicted.

And yet there were so many reasons to feel complacent. In October 2019, the Nuclear Threat Initiative, together with the Johns Hopkins Center for Health Security, and the Economist Intelligence Unit, compiled the first-ever "Global Health Security Index," a sober report of a world largely unprepared to deal with a pandemic. "Unfortunately, political will for accelerating health security is caught in a perpetual cycle of panic and neglect," the authors observed. "No country is fully prepared." Yet one country stood above all others in its readiness to confront a novel disease: the United States.

During the transition to the Trump administration, the Obama White House handed off a sixty-nine-page document called the "Playbook for Early Response to High-Consequence Emerging Infectious Disease Threats and Biological Incidents." A meticulous, step-by-step guide for combatting a "pathogen of pandemic potential," the playbook contains a directory of the government's resources in time of need and is meant to be pulled off the shelf the moment things start to go haywire.

At the top of the list of dangerous pathogens are the respiratory viruses, including novel influenzas, orthopoxviruses (such as smallpox), and coronaviruses. The playbook outlines the conditions under which various government agencies should be enlisted. With domestic outbreaks, the playbook specifies that "[w]hile States hold significant power and responsibility related to public health response outside of a declared Public Health Emergency, the American public will look to the U.S. Government for action when multi-state or other significant public health events occur." Questions concerning the severity and contagiousness of a disease, or how to handle potentially hazardous waste, should be directed to the Department of Health and Human Services (HHS), the Federal Emergency Management Agency (FEMA), and the Environmental Protection Agency (EPA). Is there evidence of deliberate intent, such as a terrorist action? The FBI has the lead. Have isolation and quarantine been implemented? How robust is contact tracing? Is clinical care in the region scalable if cases explode? There are many such questions, with decisions proposed and agencies assigned. Because the playbook was passed to a new administration that might not be familiar with the manifold resources of the federal government, there are appendices describing such entities as the Surge Capacity Force in the Department of Homeland Security, consisting of a group of FEMA reservists and others that can be called upon as "deployable human assets." The Pentagon's Military Aeromedical Evacuation Team can be assembled to transport patients. HHS has a Disaster Mortuary Operational Response Team, with the dry acronym DMORT, consisting of "intermittent federal employees, each with a particular field of expertise," such as medical examiners, pathologists, anthropologists, dental assistants, and investigators.

The Trump administration jettisoned the Obama playbook. In 2019, HHS, headed by Alex M. Azar Jr., conducted an exercise called Crimson Contagion. It involved a number of government agencies, including the Pentagon and the NSC; healthcare organizations and major hospitals, such as the Mayo Clinic; public groups with a specific interest in health-care, including the American Red Cross; and twelve state governments. The exercise scenario envisioned an international group of tourists visiting China who become infected with a novel influenza, and then spread it across the world. One of the tourists, a middle-aged man, returns to Chicago with a dry cough. His son attends a crowded public event, and the contagion races through America. There's no vaccine and antiviral drugs are ineffective. Within a few months, the hypothetical flu kills 586,000 Americans.

The Trump administration's own exercise was spookily predictive of what was to come, including how chaotically the government would respond. Federal agencies couldn't tell who was in charge; there was a lack of production capacity for personal protective equipment (PPE); ventilators were in short supply; and states were frustrated by their attempts to secure enough resources. Cities defied a CDC recommendation to delay opening their schools. Businesses struggled to figure out how to keep their employees working from home. The longer the hypothetical contagion went on, the more bollixed the government response became. The Public Health Emergency Fund was dangerously depleted; needles, syringes, hospital-grade N95 masks, and other medical essentials were in limited supply and difficult to restock because of an absence of domestic manufacturing capacity. The report on the exercise was briefed to Congress but kept under wraps. By the time Covid-19 arrived in America nothing meaningful had been done to address these shortcomings.

One could say that the Trump administration was in an enviable spot at the beginning of the pandemic. It had a step-by-step playbook that could serve as a guide through bureaucratic snares that accompany such a disaster. It had been alerted to its own failings by the Crimson Contagion exercise. And it was blessed with institutions that were envied and admired throughout the world. Beyond the matchless government medical and research institutions such as the CDC, National Institutes of Health, Walter Reed National Military Medical Center, the U.S. Army Medical Research Institute of Infectious Diseases, and the Biomedical Advanced Research and Development Authority, America also commands the world's top medical schools and many of the largest pharmaceutical companies. When the Trump administration came into office, it was handed the keys to the greatest medical-research establishment in the history of science.

Robert Kadlec, the assistant secretary of HHS in charge of preparedness and response, had led the Crimson Contagion exercise. He would later admit, "We knew before the movie started it was going to have a bad ending."

2

The Trickster

I JUST LOVE infectious diseases," John Brooks, the chief medical officer of the Covid-19 response team at the Centers for Disease Control and Prevention, admitted. "I know diseases are terrible. They kill people. But something about them just grabs me."

Each generation has its own struggle with disease. Brooks's mother, Joan Bertrand Brooks, developed polio in 1939, which left her with a lifelong limp. Like many survivors her symptoms improved in her young adulthood and then returned, forcing her to rely on an electric scooter. Her legs were covered with surgical scars, and her right leg was noticeably shorter than her left. "She spoke about that experience often, and how she was teased, stigmatized, or blatantly discriminated against outside of that community," Brooks recalled.

For Brooks, who is gay, the disease of his generation was HIV/AIDS. He grew up in Washington, D.C., in the Logan Circle neighborhood, which had a large gay population, and watched men he knew disappear. "Guys would get thin and develop lesions and then be gone. It was scary." The fact that science offered no solution was on Brooks's mind when he decided to become a doctor. The day he was accepted at Harvard Medical School, he and his mother went to lunch on K Street to celebrate. Afterwards, they dropped in on a ten-dollar palm reader, who said she saw him marrying a tall Swedish woman and flying around the world with their three children in their private jet. "We had a good laugh," he said. "I should have asked for a refund."

In 2015, Brooks became chief medical officer of the HIV/AIDS division at CDC. Every researcher who has dealt with HIV has been humbled by the various manifestations of this horrid disease. "At every turn, there was something different," Brooks marveled. "All these opportunistic infections show up. What in the world is this all about? Very cool." The experience helped prepare him for the many tricks that Covid-19 would present.

THE CDC WAS FOUNDED in 1946, as the Communicable Disease Center. Atlanta was chosen as the site because it was in the heart of what was called "the malaria zone." Five years later, America was declared malaria-free. The organization's mission broadened to attack other diseases, including typhus and rabies; it led the charge that wiped out polio in the U.S. In 1981, the CDC reported the first cases of AIDS in Los Angeles. The CDC also addressed workplace safety, and it joined with the National Institute of Justice to create the first survey, in 1994, of violence against women. Year after year, the organization—rechristened the Centers for Disease Control and Prevention—maintained a reputation as the gold standard for public health, operating above politics and proving again and again the value of enlightened government and the necessity of science for the furthering of civilization. During the twentieth century, the lifespan of Americans increased by thirty years, largely because of advances in public health, especially vaccination.

When I was a young reporter, I wrote several stories that took me to the CDC. It sits on the edge of the campus of Emory University. I was awed by the recondite learning of the scientists I met there. I attended an annual meeting of the Epidemic Intelligence Service, a swaggering group of Ivy League postdocs and buckaroos in bolo ties who journeyed into hot zones to investigate outbreaks of diseases that could cripple civilization. They struck me as courageous, ingenious, and noble, and they regarded the institution they worked for as somehow sacred.

The CDC has expanded from the days when I used to haunt it; it's now like a midsized college with numerous departments and more building underway, including a new high-containment facility to store all the most dangerous diseases in the world. Lab animals—mice, ferrets, monkeys—inhabit the cages inside the Biosafety Level 4 chambers. Humans move around like deep-sea divers in inflated suits, tethered to an overhead airflow system. The Emergency Operations Center—a large, bright room, with serried rows of wooden desks facing a wall of video screens—exudes a mixture of urgency and professional calm.

Brooks directed the Covid-19 task team with Greg Armstrong, a fellow epidemiologist. Armstrong oversaw the Office of Advanced Molecular Detection, a part of the CDC's center for emerging and zoonotic diseases—those diseases that come from animals, as coronaviruses typically do. Humanity's encroachment into formerly wild regions, coupled with climate change, has forced animals to migrate from traditional habitats. That has engendered a host of new diseases, including Ebola, Zika, West Nile, Nipah—just to mention a few that have arisen fairly recently. At first, SARS-CoV-2 presented itself as a typical coronavirus, like the common cold, spreading rapidly and symptomatically. In fact, this new virus was more like polio, in which most infections are asymptomatic or very mild, with fever and headaches. The cases that doctors actually see are about one in every two hundred infections. Stealth transmission is why polio has been so hard to eradicate.

Armstrong was in Salt Lake City conducting a training on genetic sequencing when he happened to read an article on the website of the *New England Journal of Medicine* titled "Early Transmission Dynamics in Wuhan, China, of Novel Coronavirus-Infected Pneumonia." The authors, mostly associated with the Chinese CDC, were among the first to describe the means of human contagion of the new virus, a development that didn't surprise Armstrong: "Anybody with any experience could tell you it was human-to-human transmission." Then he took a look at Table 1, "Characteristics of Patients," which noted the original source of their infection. Of the Chinese known to have contracted the virus before January 1, 26 percent had no exposure to the Wuhan wet market or to people with apparent respiratory symptoms. (In the following weeks the proportion of people with no obvious source of infection surpassed 70 percent.) Armstrong realized that, unlike SARS or MERS, there were probably a lot of asymptomatic or mild infections with the

SARS-CoV-2 virus. That spelled trouble. Contact tracing, isolation, and quarantine were probably not going to be enough. These telling details were buried in Table 1.

Viruses circulate in our bodies all the time, but not until a virus causes an infection do we begin to talk about disease—when HIV becomes AIDS, or SARS-CoV-2 becomes Covid-19. Confoundingly, a person can be infected and show no symptoms; that person still does not have the disease but he is carrying the virus, which is how Covid spreads asymptomatically. The moment the carrier starts to cough or run a fever because of the virus, we can say he has Covid-19 disease.

It wasn't clear yet how infectious SARS-CoV-2 was, but because it is genetically related to SARS and MERS, the immediate assumption had been that, as with those diseases, people would not be contagious unless they were symptomatic, and that anyone who got infected would manifest some kind of illness. SARS had spread slowly. The time between infection and the onset of symptoms, called a serial interval, was about eight days, and the carrier wasn't contagious until then. SARS-CoV-2 spread twice as fast, which was alarming, but what was totally confounding was the discovery of a "negative serial interval," which meant that some people were showing symptoms before the person who infected them.

CDC's early guidance documents didn't mention that possibility, because the evidence of asymptomatic spread in January and most of February was deemed insufficient. "Frankly, from a public health perspective, you want to lead with facts that reassure people," said Brooks. "It scares people if it sounds like you don't know anything." Later, many people at CDC would wish that they had been able to better explain their early directives. "In the beginning, for every mathematical analysis that indicated a shorter serial interval than incubation period, others reported no difference," Brooks observed. "When the science changed, we changed. And our recommendations changed, too." But by that time, the CDC had been muzzled by the Trump administration.

"THERE ARE THREE THINGS this virus is doing that blow me away," said Brooks, marveling at the resourcefulness and agility of his adversary. "The first is that it directly infects the endothelial cells that line our blood vessels. I'm not aware of any other respiratory viruses that do this. This causes a lot of havoc." Endothelial cells provide a protective coating inside the blood vessels, sealing off the cell like a Ziploc bag. They modulate blood pressure and serve as traffic cops, using sticky proteins to nab passing immune cells and direct them where they are needed when a threatening virus is present.

With coronaviruses, the vulnerable spot for infection in humans is the ACE2 receptor. If the virus is the key, the receptor is the lock it's looking for. ACE2 receptors are enzymes found in the lungs and kidneys as well as in the gut and the brain, accounting for the many manifestations of the disease in humans. They are also abundantly present in the endothelial cells. The virus binds to these receptors, hijacking the cell's machinery to make copies of itself, thereby killing the cell and scouring the thin cell wall, which generates turbulent blood flow. Powerful chemical contents get dumped into the bloodstream, stirring up inflammation elsewhere in the body. Brooks had never seen that condition before.

The second surprise was hypercoagulability—a pronounced tendency to develop blood clots. Brooks was reminded of Michael Crichton's 1969 best-selling thriller, *The Andromeda Strain*, in which a pathogen causes instant clotting, striking down victims in midstride. "This is different," Brooks continued. "You're getting these things called pulmonary embolisms, which are nasty. A clot forms; it travels to the lung, damaging the tissues, blocking blood flow, and creating pressures that can lead to heart problems." These clots can cause strokes, even in previously healthy young people. Brooks referred to an early report documenting autopsies of victims. Nearly all of them had pulmonary thromboses—clots in the lung—but until the autopsy, no one had suspected the clots were even present, let alone the probable cause of death.

"And the last one is this hyperimmune response," said Brooks. Infectious diseases frequently kill by triggering an excessive immune-system response. Brooks gave the example of pneumonia: The body doesn't die because the bacteria eats the lung; it's because the body overreacts by flooding the lung with white blood cells, which carry antibodies but also clog up the lungs with fluid, "and you drown."

Some patients require kidney dialysis or suffer liver damage. The disease can affect the brain and other parts of the nervous system, causing delirium and lasting nerve damage. Covid can also do strange things to the heart. Hospitals began admitting patients with typical symptoms of heart attack, including chest pains and trouble breathing. "They do the EKG, and the EKG says this person is having a heart attack," said Brooks, "but their coronary vessels are clean. There's no blockage." Instead, an immune reaction has inflamed the entire heart muscle, a condition called myocarditis. "And there's not a lot you can do but hope they get through it." A German study of 100 recovered Covid patients with the average age of 49, found that 22 of them had lasting cardiac problems.

Even after Brooks thought SARS-CoV-2 had no more tricks to play, a sneaky aftereffect totally confounded him. "You get over the illness, you're feeling better, and it comes back to bite you again." In adults, it might just be a strange rash. But some children develop a multi-organ inflammatory syndrome. "They have conjunctivitis, their eyes get real red, they have abdominal pain, and then they can go on to experience cardiovascular collapse." Some of the children don't even remember being ill until then. "They were asymptomatically infected," Brooks said. "So it's weird."

3

Spike

WHEN I WAS around six years old, I woke up one morning and couldn't get out of bed. My legs wouldn't move. I was paralyzed from the waist down.

This was during the polio era, in the early 1950s. My mother came in because I wasn't ready for school. I remember the alarm in her eyes. In those days, doctors made house calls, and he entered my room carrying his black physician's bag, sat on the edge of the bed, stuck a thermometer under my tongue, and checked my pulse. There was little else he could do. The terror of polio haunted children and parents everywhere. It was common to see young people in leg braces or wheelchairs; those imprisoned in iron lungs we only heard about.

I was lucky. It wasn't polio; it was possibly a severe allergic reaction to a tetanus shot I had had a few days before, caused by the tetanus antitoxin, which is harvested from horse blood. Horses were so important to the production of antibodies that many of the great pharmaceutical companies began as horse farms. It might also have been a dangerous disease called Guillain-Barré syndrome, an autoimmune disorder sometimes associated with infections such as influenza, Zika, and dengue fever—but so far not Covid-19. After a day or two, I could move my legs, but the memory was searing. Naturally, I have a wariness about vaccines. I'm not supposed to take flu shots, for instance, which in rare instances are associated with Guillain-Barré.

I remember, as a child, collecting coins for the March of Dimes, which was founded by President Franklin D. Roosevelt, who was crippled by polio (although more recent scholarship suggests he may have been misdiagnosed, and that he actually had contracted Guillain-Barré syndrome). Millions of dimes, many of them contributed by schoolchildren, established the National Foundation for Infantile Paralysis and led to FDR's profile being put on the dime.

Since 1796, when Edward Jenner created the first vaccine, for smallpox, the field of public health has been dogged by anti-vaccination movements. They are sometimes inspired by moral or religious sentiments, citing the use of animals or fetal tissue; or they may be swayed by political notions of individual liberty; but the main argument is the threat of disease caused by the vaccine itself. In 1998, there was a paper published in *The Lancet*, one of the world's oldest and most respected medical journals, by Andrew Wakefield, a British doctor, that purported to show a link between the Measles Mumps Rubella (MMR) vaccine and the development of autism. Numerous other studies have contradicted the findings, and *The Lancet* withdrew the paper in 2010, after investigations showed the original study was fraudulent and that Wakefield had been bankrolled by a lawyer trying to raise a class-action suit against vaccine manufacturers.

Wakefield's medical license was revoked. The disgraced British doctor did what so many have done: he moved to Austin, my town. Texas was a fertile field for anti-vaccination propaganda. In 2003, lawmakers passed new rules allowing anyone to refuse to vaccinate their children. The number of unvaccinated children in Texas is estimated to be more than 100,000.

The anti-vaxxers have prompted an upsurge in childhood diseases, especially measles, one of the most contagious diseases ever known. It used to infect nearly every child in America by the age of fifteen, killing from 400 to 500 of them, and hospitalizing about 48,000, some with serious secondary infections, such as encephalitis. Thanks to an effective vaccine, the United States was declared free of measles in 2000. And then it came back. In 2019, nearly 1,300 cases were reported, many of them in religious communities, such as among the Amish and ultra-Orthodox Jews.

In 1955, more than 200,000 American children received a polio vaccine containing a live virus that had not been properly inactivated; 40,000 of them got polio, 200 were paralyzed, and 10 died. The legacy of that awful disaster led to more effective government oversight of vaccines, but it also generated a flood of lawsuits that caused many pharmaceutical companies to back away from vaccine development. A heroic international effort over decades has led to the point that this incurable disease is on the verge of extinction. Vaccines did that. And yet, of the cases that still occur each year, most of them are the result of vaccination. Only a few cases of wild poliovirus continue to turn up—169 in 2019—primarily in Afghanistan and Pakistan, where vaccination rates remain low. The conundrum is this: The oral polio vaccine, which is easy to dispense, consists of three attenuated polio viruses, and a child receiving the vaccination may infect other children who haven't been vaccinated. There is an injectable vaccine made of an inactivated virus, which is safer, but until polio is fully eradicated, oral vaccines will continue to be administered. The only way to stop the spread is to vaccinate more children.

Robert F. Kennedy Jr., an environmental lawyer who is the nephew of the former President John F. Kennedy, has become perhaps the most prominent voice of the anti-vaccine movement in the U.S. He has championed Judy Mikovits, a former researcher at the National Cancer Institute, who made a number of discredited assertions in a documentary called *Plandemic*. It was released on May 4, 2020, and raced across the internet with its sensational claims—among them, that Anthony Fauci and other researchers were responsible for the death of millions of AIDS victims who were given the wrong therapy, while the scientists reaped fabulous profits from the patents on the faulty medicines. (According to the *British Medical Journal*, Dr. Fauci's colleague at NIAID, Dr. Clifford Lane, said he received about $45,000 from the patents; Fauci donated his entire portion to charity.) Mikovits asserts that SARS-CoV-2 was created in laboratories at the University of North Carolina, the U.S. Army Medical Research Institute of Infectious Diseases in Fort Detrick, Maryland, and the Wuhan Institute of Virology, without offering proof or saying why they would do this. Boosted by QAnon and anti-vaccine advocates, *Plandemic* was liked, shared, or commented on nearly 2.5 million times on Facebook before it was taken down. The contest between science and conspiracy would constantly undermine efforts to coordinate a national response to the Covid-19 pandemic.

THE ROOTS OF the modern anti-vaccine movement are in the swine flu scare of 1976. It was a strain of influenza, H1N1, similar to the 1918–19 Spanish flu that killed an estimated 670,000 Americans. The return of H1N1 was the nightmare that haunted the world of public health, and when it happened, the CDC was the lead agency in dealing with it.

I played a small, inconclusive role in the fiasco it became. In February 1976, at Fort Dix, New Jersey, a nineteen-year-old Army recruit named David Lewis collapsed during a training march and died. Isolates from Lewis's body were sent to Gary Noble, a virologist at the CDC. Noble compared it to historic strains, but they only went back a few decades. It wasn't until he tested it for a swine strain of H1N1 that he found a match. Pigs had probably gotten the disease from humans and it remained in them as a reservoir.

Eventually, investigators would find 273 men on the base who tested positive for swine flu, so it was transmissible, but David Lewis was the only person who died. Was it really something to worry about? Or were we facing 1918 again? In that case, a vaccine had to be compounded immediately and gotten into the arms of every American.

There were side effects to consider, including fevers, malaise, nausea, and sore arms. The director of the CDC at the time, David Sencer, decided that the safest route was to go "whole hog," as he jokingly put it, and vaccinate the entire country. President Gerald Ford signed on. "We cannot afford to take a chance with the health of our nation," he said gravely, with Jonas Salk and Albert Sabin, the inventors of the polio vaccines, standing beside him. At that point I went to Fort Dix to write about what appeared to be the most consequential public health decision since polio was eradicated by the genius of those two men.

At the military base, I happened to mention to the health and environment officer that I had spoken to David Lewis's mother, a nurse. He smirked and said, "Did she tell you about the pig?"

"What pig was that?"

"Oh, some story about how David ran into a pig over Christmas." Mrs. Lewis had suggested that might have been how David got the flu.

There have been occasional cases of farmers getting infected with swine flu from animals. Suppose Lewis was Patient Zero, the first documented case in an epidemic. He got a virulent infection from a pig, which is what killed him, but the disease he transmitted was not so fatal and was never well enough adapted to humans to escape the military base. In that case, there would be no reason to vaccinate millions of Americans.

I met David Lewis's fiancée, a vibrant young woman named Peg Lapham, a nursing student and pilot. She and David had planned to go into the mission fields when he got out of the Army. She recalled that they were driving from her house in the Catskills to his home in Massachusetts. It had been snowing hard and the road was narrowed down to a single lane. Then, in the middle of the road, they came upon a shivering pig. It had apparently tumbled out of the bed of a pickup into the snow. Peg estimated that it weighed at least two hundred pounds. David nudged it with the car to see if it would move out of the way. Finally, he got out and grabbed the pig by the ears and tugged it aside.

In that fateful moment, did the pig cough in his face?

Peg and I retraced their steps, stopping at farmhouses along the way. We finally found the owner of the pig, who was not happy to hear my theory that his pig may have been the source of a disease that could potentially kill millions. I told him I just needed a little blood from his pig, which was actually a house pet, to send to the CDC.

The owner turned to this still grieving young woman sitting on his couch and said, "I know you. I know where you live. You fuck with my pig and I'll burn your house down."

Wow, welcome to epidemiology.

I finally negotiated a deal in which his veterinarian would draw the blood and send it to Gary Noble at the CDC. I was pretty sure that the blood would show antibodies to swine influenza, and that the vaccination program would be put on ice until other infections surfaced, if they ever did.

The pig had never been sick a day in its life. The vaccination program went ahead, "whole hog." It was inaugurated in October 1976, at the Indiana State Fair, in the middle of a presidential election campaign. Forty-eight million Americans were vaccinated; 532 of them got Guillain-Barré syndrome and 25 died. The inoculations were suspended. No one else got swine flu. Gerald Ford lost the election. History might have been different if that pig had been sick.

BUILDING 40 OF the main campus of the National Institutes of Health, in Bethesda, Maryland, houses the National Institute of Allergy and Infectious Diseases. On the second floor is the laboratory of Dr. Barney Graham, deputy director of the Vaccine Research Center and chief of the Viral Pathogenesis Laboratory and Translational Science Core. He studies how viruses cause disease and designs vaccines to defeat them.

The first thing you notice about Barney Graham is that there's a lot of him. He's six-foot-five, with a gray goatee and a laconic manner. Graham's boss at NIAID, Dr. Anthony Fauci, said, "He understands vaccinology better than anybody I know."

Bookshelves in Graham's office hold colorful 3-D printouts of viruses that he has worked with, including Ebola, Zika, and influenza. When I was researching *The End of October*, a novel about a pandemic, which coincidentally appeared at the peak of the first wave of the Covid contagion, in April 2020, Graham helped me design the virus and then rescued the plot by concocting a vaccine for the disease he had cooked up. I came to understand that researchers like Barney Graham are essentially puzzle solvers. When the actual pandemic struck, he solved one of the most consequential puzzles in modern science: He is the chief architect of the first Covid vaccines to be authorized for emergency use. Manufactured by Moderna and Pfizer, they differ only slightly in their delivery systems.

On Graham's wall is a map of Kansas, where he grew up. His dad was a small-town dentist and his mother was a teacher. For part of his childhood, they lived on a hog farm in the eastern part of the state. By working with animals, Barney learned a lot about veterinary medicine, and at Rice University, he switched his major from math to biology. He earned his medical degree at the University of Kansas, where he met the woman who would become his wife, Cynthia Turner. She was studying to be a pediatrician (she is now a psychiatrist). In 1978, on an infectious disease rotation while still in medical school, Barney spent time at the NIH, where he first encountered Dr. Fauci. "Cynthia noticed when I came back how excited I was," Graham recalled. "There was no intellectual laziness. People were willing to battle each other's ideas. She thought I would end up here."

First, he and Cynthia had to complete residencies. They wanted to be in the same town, a problem many professional couples face, but additionally complicated in their case because Cynthia is Black. She suggested Nashville: he could apply to Vanderbilt Medical School and she to Meharry Medical College, a historically Black institution. Tennessee had only just repealed its ban on interracial marriages, more than a decade after the Supreme Court struck down miscegenation laws, but attitudes were slow to change.

Driving back to Kansas on Christmas Eve, Graham stopped in at Vanderbilt. He asked for an application form and was surprised to find that the director of the residency program, Dr. Thomas Brittingham, was at his desk and willing to interview him right then. Afterwards, as Graham was leaving, he said to Brittingham, "I know this is the South. I'm going to marry a Black woman, and if that makes a difference, I can't come here."

"Close the door," said Brittingham. He turned out to be a closet integrationist and an ardent proponent of interracial marriage. He welcomed Graham on the spot. Cynthia was accepted at Meharry, and so they made a home in Nashville.

By 1982, Graham had become the chief resident at Nashville General Hospital. That year he saw a patient suffering from five different opportunistic infections simultaneously. Most infections are solitary events, but this patient was riddled with cryptococcal meningitis and herpes simplex, along with an array of other rare infections. It was puzzling, not just because of the gruesome manifestations of disease but also because, in Graham's experience, it didn't make any sense. The medical staff, which didn't have the kind of PPE available now, was terrified. As it turned out, they were treating Tennessee's first AIDS patient. They kept him alive for three weeks.

So many lives would be changed, and so many ended, by this remorseless, elusive disease. Immunology, then a fledgling field, was transformed by the battle, although the war still has not been won. Graham started an AIDS clinic in Nashville and began running vaccine trials. "It took us a couple years to figure out that HIV was a virus," he said. "It was not till the mid-nineties that we had decent treatments. There were some really hard years. Almost everyone died."

In 2000, NIH recruited Graham to evaluate vaccine candidates. He insisted on keeping a research lab. With space for two dozen scientists, his lab focused on creating vaccines for three categories of respiratory viruses: influenza, coronaviruses, and a highly contagious pathogen called respiratory syncytial virus (RSV), which ended up playing a key role in the development of a Covid vaccine.

RSV causes wheezing pneumonia in children and sends more kids under five years old to the hospital than any other disease. One of the last childhood infectious diseases without a vaccine, RSV also kills about as many of the elderly as influenza. It's wildly infectious, spreading through particle droplets and contaminated surfaces. In order to stop its spread in a hospital pediatric ward, staff must wear gloves, masks, and goggles; if any of these items is omitted, RSV will surge. In the 1960s, a clinical trial of a potential RSV vaccine made children sicker and led to two deaths—a syndrome called vaccine enhanced disease. Graham spent much of the first twenty-five years of his career trying to solve the riddle of what causes RSV disease and how to create a safe vaccine, but the technology he needed was still being developed.

In 2008, Graham had a stroke of luck. Jason McLellan, a young post-doc, got squeezed out of a structural biology lab upstairs, where HIV research was done. HIV had so far proved invulnerable to a vaccine solution, despite extraordinary technological advances and some very elegant new theories for designing one. "I thought, let's try them out on a more tractable virus," McLellan recalls. "Barney suggested RSV would be perfect for structure-based vaccine." It would prove to be the first step in countering what was not yet a human disease, SARS-CoV-2.

A vaccine trains the immune system to recognize a virus in order to counter it. Using modern imaging technology, structural biologists can intuit the contours of a virus and its proteins, then reproduce those structures in order to make more effective vaccines. McLellan said of his field, "From the structure, we can determine function—it's similar to how seeing a car, with four wheels and doors, implies something about its function to transport people."

The surface of the RSV particle features a paddle-shaped protein, designated F. On top of that protein, there is a spot called an epitope that serves as a kind of landing spot for antibodies. As long as it stays in its original conformation, antibodies can repel it. But something extraordinary happens when the virus invades a cell. The F protein swells, like an erection, burying the vulnerable epitope and effectively hiding it from the antibodies. McLellan's challenge was to keep the F protein from getting an erection.

Classically, vaccines are made from real viruses. One way is to weaken them to the point that they no longer cause illness but can still stir up an antibody response; that is how Louis Pasteur, one of the founding figures of microbiology, created a vaccine for cholera in chickens. Chemically inactivated viruses can fool the body into believing it is being infected; such vaccines have been used for encephalitis and rabies. But there was uncertainty. Immunologists were handicapped because they couldn't clearly see what they were doing. Until recently, one of the main imaging tools used by vaccinologists, the cryogenic electron microscope, wasn't powerful enough to visualize viral proteins, which are incredibly tiny. "The whole field was referred to as 'blobology,'" said McLellan.

As a work-around, McLellan developed expertise in X-ray crystallography. With this method, a virus, or even just a protein on a virus, is crystallized, then hit with an X-ray beam that creates a scatter pattern, like a shotgun blast; the structure of the crystallized object can be determined from the distribution of electrons. McLellan showed me an "atomistic interpretation" of the F protein on the RSV virus. The visualization looked like a pile of Cheetos. It required a leap of imagination to sketch an armature of amino acids inside a projection of a protein they could not actually see. But inside that near-invisible world, Graham and McLellan and their team were able to manipulate the F protein, essentially by cloning it and inserting mutations that kept it strapped down. "That's what structure-based design is," said McLellan. "There's a lot of art to it."

In 2013, Graham and McLellan published "Structure-Based Design of a Fusion Glycoprotein Vaccine for Respiratory Syncytial Virus" in *Science*, demonstrating how they stabilized the F protein in its pre-erect form in order to use it as an antigen—the part of a vaccine that sparks an immune response. Antibodies could now attack the defenseless F protein, vanquishing the virus. Graham and McLellan calculated that the vaccine could be given to a pregnant woman and provide enough antibodies to her baby to last for the first six months of its life—the critical period. Their paper opened a new front in the endless war against infectious disease. In a subsequent paper in *Science*, the team declared that they had established "clinical proof of concept for structure-based vaccine design," portending "an era of precision vaccinology."

IN 2012, the MERS coronavirus emerged in Saudi Arabia. Humans initially caught it from camels—perhaps in the slaughterhouse or by drinking camel's milk. MERS was unstable and terribly dangerous to work with. Ominously, it was the second novel coronavirus in ten years. Coronaviruses have been in humans for as long as eight centuries, but before SARS and MERS, they only caused the common cold. It's possible that, in the distant past, cold viruses were far more deadly, and that humans developed resistance over time. That may be the destiny of SARS-CoV-2.

One of Graham's postdocs happened to go on hajj, and he returned from Saudi Arabia with a coronavirus infection. "We thought he might have MERS," Graham remembered. They took a swab of snot from the postdoc's nose. It turned out he had a cold. The coronavirus that caused it was called HKU1, for Hong Kong University, where it was first described. Graham figured it would be safer to work on than MERS.

Like RSV, coronaviruses have a protein that elongates when invading the cell. "It looks like a spike, so we just called it Spike," said Graham. Spike was large, flexible, and encased in sugars, which made it difficult to crystallize, so X-ray crystallography wasn't an option. Fortunately, around 2013, what McLellan called a "resolution revolution" in cryogenic electron microscopy allowed scientists to visualize microbes down to angstrom level, one ten-billionth of a meter. Finally, vaccinologists could truly see what they were doing.

Andrew Ward at Scripps Research had one of the massive cryo-EM machines. Once the team was able to stabilize the spike of the HKU1, they applied the same procedure to MERS. Their model vaccine worked well in mice, and Graham and McLellan were on the way to making a human version, but after killing hundreds of people, MERS petered out as an immediate threat to humans—and interest in vaccine development petered out as well, a pattern repeated endlessly in science. "We kept having to respond to these epidemic threats, like MERS and chikungunya, and then Ebola and then Zika and Ebola again, and now SARS again," Graham said, betraying a hint of the frustration he must have experienced. "We just had to get a better way of dealing with this."

He understood the rules. "Science is all about making incremental advances toward a larger goal," he said. "It would be rare for institutions to invest in things that might not happen." But he had a dream. About two dozen virus families are known to infect humans, and the modified protein that Graham's lab had developed to deal with RSV might be transferable to many of them.

Then there was the question of how to deliver the vaccine.

Graham knew that Moderna, a biotech startup in Cambridge, Massachusetts, had encoded a modified protein on strips of genetic material known as messenger RNA. The company had never brought a vaccine to market, concentrating instead on providing treatments for "orphan diseases"—rare disorders that aren't profitable enough to interest Big Pharma. But its mRNA platform was potent. It was designed to easily slip into the cell nucleus and begin manufacturing spike proteins that would elicit antibodies—that was the theory. If it worked, the vaccine could be produced rapidly and relatively cheaply. It would be a revolutionary platform for vaccines of the future.

Graham had already proved the effectiveness of structure-based vaccine for RSV, and had applied similar approaches to MERS. He had arranged a demonstration project for Nipah, a particularly fatal virus that has no cure, using Moderna's mRNA platform. He was about to prepare enough protein to take the Nipah vaccine through the first phase of human trials when he heard the news from Wuhan.

Graham called McLellan, who was in a Park City, Utah, resort shop getting snowboard boots heat-molded to his feet. By then, Jason McLellan was a recognized star in the field of structural biology and had been recruited to the University of Texas at Austin and given a lab of his own, along with access to the latest cryogenic electron microscopes.

It took someone who knew Graham well to detect the urgency in his voice. Graham said he suspected that China's cases of atypical pneumonia were caused by a new coronavirus, and he was trying to obtain the genetic sequence. It was a chance to test their concept in a real-world situation. Would McLellan and his team like to get "back in the saddle" and create a vaccine?

"Of course," McLellan said.

"We got the sequences Friday night, the tenth of January," Graham recalled. "We woke up on the eleventh and started designing proteins."

Nine days later, the coronavirus officially arrived in America.

GRAHAM AND MCLELLAN designed the modified proteins within a day after downloading the sequence for SARS-CoV-2. The key accelerating factor was that they already knew how to alter the spike proteins of other coronaviruses. On January 13, they turned their modified spike protein over to Moderna, for manufacturing. Six weeks later, Moderna began shipping vials of vaccine for clinical trials. Typically it takes months to years, if not decades, to go from formulating the vaccine to making a product ready to be tested, a process that privileges safety and cost over speed. The FDA required another twenty-four days to approve the product for trials, for a total of sixty-five days from inception to trials, "an all-time record," said Graham.

Graham had to make several crucial decisions while designing the vaccine, including where to start encoding the spike-protein sequence on the mRNA. Making bad choices could render the vaccine less effective—or worthless. He solicited the advice of his colleagues. They all said the final decisions were up to him—nobody had more experience in designing vaccines. Graham made his choices. Then, after Moderna had already begun the manufacturing process, the company sent back some preliminary data that made him fear he had botched the job.

Graham had a panic attack. Cynthia was alarmed by his mood. "It was a crisis of conscience that I just never see in him," she said. "He was beside himself." His expertise and judgment had been called into question. So much depended on the prompt development of a safe and effective vaccine. The candidate generated in Graham's lab was off to a fast start. If his vaccine worked, millions of lives might be spared. If it failed or was delayed, it would be Barney Graham's fault.

After the vaccine was tested in animals, it was clear that his design choices had been sound. The first human was inoculated on March 16, beginning the Phase 1 trial. A week later, Moderna began scaling up production to a million doses per month.

4

"An Evolving Situation"

THE CHAMBER OF the U.S. Senate is fusty, dignified, subdued, intimate, and usually vacant. Members drift in for votes and quickly leave. He or she who stands before the marbled dais to make a speech usually addresses a hundred vacant chairs. The intended audience is the local news back home, or the *Congressional Record,* or Twitter. The camera never wheels about to show the vacancy, but you can hear it in the hush.

Rarely, in modern times, has the chamber been full, every seat taken; but on January 23, 2020, members gathered for the second day of opening arguments in the first impeachment trial of Donald Trump. The spacious room now felt stuffed and cramped. The gallery was packed with press and dignitaries leaning over the rail. Members who rarely see each other were elbow to elbow.

On its face, the impeachment was an empty exercise with a foreordained result. Conviction required a two-thirds majority; there were only forty-five Democrats and two independents in the Senate. The goal of the House managers was to chip off at least a handful of votes from the flinty Republican wall that faced them, but never in history had a senator voted to convict a president of his own party. The Democrats targeted Mitt Romney of Utah, Lisa Murkowski of Alaska, Susan Collins of Maine, and the retiring Lamar Alexander of Tennessee—the four Republicans who supported allowing a vote on whether additional evidence would be needed. Senate Majority Leader Mitch McConnell had already announced that he was going to roll over Democratic attempts to introduce witnesses and new evidence. "We have the votes," he curtly decreed, but Alexander insisted, "We have a constitutional duty to hear the case."

"The House managers had prepared as if it was the trial of their lifetime, and the president's lawyers hadn't prepared at all," Senator Michael Bennet, a Democrat of Colorado, lamented. "It was overwhelmingly depressing." Like three other senators in the room—Bernie Sanders, Elizabeth Warren, and Amy Klobuchar—Bennet was still running for the Democratic presidential nomination. Kamala Harris had dropped out of the race in early December, followed by Cory Booker in January. For the remaining candidates, impeachment created havoc, coming as it did right before the Iowa caucuses. As soon as the trial recessed on Friday evenings they would race off to campaign every moment of the weekend. "I was doing planetariums in small towns at midnight," Klobuchar recalled. Then it was back to Washington for another week in the stuffy chamber to listen to an argument only one side could win.

The House managers took turns laying out their case. "We will show that President Trump abused his power when he used his office to solicit and pressure Ukraine to meddle in our elections for his personal gain," Representative Jerrold Nadler of New York promised. "We will show that he betrayed vital national interests . . ." The senators struggled to stay alert; the proceedings had lasted until one in the morning the night before.

For Republicans like Marco Rubio, impeachment was a dangerous distraction. He didn't doubt the truth of the charges against Trump. He knew what the president was capable of, having faced him in the Republican primaries four years before, when he called Trump a "con artist." There might be some personal satisfaction in casting his vote for conviction, but there were larger concerns. South Florida, where Rubio lives, is closer to his parents' native Cuba than it is to Orlando. Haiti, Venezuela, and Nicaragua are near neighbors, and their violent politics waft through the cafés of Miami's Little Havana. One of the lessons Rubio took from the experience of growing up there was that societies are not as stable as they might seem. America may appear to be immune to coups and revolutions, but to actually remove a president, for the first time in the nation's history, in such a fractious environment, was a test he wasn't sure the nation could survive.

While the managers were making their case, Lamar Alexander sometimes roamed about. At the age of seventy-nine, in his final term, he was liberated as few political figures in the room could allow themselves to be. The Tennessee Republican had a history as a centrist who cherished the more bipartisan era that prevailed when he entered the Senate in 2003; since then, he had watched the body become increasingly acrimonious and ineffectual. "The Senate reflects the populace it serves and the society in which it exists," he said wistfully. "Society is more partisan and divisive, and so are we."

Although not formally a part of Republican leadership, Alexander was seen by members of both parties as a conduit to McConnell, his close friend, which is probably why Cory Gardner of Colorado approached Alexander during the trial. "This virus in China is a serious thing. We ought to get a briefing on it," Gardner said. That evening, after a short break, McConnell announced to the senators, "In the morning, there will be a coronavirus briefing for all members at ten thirty." It was the first mention of Covid-19 in Congress.

The briefing took place on January 24, in the hearing room of the Health, Education, Labor and Pensions Committee, which Alexander chaired. Senator Patty Murray was the ranking Democratic member. A former preschool teacher, sporting a silvery blond bob with bangs, she had been in the Senate for twenty-seven years. Her father had managed a five-and-dime store until he developed multiple sclerosis and was unable to work. Patty was fifteen. The family went on welfare. She knew how illness can flatten people economically, and how government can help.

A few days earlier, she had heard about the first confirmed case of Covid-19 in the U.S.—the man who had traveled from Wuhan to Washington, her state. Murray contacted local public health officials, who seemed to be doing everything right: the traveler was hospitalized and officials were tracing a few possible contacts. Then almost overnight they were tracking dozens of people. Murray thought, "Wow, this is kinda scary. And this is in my backyard."

About twenty senators showed up to hear Dr. Fauci and Dr. Redfield speak at the hour-long briefing. Murray was alarmed by the casual nature of their presentations. Senator Alexander was more circumspect. After all, there were still only two cases in the U.S., and both were people who had been in China. The health authorities were reassuring. "We are prepared for this," Redfield promised.

No one realized at the time how widely the disease had already seeded itself. Dr. Fauci said in a radio interview that Covid-19 "isn't something the American people need to be worried or frightened by," although he added that it was "an evolving situation. Every day, we have to look at it very carefully."

WHILE THE SENATORS were being briefed, Matt Pottinger convened an interagency meeting of forty-two people, including NSC staffers as well as cabinet-level officials and their deputies. China had just announced its lockdown of Wuhan, which could only mean that sustained human-to-human transmission was occurring. Indeed, Pottinger's staff reported that another city, Huanggang—population over seven million—was also locked down. There was a decision to require anyone who had been to Wuhan to land at one of five airports in the U.S., where CDC teams would be waiting to screen them. That would turn out to be a worthless exercise: only one passenger turned up positive, but many of the screeners caught the disease, possibly from hanging around airports.

Pottinger attended a Chinese New Year party in Washington at the Capitol Hill home of Dimon Liu, an architect and human rights activist, on January 25, the first day of the Year of the Rat. The party had become a kind of annual rallying spot for émigrés, journalists, diplomats, and notable Chinese dissidents. Liu had been cooking for days, a typical New Year's banquet with twenty-five main courses, including three kinds of pork, a baked salmon, and turkey done Peking Duck style. The guests were subdued, relaying stories from frightened friends and family members back in China. It sounded like SARS all over again.

Pottinger went home and dug up some old files from his reporting days, and began calling former sources. He also phoned his brother, Paul, who is an infectious-disease doctor in Seattle and a professor at the University of Washington Medical Center. Paul had been reading about the new virus on infectious disease email lists, but until the first case arrived in Washington State, he thought it was "a flash in the pan."

If flights from China were halted, Matt asked, could America have more time to prepare?

Paul was hesitant. Like most public health practitioners, he held that travel bans have unintended consequences. They stigmatize countries contending with contagion. Doctors and medical equipment need to be able to move around. And by the time restrictions are put in place, the disease has usually slipped across borders anyway, making the whole exercise irritating and pointless. But Matt spoke with resolve. Little was known about the virus except for the fact that it spread like wildfire, embers flying from city to city, country to country. First Wuhan, now Seattle. Paul said yes, do whatever you can to slow the advance. It will give us a chance to do the testing and the contact tracing we need in order to keep this disease under control. Otherwise the year ahead might be calamitous.

DR. RICK BRIGHT HAD run the Biomedical Advanced Research and Development Authority since 2016. A division of HHS, BARDA was created in reaction to 9/11 as the government agency responsible for medical countermeasures in the event of bioterrorism or a pandemic. After Trump became president, Bright often clashed with political appointees over what he saw as their attempts to overlook scientific merit and to award lucrative contracts based on political connections.

Bright received an email on January 22 from Mike Bowen, an executive at the Texas-based firm Prestige Ameritech, the country's largest maker of surgical masks. Bowen wrote that he had four N95 manufacturing lines that weren't in use. "Reactivating these machines would be very difficult and very expensive but could be achieved in a dire situation with government help," he wrote. In another message, Bowen noted, "We are the last major domestic mask company. . . . My phones are ringing now, so I don't 'need' government business. I'm just letting you know that I can help you preserve our infrastructure if things ever get really bad. I'm a patriot first, businessman second."

Bright was already worried about the likely shortage of personal protective equipment in the Strategic National Stockpile. He also felt that not enough was being done to develop diagnostics for the virus from Wuhan. On January 23, at an HHS leadership meeting with Secretary

Azar, he warned that the "virus might already be here—we just don't have the tests to know." He became one of the many scientists who fell out of favor after sharing bad news in the Trump administration.

On January 25, Bowen wrote Bright again, saying that his company was getting "lots of requests from China and Hong Kong" for masks. This was a stunning piece of intelligence. Half the masks used in the U.S. came from China; if that supply stopped, Bowen warned, American hospitals would run out: "No way to prevent it."

Prodded by Mike Bowen, Rick Bright continued to advocate for immediate action on masks and other critical equipment, but he claimed that HHS was unresponsive and even hostile to his pleas. On January 27, Bowen wrote, "Rick, I think we're in deep shit. The world."

There was an op-ed in *USA Today* that morning. "I remember how Trump sought to stoke fear and stigma during the 2014 Ebola epidemic," Joe Biden wrote. "Trump's demonstrated failures of judgment and his repeated rejection of science make him the worst possible person to lead our country through a global health challenge." The former vice president cited Trump's proposed cuts to NIH, CDC, and the Agency for International Development—"the very agencies we need to fight this outbreak and prevent future ones." Trump had dismantled the White House team in charge of global health security. "And he has treated with utmost contempt institutions that facilitate international cooperation, thus undermining the global efforts that keep us safe from pandemics and biological attacks. "To be blunt, I am concerned that the Trump administration's shortsighted policies have left us unprepared for a dangerous epidemic that will come sooner or later."

THAT SAME DAY, Pottinger convened another interagency meeting. The people in those early meetings fell into four camps. There was the public health establishment—Redfield, Fauci, Azar—data-driven people who at the moment had no data. Another group—the acting White House chief of staff, Mick Mulvaney, along with officials from the Transportation Department and the Office of Management and Budget—were preoccupied with the economic damage that would result if drastic steps were taken. A State Department faction was mainly concerned with logistical issues, such as extracting Americans from Wuhan. And finally, there was a group of one, Matt Pottinger, who saw the virus not just as a medical and economic challenge but also as a national security threat. He wanted dramatic action now.

For three weeks, the U.S. had been seeking permission to send medical experts into China, requests that Chinese authorities rejected. The public health contingent in the meeting didn't want to make decisions about quarantines or travel bans without definitive intelligence, but that's exactly what the Chinese refused to supply. The State Department had just heightened its travel advisory for travelers to the Wuhan region. The Chinese were enraged by the implications of the evacuation of Americans, especially the diplomatic staff at the consulate in Wuhan. Tedros Ghebreyesus, the director-general of the WHO, complained that the U.S. was overreacting. In part to placate the Chinese, the 747s that were sent to collect Americans were filled with eighteen tons of PPE, including masks, gowns, and gauze. It was a decision that many came to regret—especially when inferior substitutes were sold back to the U.S. at colossal markups.

When Pottinger put on the table his proposal to curtail travel from China, the economic advisers derided it as overkill. Think of the damage to the airlines. Travel bans were death on trade—a serious consideration with China, which, in addition to PPE, manufactured much of the vital medicines the U.S. relied on. Their view was "It's going to hurt the economy and it's totally unnecessary." Predictably, the public health representatives were resistant, too: viruses found ways to travel no matter what. Moreover, at least 14,000 passengers from China were arriving in the U.S. every day; there was no feasible way to quarantine them all. These arguments would join a parade of other public health verities that would be jettisoned during the pandemic. Countries that quickly imposed travel restrictions, such as Vietnam and New Zealand, kept contagion at manageable levels.

The next morning, Pottinger spoke to a doctor in China who was treating patients. Transmission was so widespread that contact tracing was no longer possible, the doctor told him. People were getting sick and there was no way to know how and where the infection happened—a stage of contagion called community spread.

Pottinger asked, "Is this going to be as bad as SARS?"

"Don't think SARS, 2003. Think flu, 1918," the doctor said. "SARS had

9,600 cases. Only one was ever shown to be asymptomatic. In China, 50 percent of the cases of this new disease are asymptomatic. And they spread."

Later that day, the national security adviser, Robert O'Brien, brought Pottinger into the Oval Office, where the president was getting his daily intelligence briefing. Far down the list of threats was the mysterious new virus in China. The briefer didn't seem to take it seriously. O'Brien did. "This will be the biggest national security threat you will face in your presidency," he warned.

"Is this going to be as bad or worse than SARS in 2003?" Trump asked.

The briefer responded that it wasn't clear yet.

Pottinger, who was sitting on a couch, jumped to his feet. He had seen enough high-level arguments in the Oval Office to know that Trump relished clashes between agencies. "Mr. President, I actually covered that," he said, recounting his experience with SARS and what he was learning now from his sources—most shockingly, that more than half of the spread of the disease was by asymptomatic carriers. China had already curbed travel within the country, but every day thousands of people were traveling from China to the U.S.—half a million in January alone.

"Should we shut down travel?" the president asked.

"Yes," Pottinger said unequivocally.

Pottinger walked out of the Oval Office to the Situation Room, where the improvised task force was meeting. People were annoyed with him. "It would be unusual for asymptomatic persons to drive the epidemic in a respiratory disorder," Dr. Fauci told him. That was certainly true of SARS. Fauci was still demanding that U.S. scientists be dispatched to China in order to get more data. Redfield considered it too early for disruptive actions, noting there were only a handful of cases outside of China, and it did not seem to be a fast-moving pathogen. The public health contingent was united. "Let the data guide us," they advised.

Pottinger pointed out that the Chinese continued to block such efforts: "We're not getting data that's dependable!"

The economic advisers, meantime, were horrified—a travel ban would be the death of the airline industry and shut down the supply chain. Larry Kudlow, the president's chief economic adviser, had been questioning the seriousness of the situation. He couldn't square the apocalyptic forecasts with the bouyant stock market. "Is all the money dumb?" he wondered. "Everyone's asleep at the switch? I just have a hard time believing that."*

Pottinger, sensing he'd need backup, had brought along Peter Navarro, an abrasive economic adviser who had been part of the trade negotiations with China. Navarro was warily regarded in the White House, thought by many to be a crackpot but known to be one of Trump's favorites because of his advocacy for tariff wars and his dire portrayals of China as an existential threat to American dominance. Navarro warned the group, "We have got to seal the borders now. This is a black-swan event, and you're rolling the dice with your gradualist approach."

Within minutes, Navarro was at odds with everyone in the room. He argued that the new virus was spreading faster than seasonal flu or SARS. The possible economic costs and loss of life were staggering. A travel ban might stem the spread. Azar countered that blocking travel from China would be overreacting. Nothing changed in that meeting except that Navarro was so strident that Mulvaney barred him from future sessions.

Then a piece of data surfaced that shifted the argument. In mid-January, a Chicago woman returned from China. Within a week, she was hospitalized with Covid—the first in Illinois. On January 30, her husband, who had not been in China, also tested positive. Fauci, Redfield, and others in the public health contingent abruptly changed their minds: human-to-human transmission was definitely happening in America.

Trump received the news soberly. The timing couldn't have been worse for him. The curtain had risen on election season. The bitter trade war he provoked with China had just reached a tentative pause, after inflicting considerable damage to both economies. Since then, he had been touting his great friendship with Xi Jinping and praising the Chinese president's handling of the contagion, despite evidence of a cover-up. A travel ban would reopen wounds. But the president made the decision and announced it the next day. Pottinger thought it was a bold stroke, one that the president deserved credit for.

---

* Kudlow said he doesn't recall this remark, which was in contemporaneous notes of the meeting.

The administration blocked non-American travelers coming from China, but U.S. citizens, residents, and their family members were still free to come and go. Three major U.S. carriers had already suspended service on their own, but dozens of direct and one-stop flights from China continued into the U.S. A two-week quarantine was imposed on travelers coming from the Wuhan region, but the U.S. did little to make sure incoming passengers actually isolated themselves—unlike Taiwan, Hong Kong, Australia, and New Zealand, which rigidly enforced quarantines. In each of those countries, the travel ban plus the mandatory quarantine helped get the contagion under control.

Trump said repeatedly that he made the decision alone, "against the advice of almost everybody." His decision was controversial, even in his own cabinet, but that day in the Oval Office his top advisers were clear. Something needed to be done to slow the spread. At the time, there were only six confirmed cases in the U.S., a small number, but triple what it had been three days earlier. Exponential growth begins modestly, 2 times 2 becomes 4, times 4 becomes 16, times 16 becomes 256, times 256 becomes 65,536, times 65,536 becomes . . .

BEFORE THE VOTE on allowing witnesses in the impeachment trial of President Trump, Lamar Alexander, one of the four senators the House managers were appealing to, made his position clear in a series of tweets. "It was inappropriate for the president to ask a foreign leader to investigate his political opponent and to withhold United States aid to encourage that investigation," he conceded. However, he added: "If this shallow, hurried and wholly partisan impeachment were to succeed, it would rip the country apart, pouring gasoline on the fire of cultural divisions that already exist. It would create the weapon of perpetual impeachment to be used against future presidents whenever the House of Representatives is of a different political party." There was an election on the horizon, he noted, and that would provide its own remedy. "Let the people decide," Alexander concluded.

The trial was effectively over at that point. Marco Rubio followed up with a statement that reflected the thinking of many Republican senators: "Just because actions meet a standard of impeachment does not mean it is in the best interest of the country to remove a President from office. . . . Can anyone doubt that at least half of the country would view his removal as illegitimate—as nothing short of a coup d'état?"

On February 4, the president strode into the House chamber to deliver the last State of the Union address before he faced the voters. He had on his battle face. When he approached the dais and handed copies of his speech, first to Vice President Pence and then to Speaker Nancy Pelosi, he turned his back on her offered hand. Nor did she say, as is traditional, "I have the high privilege and distinct honor of presenting to you the president of the United States." She simply said, "Members of Congress, the president of the United States."

The contempt between them reflected the division in the country, which was fierce and irreconcilable. The president paced back and forth, synchronizing the applause with his own clapping, as the Republicans in the chamber chanted "Four more years!" Thanks in part to his impeachment, Trump was at the peak of his popularity, reaching a 49 percent approval rating, with 48 percent disapproving. The terrain of undecideds was uninhabited.

"Three years ago, we launched the great American comeback," the president began. "Tonight, I stand before you to share the incredible results. Jobs are booming, incomes are soaring, poverty is plummeting, crime is falling, confidence is surging, and our country is thriving and highly respected again. America's enemies are on the run, America's fortunes are on the rise, and America's future is blazing bright." His administration did achieve some notable accomplishments, of which the president rightfully boasted: "The net worth of the bottom half of wage earners has increased by 47 percent—three times faster than the increase for the top one percent. . . . wages are rising fast—and, wonderfully, they are rising fastest for low-income workers, who have seen a 16 percent pay increase since my election . . . Real median income is now at the highest level ever recorded. . . . U.S. stock markets have soared 70 percent . . ." He concluded: "My fellow Americans, the best is yet to come."

He was uttering these words at the very moment that each item in his summation was about to plummet, like pigeons shot out of the air.

5

"Flatten the Curve"

I N 1989, Howard Markel was in graduate school at Johns Hopkins, specializing in both pediatrics and the history of medicine. It was in the thick of the AIDS pandemic. Markel began volunteering in an AIDS clinic, where he saw a lot of gay men and intravenous drug users. He had just lost his wife to cancer, one month after their first anniversary. His friends were worried about him—still in mourning—being surrounded by so much death, and yet he found that helping men his own age who were facing their mortality, or their partner's, was immensely consoling, "the most spiritually uplifting work I did in my entire clinical career."

Markel's patients often asked him, "Doc, do you think I'll be quarantined because I have HIV?" He'd reply that it wasn't appropriate for that disease. But, realizing how worried these young men were that they would be permanently shut away, like victims of leprosy, he began to study what he calls "the uses and misuses of quarantine."

His first book was about two epidemics in New York City in 1892, one of typhus and one of cholera, both blamed on Jewish immigrants because they were thought to be "dirty, unkempt, awful people who brought diseases." Many were sent to the artificial islands in New York's Lower Bay that had been built especially for quarantine. Markel's own grandparents were Jewish immigrants, and he related to the stigma experienced by the dying gay men. His book was published in 1997. Markel would go on to become the director of the University of Michigan's Center for the History of Medicine.

Then, in 2005, on the Fourth of July weekend, Markel got a mysterious call from a physician at the Pentagon named Cleto DiGiovanni, who worked for the Defense Threat Reduction Agency. "He knew all about me," Markel said. DiGiovanni had an assignment. Secretary of Defense Donald Rumsfeld had become concerned about a possible pandemic strain of influenza, H5N1, circulating in avian populations in East and Southeast Asia. It was highly contagious among birds and terribly fatal to people who got infected. Suppose it mutated and became transmissible among people? A distinguished virologist, Robert G. Webster, had warned that such a pandemic could possibly kill "a large fraction of the human population."

That got Rumsfeld's attention. It led to DiGiovanni's idea that Markel should study "escape" communities in the 1918 Spanish flu pandemic, which had essentially closed their doors against the rest of the world and survived the contagion virtually unscathed. They included Gunnison, Colorado; Princeton University and Bryn Mawr College; a school for the blind in Pittsburgh; the naval training station on Yerba Buena Island, California; a tuberculosis sanitorium in upstate New York; and the town of Fletcher, Vermont. The Pentagon had come up with the idea that, in the event of a pandemic, members of the armed forces could be crowded onto naval ships, which would become floating escape communities.

Six months later, Markel and his team presented their findings to a group of military brass, along with state and local health officials. Escape communities were very successful if they were situated on islands or in a tiny town in the Rockies, but they were not useful for society at large, and they were unlikely to work on naval ships. Even if the plan succeeded it would require sequestering the very people needed to protect society. While the subject was being debated, Markel fell into conversation with Martin Cetron, at the time a captain in the commissioned corps of the U.S. Public Health Service (he later became director of the Division of Global Migration and Quarantine at CDC). They had much in common, sharing a fascination with quarantine and a background of East European Jewish ancestry. Cetron was working on a comprehensive pandemic preparedness initiative for the George W. Bush administration. His specific job was to figure out how to manage the early waves of a hypothetical pandemic that has no medical solutions. During a break, they grabbed a sandwich, and Markel pitched the idea of studying the experience of American cities during the 1918 pandemic. Some had fared far better than others, despite the absence of a vaccine or any effective treatment. What had they done that succeeded? Markel and Cetron decided to look at the interventions that were used in 1918 and plot the epidemic curves city by city. They would take into account school closures, public gathering bans, business shutdowns—traditional tools of public health. Markel's team would gather the raw data and Cetron's would do the statistical analysis.

Markel assembled a dozen researchers—"which was like the Manhattan Project for historians," he joked—who spread out across the country, looking through more than a hundred different archives and haunting newspaper morgues. To make sure the data included material from different political perspectives, the team studied at least two papers a day for every city between September 1918 and April 1919 (in the early twentieth century, most American cities had Democratic and Republican newspapers). There was a weekly health index for major American cities during that pandemic, compiled by the U.S. Census Bureau, but it seemed to have vanished. Markel finally discovered it on a microfilm reel in the basement of the New York Public Library. Forty-three cities had reported to the index, the most complete compilation of mortality data available. It became the Rosetta Stone for the study.

IN 1918, Americans were facing the same confounding choices they would a century later. Twenty-five cities shuttered their schools; fourteen did so twice, and Kansas City three times. More than half of the cities were "double-humped," suffering two waves of flu. "They raised the bar too early because the natives got restless," said Markel. "When the measures were in effect, the cases went down; when the measures were lifted, the cases went up. They each acted as their own control group. So that was really kinda cool."

The graphs the modelers put together differ in surprising ways. New York City was the first to respond to the crisis, on September 18, before anyone in the city had died. New York's health department was renowned all over the world for its strict quarantine and mandatory case reporting. The health commissioner, Dr. Royal S. Copeland, enforced compulsory isolation and staggered business hours. He allowed individual theaters and cinemas to remain open, but only if they were well ventilated and banned coughing, sneezing, and smoking. Sanitary police stood guard to yank anyone out of the audience if they violated the rules. Broadway largely shut down that fall in any case, because people were too fearful to go to shows.

Copeland's protocols were enforced for seventy-three days. New York achieved the lowest death rate on the East Coast, but it failed to "layer" its response by simultaneously imposing nonpharmaceutical interventions, such as social distancing and public-gathering bans. Copeland didn't close the schools because he thought kids would be safer with district doctors and school nurses on the lookout for signs of infection. The graph tells the story. Mortality shoots up to a startling peak in mid-October, before plummeting back to near normal in early December. There's a smaller bump in January and February of the following year. The total excess death for the city was 452 per 100,000. The graph looks similar to what New York experienced from March to May 2020; in both cases, there is a large bump in the epidemiological curve, when not enough is being done to mitigate the contagion, followed by a flattening out as the interventions take effect.

Philadelphia recorded the earliest case of influenza of the cities studied, in late August. By mid-September, the contagion was out of control, but the public health director, Dr. Wilmer Krusen, remained convinced that the mortality would be low. It was wartime, and all cities, but particularly Philadelphia, the birthplace of American independence, were imbued with patriotic spirit. Families crowded the train stations as they saw their sons off to war. There were parades all over the country to sell Liberty Loans to support the war effort, and one was scheduled for Philadelphia. Dr. Krusen did not dare to stand in the way of such a popular cause. In any case, most of the afflicted were thought to be in the nearby Navy Yard. No one realized how widely the infection had seeded itself throughout the city.

And so on September 27, about 200,000 Philadelphians crowded along Broad Street to watch the parade, which was led by the "March King," John Philip Sousa. Within a few days, infections skyrocketed.

Finally, on October 3, the city closed the schools, but it was too late to stop the deluge of death. The coroner's office was so overwhelmed that it suspended issuing death certificates; bodies were summarily loaded into trucks and buried in a potter's field. Philadelphia had the second-worst mortality rate in the nation.

It was exceeded only by Pittsburgh. That city didn't record its first case until October 1, a day when Philadelphia, on the other side of Pennsylvania, recorded 635 deaths in twenty-four hours. With the specter of Philadelphia as a reminder, the acting state health commissioner, Dr. Benjamin Franklin Royer, banned public gatherings; closed the theaters, bars, and movie houses; and ended parades and public funerals. He left the tricky political question of closing churches and schools up to the local authorities. Despite these efforts, the rate of infection in Pittsburgh leaped up. New measures were implemented: suspending jury trials, limiting the number of passengers on an elevator, and ending church services altogether. Alcohol sales were banned, except in drugstores. School attendance dropped dramatically, and finally, on October 24, schools were closed.

Business interests were furious at the shutdown—saloon owners in particular—and under pressure, the mayor declared the city open for business on November 9. As a result, the epidemic dragged on, month after month. Pittsburgh would not celebrate forty-eight hours without the flu until April 21, 1919, tallying a staggering death rate of 806 people per 100,000. Together, Philadelphia and Pittsburgh contributed many of the 40,000 to 50,000 orphans that the flu left behind in its march through Pennsylvania.

Practically alone among American cities, San Francisco ordered the mandatory use of face masks. Most masks worn by healthcare workers were strips of gauze offering little protection. Chiffon veils were touted as being effective for fashion-conscious women, and some folks wore what appeared to be "extended muzzles." Shirkers were arrested and fined. In truth, none of these masks were very effective, but the city's public health officer, Dr. William C. Hassler, repeatedly boasted that San Francisco was the only large city in the entire world to quickly contain the contagion. Still, mutinous sentiments arose, even among the politicians who had imposed the rules. Both Hassler and Mayor James Rolph were caught maskless while attending a boxing match; they sheepishly paid their fines. On November 21, the order was rescinded, and at noon San Franciscans ceremonially removed their masks. A second wave engulfed the city after the turn of the year. Masks returned, along with complaints. An "Anti-Mask League" formed, including doctors and civic leaders. They held a public meeting attended by two thousand maskless people. As it turned out, San Francisco's death rate was among the worst of American cities.

So what did St. Louis do right? Like Pittsburgh, the city had time to prepare. The city health commissioner, Dr. Max C. Starkloff, had followed the devastation the contagion inflicted on the East Coast. In September, before the flu reached his city, he directed doctors to report any suspected case, and he wrote an editorial in the *St. Louis Post-Dispatch* alerting the citizens to the threat and giving them guidelines about how to avoid it.

The first seven cases in St. Louis were reported on October 5, all in a single family. The next day there were fifty. Dr. Starkloff shut down the scheduled Liberty Loan parade. Two days later, he convened a meeting of city officials and business leaders, along with school and hospital administrators, to discuss how to handle the forthcoming crisis. They put him in charge. Right away Starkloff closed the city's entertainment places, banned public gatherings, and shuttered the schools. Nurses attended patients in their homes, sparing the overcrowded hospitals. The St. Louis Tuberculosis Society passed out educational brochures. Police conducted surveys of the afflicted in their districts and made sure they received care. Teachers, no longer in their classrooms, volunteered at the health department. To make sure the city spoke with one voice, Starkloff created a Bureau of Information. The city was rewarded with a slow rise in infections through October that began to slope down in November.

On November 11, the war ended. There were celebrations all over the U.S. and Europe, but Starkloff maintained public closures, forcing celebrants to remain outside, where he intuited the chance of contagion was less likely. Schools opened on November 14, but thirteen days later a spike in infections prompted Starkloff to shut them again. They were not fully opened again until January 2. St. Louis had one of the lowest death rates in the country, 358 out of 100,000.

The lesson was that, by imposing several nonpharmaceutical interventions quickly, a city could dramatically lower the peak infection, making a shape on a graph more like a rainbow than a skyscraper. Thousands of lives were saved in St. Louis. Determined and unified leadership, and transparent communication, stirred to life an engaged citizenry, who were willing to endure the sacrifices and setbacks any such struggle against a lethal new disease is bound to impose. Markel compared each intervention to a slice of Swiss cheese; one layer by itself was too riddled with holes to be effective, but a layer upon a layer made a profound difference. Cities that acted early, for an extended period of time, did far better in terms of cases and deaths. "Early, layered, and long" was the formula for success.

"Nonpharmaceutical Interventions Implemented by US Cities During the 1918–1919 Influenza Pandemic" was published in *JAMA: The Journal of the American Medical Association* in August 2007. "The Influenza pandemic of 1918–19 was the most deadly contagious calamity in human history," the paper begins. "We found no example of a city that had a second peak of influenza while the first set of nonpharmaceutical interventions were still in effect." When the measures were withdrawn, "death rates increased."

October 1918 remains the most mortal month in American history. But America was a different country a century ago. More people lived in rural areas. Trust in government and the medical profession was high. Trains and automobiles made America mobile, but they scarcely compared to the rapidity and volume of present-day air travel, which links the whole world in a single ecosphere. In 1918, scientists had a poor understanding of viruses, which were murderous phantoms too small to see. Although the curtain that concealed the viral world has been pulled open, the tools for curbing a novel pandemic haven't changed. Nonpharmaceutical interventions—traditional public health measures—are still the only reliable way of slowing contagion until effective treatments or vaccines can be put into play. The only real difference in a hundred years is that face masks are more effective.

Whenever Markel was in Atlanta, he and Cetron would go to a Thai restaurant for dinner and talk over their study. One night they were working late at the hotel and ordered out. Finally, when dinner arrived, Markel opened his Styrofoam container. Inside, was a mass of noodles, which instead of a fluffy mound was a level, gelatinous mass. "Oh, look,"

said Markel. "They've flattened the curve, just like we're trying to do."
A slogan was born.

ON JANUARY 31, Markel was driving home, listening to *All Things Considered* on NPR. Just as he pulled into his driveway, a report came on about 195 Americans who had been evacuated from Wuhan. They were under a mandatory two-week quarantine at an air base in California after one of them had tried to leave. It was the first time in more than fifty years that the CDC had issued a mandatory quarantine order.

Markel listened in his car, expecting that Marty Cetron would come on the air. He did. "The best way to enforce a quarantine is to educate people on its purpose," he said of the evacuees. "These are American citizens who clearly want to do the right thing."

While the report was going on, Markel texted Cetron: "Hey, I'm listening to you on NPR!"

Cetron immediately texted back. "It's history repeating itself all over again," he said.

Markel got a chill. "That's the moment when I first realized a storm of contagion was upon us."

MATT POTTINGER HANDED out a study of the 1918 flu pandemic to his colleagues in the White House, indicating the differing outcomes between the experiences of Philadelphia and St. Louis—a clear example of the importance of leadership, transparency, and following the best scientific counsel. His brother, Paul, the infectious-disease doctor at the University of Washington Medical Center, kept him apprised of the ravaging infection in the nursing homes in the Seattle area. "I'm watching [a patient] die of this now," Paul texted from a nursing home. "He beshat himself, flooded his toilet, caused a flood, and the shitwater dripped into the floor below. . . . A literal deadly shitshow."

Matt asked, "You getting enough test kits?"

"We use none of the CDC kits," Paul responded. "They have been way too slow in coming. . . . Instead, we are using a homemade platform. It works well . . . but, today we ground to a halt because our capacity is still way less than demand."

CDC tests weren't yet approved for screening nonsymptomatic patients and non-CDC tests weren't authorized for emergency use. Paul was especially frustrated because the University of Washington is renowned for its testing capability. He was frantically setting up triage procedures, guessing which cases were Covid, trying to separate them from influenza patients, and ensuring that respiratory wards were established in separate areas in an effort to keep the Covid patients from infecting the whole hospital.

6

"It's Coming to You"

AMERICA WOULD HAVE three distinct opportunities to curb the Covid contagion before it got out of hand. The first was lost when the Chinese rejected U.S. offers to send a team of disease detectives to investigate the outbreak in Wuhan. Had CDC specialists been allowed to visit China in early January, Redfield believes, they would have learned exactly what the world was facing. The new disease was a coronavirus, and as such it was thought to be only modestly contagious, like its cousin the SARS virus. This assumption was wrong. The virus in Wuhan was far more infectious, and it spread in large part by asymptomatic transmission. "That whole idea that you were going to diagnose cases based on symptoms, isolate them, and contact-trace around them was not going to work," Redfield told me. "You're going to be missing 50 percent of the cases. We didn't appreciate that until late February."

The testing fiasco marked the second failed opportunity America had to control the Covid contagion. At a Coronavirus Task Force meeting, Redfield announced that the CDC would send a limited number of test kits to five "sentinel cities." Pottinger was stunned: five cities? Why not send them everywhere? He learned that the CDC makes tests, but not at scale. For that, you have to go to a company like Roche or Abbott—molecular-testing powerhouses which have the experience and capacity to manufacture millions of tests a month. The CDC, Matt realized, was "like a microbrewery—they're not Anheuser-Busch."

By that time, Secretary Azar, a former top executive of Eli Lilly, was leading the Coronavirus Task Force. He agreed with Pottinger that test kits needed to be broadly distributed, yet nothing changed. Everyone on the task force understood the magnitude of the crisis; they were diligent, meeting every weekday, with conference calls on weekends. North Korea and Iran didn't merit such concentrated attention. The real problem was that the administration was simply not executing the tasks that needed to be done to limit the pandemic. There was also a telling disparity between what Azar said in private or in the task force meetings and what he told the president. He was hammering Redfield and the CDC relentlessly on testing delays; meanwhile, he was assuring Trump that the coronavirus epidemic was under control.

The confusion of authority that would characterize every step that the Trump administration took in the pandemic was evident from the beginning. The CDC turned its test over to the Food and Drug Administration on January 20. (A functional test had been developed in Germany a few days before.) It was "the fastest we've ever created a test," Azar boasted to Trump. It took the FDA until February 4 to approve it. Then everything went to pieces.

A bottleneck of constraints imposed by the CDC meant that testing was initially limited to symptomatic patients who had come from China, or who had been in close contact with an infected person. Even health-care workers who'd fallen ill with Covid-like symptoms while treating patients had trouble getting tests, because the CDC's capacity was so limited. For people who did get the test, the results took as long as two weeks to be processed. But that wasn't the main problem.

Microbiologists are acutely aware of the danger of contamination. Viral DNA can linger for hours or days on surfaces, adulterating testing materials. CDC scientists wipe down their instruments every day. Chin-Yih Ou, a Taiwanese microbiologist who retired from the CDC in 2014, recalled how, when he was creating a test for HIV in infants, he refused to let janitors into his lab, choosing to mop the floor himself. In some labs, the last person to leave at night turns on ultraviolet lamps to kill any stray bits of DNA that might have drifted onto the floor or a lab bench. A new pathogen is like an improvised explosive: one wrong decision can be fatal.

Because of the backlog at the CDC in dealing with the samples coming in from labs all over the country, the agency decided to manufacture test kits so that state health labs could perform the testing themselves. This project was overseen by Stephen Lindstrom, an experienced microbiologist from Saskatchewan who was known for his ability to function under pressure. CDC scientists began working sixteen-hour days, trying to make the test kits as quickly as possible. For a diagnostic test to be properly validated, virus samples from an actual patient are required, but the Chinese refused to provide them. A human sample wasn't available until the first reported case in Washington State, on January 21, and then it had to be isolated and propagated in a special lab, which took until February 12. By then, the German test had been distributed to seventy laboratories around the world.

The CDC's Biotechnology Core Facility Branch is in charge of producing the components used to detect such pathogens as flu, HIV, and SARS. To save time, Lindstrom asked the branch to produce both the components and a template of a coronavirus fragment, which would be used to generate the positive control for the CDC test. Doing these procedures together risked the possibility of contamination, which is why they are normally done in separate facilities. Just as the test kits were being boxed up and mailed, a last-minute quality-control check found a problem that could cause the test to fail a third of the time. A decision was made—perhaps by Lindstrom, perhaps by his superiors—to send the test anyway. Lindstrom reportedly told his colleagues, "This is either going to make me or break me."

Almost immediately, public health labs realized something was wrong with the kits. The labs are required to do a negative control on the test—typically using sterile water—and the tests were turning up false positives at an alarming rate.

The CDC kit contained three sets of primers and probes, which are tiny bits of nucleic acid that find a segment of RNA in the virus and replicate it until it gets to a detectable level. They were enumerated N1, N2, and N3. The first two targeted SARS-CoV-2 and the third would detect any coronavirus, in case a mutation occurred. That was the element that failed. Public health labs figured this out quickly. On their behalf, Scott

Becker, the CEO of the Association of Public Health Laboratories, communicated with the CDC on February 9, seeking permission to use the test without the third component. "I got radio silence," he said. Later, he learned about an internal CDC review showing that the test passed a quality-control check before the kits were sent out. "That was a gut punch."

IN THE FALL OF 2009, Matt Pottinger was in Kabul, in his final deployment as a Marine officer. As he was walking through a tunnel connected to the U.S. Embassy, he passed a young woman. He took a few more steps then abruptly wheeled around.

Her name was Yen (pronounced "Ing") Duong. She was working with the Afghan government on improving its HIV testing. "It was like seven o'clock at night," Yen remembers. "He came up to me and asked if I knew where So-and-So's office was. I was thinking that I'm pretty sure So-and-So's office is closed right now. It was just a ploy to talk." They kept in touch but didn't see each other for another two years, when Matt flew down to Atlanta to get reacquainted. They married in 2014.

Matt and Yen have lived two very different American lives. He grew up in Massachusetts. His parents divorced when he was very young, and he lived mostly with his mother and stepfather. His father, J. Stanley Pottinger, was a lawyer in the Nixon administration. Matt had an ear for languages. He studied Mandarin in high school and planned to take a year abroad in China in 1989. Just before his departure, pro-democracy demonstrators took possession of Tiananmen Square in Beijing. The protests spread to hundreds of cities in China, led by students, many of them Matt's age. The government declared martial law and, on June 3, sent as many as 250,000 troops into Beijing. Hundreds, if not thousands, of protesters were massacred.

That incident set a hook in Matt Pottinger. After graduating from the University of Massachusetts, Amherst, in 1996, he soon found his way to China, reporting for Reuters and then the *Wall Street Journal*. He felt the need to defend liberty, not just report on repression, and that's what prompted him to join the Marines. When he met Yen, he was wondering what to do with the rest of his life.

Yen was six months old when her family fled Vietnam, in 1979, in a boat that her father had secretly built in his sugar factory. They were a part of one of the great migrations in history. Some 800,000 Vietnamese made the journey out of their homeland in overcrowded vessels. No one knows how many died, but the UN High Commission for Refugees estimates 200,000 to 400,000. The Duong family—68 in all—set sail in the middle of the night. They were shot at. A fierce storm nearly capsized the vessel. Pirates robbed them and threw the navigation equipment overboard. When the Duongs approached Malaysia, a government boat came out to meet them. Instead of towing them to land, the sailors tied a line to the family's battered boat and took them far out to sea, warning that they wouldn't be spared if they tried to come again.

Finally the family reached a Red Cross refugee camp in Indonesia. Six months later, the Duongs were sponsored by four American churches on Long Island, which is how they suddenly found themselves living in the Hamptons. Yen's mother cleaned houses and took in sewing and then found a job in a bakery. Yen's father painted houses and worked in construction. They supplemented their food by fishing and collecting watercress under bridges. Eventually they saved enough money to send their daughter to a private boarding school in upstate New York.

Because of their courage and resourcefulness, their daughter flourished. Yen was drawn to science, and along the way fell in love with viruses. She saw them as the major threat to the future of humanity, but she also thought they were amazing. She got a doctorate in pharmacology at the University of California, Davis, and in 2007 became a virologist at the CDC. She worked under Bharat Parekh in the global HIV branch, where she won the agency's highest award for developing what has become the standard test to measure HIV incidence. None of that would have happened if the family had stayed in Vietnam, if the boat had sunk in the storm, if the pirates had murdered them, or if they had not been taken in by Americans who wanted to help them get the opportunities that freedom allowed.

Yen Pottinger became a senior laboratory adviser at Columbia University's Mailman School of Public Health. She explained to Matt what she thought had gone wrong with the CDC test kits. "RNA and DNA are magical," she said. "On the one hand, they're very easily destroyed, and on the other, they actually survive in your lab for a really long time." SARS-CoV-2 is an RNA virus, which Yen described as "sticky," tending to cling to any surface. Once the Chinese had posted online the genetic sequence for the virus, primers would have been easy to design. But a pristine lab environment is essential, she said. "It has felled many a great scientist, by the way, this contamination issue."

ON FEBRUARY 10, the FDA learned that some of the public health labs working with CDC test kits were reporting failures. Based on CDC assurances that it could quickly fix the problem with the third component, the Trump administration—in particular, Azar—insisted on continuing with the CDC kits, despite the alternative of a workable German test and the eagerness of university scientists and researchers working in the major hospitals and the pharmaceutical giants and commercial laboratories to design their own tests. They were hampered by the bureaucratic challenge of obtaining an Emergency Use Authorization. According to Dr. Redfield, when the CDC had published the blueprint for its test, it had encouraged public health labs to apply to the Food and Drug Administration for an Emergency Use Authorization, which would allow them to do the testing themselves, without depending on Atlanta for the results. Scott Becker contends that the outside labs were waiting for the CDC to supply the tests, as it had typically done in the past.

Although FDA rules generally require that any procedure granted an EUA be used exactly as designed, the agency could have allowed public health labs to use the CDC test kits without the third component, as the labs were pleading to do. The test kits largely worked fine without it, but FDA says that it didn't have the data from the CDC to justify that simple solution. Lindstrom and the CDC insisted on sticking with the original design. Neither agency would bend.

On February 12, CDC officials estimated that it would take another week to remanufacture the third component, but six days later, Redfield told Secretary Azar that it might take until mid-March. By February 21, the test was failing in nearly every lab and the CDC admitted that it had no idea when the new test kits might be ready.

More than a month had passed since the first known patient arrived in the U.S., and in that time the CDC had conducted fewer than 500 tests. South Korea, which had its first case one day before the U.S., had already tested 65,000 people. China was reportedly testing 1.6 million per week.

The United States remained blind to the spread of the contagion, unable to fight what it couldn't see.

Officials at FDA realized that they weren't getting reliable information from the CDC, so on February 22, Dr. Timothy Stenzel, director of the agency's Office of In Vitro Diagnostics and Radiological Health, was dispatched to Atlanta to see what had gone wrong with the test. Stenzel was a microbiologist and immunologist of vast experience. He had set up the Clinical Molecular Diagnostics Laboratory at Duke University, and had developed diagnostics for breast cancer and brain tumors. He spent four years in private industry, including Abbott, where he was a senior director. He joined the FDA in 2018. He was not going to be easily fooled. When he arrived, on Saturday afternoon, there was no one to receive him, and he was turned away. The next morning, he was allowed into the building but forbidden to enter any labs. It was still the weekend. Stenzel made some calls. Finally, he was allowed into the three laboratories where the test kits were manufactured.

Stenzel instantly detected the problem: In one of the labs, researchers were analyzing patient samples in the very same room where testing ingredients were assembled. The tests are so sensitive that even a person walking into the room without changing her lab coat might carry viral material on her clothing that would confound the test, and yet the lab was processing specimens from all over the country, many of which were positive, while also creating the primers and probes for the test. It was clear to Stenzel that no one was in charge of the process. One FDA official described the lab as "filthy," and said he would have closed it down if it had been any other lab.

According to an internal FDA account, "When Dr. Stenzel toured the lab which manufactured oligonucleotides (short DNA or RNA molecules), including the primers and probes for the test, the staff indicated to Dr. Stenzel that Dr. Stephen Lindstrom—who oversaw a different lab in the manufacturing process—directed them to allow positive and negative control materials to occupy the same physical space of the lab, even though this is a violation of their written protocols."

The tests weren't failing, exactly. They were accurately detecting the presence of the virus in the kits themselves. The obvious remedy was to hand over manufacturing to two outside contractors. It was perhaps the lowest point in the history of a very proud institution. Within a week, tens of thousands of tests were available.

When asked how the contamination occurred and if anyone had been held accountable for the corrupted kits, Redfield—a round-faced man with a white Amish-style beard—replied vaguely, "One of the newer individuals hadn't followed protocol." It also could have been a design flaw that mangled results. Both mistakes might have happened, Redfield conceded. "I wasn't happy when we did our own internal review," he said, and acknowledged that the CDC should not have mass-produced the test kits: "We're not a manufacturing facility." He insisted: "At no moment in time was a Covid test not available to public health labs. You just had to send it to CDC." But the CDC couldn't process tens or hundreds of thousands of tests.

The CDC wasn't entirely responsible for the delay. According to the FDA, if China had made samples of the virus available in early January, or even December when it was first detected, the test kits could have been ready at the beginning of February. However, the FDA itself might have authorized a version of the test kit without the problematic third component and loosened the reins on tests developed by other labs. Officials say they were "fed up" with the CDC's indecision, but not until February 26 did the FDA, on its own authority, permit public health labs to use the CDC test without the third component. Three crucial weeks had been lost as the CDC and the FDA deliberated this obvious solution. Only on February 29 were other labs allowed to proceed with their own tests. The nation never recovered from its lost February. Bureaucratic inertia, compounded by scientific incompetence, handicapped America's response.

Secretary Azar held the FDA responsible for the absence of alternative tests. A senior administration official said, "Instead of being more flexible, the FDA became more regulatory. The FDA effectively outlawed every other Covid test in America." Stephen Hahn, the FDA commissioner, responded, "That's just not correct," and noted that more than three hundred tests had been authorized. But there was only one alternative test by the end of February. Whether the delay was caused mainly by the CDC or the FDA, Azar oversaw both agencies.

Without the test kits, contact tracing was stymied; without contact tracing, there was no obstacle in the contagion's path. America never had enough reliable tests, with results available within two days, distributed across the nation. By contrast, South Korea, thanks to universal health insurance and lessons learned from a 2015 outbreak of MERS, provided free, rapid testing and invested heavily in contact tracing, which was instrumental in shutting down chains of infection. By the end of 2020, the country would record some 50,000 cases in total; the U.S. was reporting more than four times that number every day.

The first two chances to curb the spread had already been lost. The third would presently appear.

FOR MOST PEOPLE, including politicians, the threat in February still appeared small. More than a month had passed between the first confirmed case in the United States and the first known death. "It's going to disappear," President Trump promised. "One day, it's like a miracle, it will disappear."

As the president was making this prediction, 175 employees of the biotech firm Biogen were heading home. They had gathered on a wintry weekend at the Marriott Long Wharf hotel in Boston Harbor. Many had traveled from other states and foreign countries. At the time, only fifteen confirmed cases of Covid-19 had been diagnosed in the U.S.—just one of them in Massachusetts. Among the international attendees were several from Italy, which was then under lockdown in the northern part of the country. The employees sat close together in the banquet rooms during sessions and socialized at the end of the day. They rode on elevators together and spent time in the gym. On Sunday, as the conference closed, they went home, carrying the virus to Boston or its suburbs; they journeyed to various states, including Florida, North Carolina, and Indiana; they flew back to Singapore, Australia, Sweden, and Slovakia. Soon, many fell ill.

Researchers affiliated with Massachusetts General Hospital, Harvard, and the Broad Institute of MIT concluded there was probably only one infected person present at the beginning of the conference. Those who contracted the virus must have become almost instantly contagious. Of the 175 attendees, about 100 would eventually test positive. Within a week, Mass General was starting to fill with suspected Covid patients, many of whom they were not allowed to test because of CDC constraints.

The particular Covid virus they contracted had mutations in its 30,000-character genetic code that allowed researchers to track its spread. By November, it had reached twenty-nine states and several foreign countries. The researchers estimate that the Biogen outbreak may have been responsible for more than 300,000 cases worldwide.

The same researchers looked at a separate outbreak at a nursing home in Boston, where 85 percent of the residents and 37 percent of the staff tested positive; this was despite masking requirements for everyone in the facility and restrictions on visitors. And yet the epidemic in the nursing home did not break free and roam the world like the Biogen strain. The authors concluded: "While superspreading events among medically vulnerable populations, such as nursing home residents, have a larger impact on mortality, our findings raise the possibility that—paradoxically—the implications may be greater, when measured as a cost to society, for superspreading events that involve younger, healthier and more mobile populations because of the increased risk of subsequent transmission."

During the initial stages of the Biogen study, in February and March, the researchers were troubled by the implications of their data. "The rapidity and degree of spread suggested it wasn't a series of one-to-one-to-one transmission," said Dr. Jacob Lemieux, the lead author of the paper in *Science*, "Phylogenetic Analysis of SARS-CoV-2 in Boston Highlights the Impact of Superspreading Events." "It was probably one or more episodes of one-to-*many* transmission events." That raised the question of airborne transmission. The researchers hesitated to broach the idea. "At the time, the idea of airborne transmission was heretical," Lemieux said. "We were afraid to consider it, because it implied a whole different approach to infection control"—one in which masks played a central role, especially indoors. But the WHO had repeatedly proclaimed that large respiratory droplets—as from a sneeze or cough—drove the spread. This conclusion wasn't based on data about the new virus, Lemieux said. "It was received wisdom on how previous respiratory viruses had behaved."

There was already a struggle going on between hospital policies, which were based on the opinion of medical authorities, and healthcare workers who feared for their lives. Under what circumstances should masks be worn, and what kind of masks would be tolerated? Hospitals had rules. They also wanted to provide a sense of security to patients and the public, but wearing PPE might raise a flag of alarm. As in China, some medical staff were reprimanded or suspended for making their own judgments about what they needed to stay safe. Doctors at the venerable Cleveland Clinic were warned not to "go rogue" by wearing masks around the hospital.

"The global public health infrastructure has egg on its face," Lemieux admitted. Science is a process of learning from mistakes, but Lemieux worried that the lessons that should have been learned hadn't been translated into policy. For more than a century, America had been spared a catastrophic pandemic, Lemieux observed. "There's a component of human nature that until you get burned, you don't know how hot the fire is."

VACCINES WERE IN development around the world, but when would they be available? Eighteen months at the earliest was the answer Pottinger was getting, and even that would be a record. A new vaccine must be subjected to three trials of increasing size, to determine safety, effectiveness, and proper dosage. Pharmaceutical companies then invest in production, ramping up from thousands of doses to millions. If we're lucky, the experts said, there might be enough vaccine for frontline workers by the fall of 2021.

On February 21, the task force conducted a brief tabletop exercise to game out the scope of the contagion. It was an eye-opener. "We're in for a disaster," Fauci realized. A Chinese report described how the new infection had spread across the entire country in thirty days despite the shutdown of entire cities. Secretary Azar agreed that there would need to be a major budget supplement to cover the cost of PPE for frontlne workers, effective therapeutics, and a speeded-up vaccine process that would pay companies to manufacture vaccine candidates that were in trials and might never be used. The tab might be as much as $3 billion.

After the meeting, Pottinger hung around and overheard a conversation between Azar and Mulvaney, Trump's acting chief of staff. They agreed that $800 million was enough for now.

Pottinger was incredulous. The administration was clearly in denial.

There were now more cases outside China than within. Italy and Iran were exploding. The absence of testing made it impossible to know how widespread the contagion was in the U.S. And yet Mulvaney and the Office of Management and Budget insisted on viewing the contagion as an overhyped influenza that could only be endured. When he got home, Pottinger complained to Yen that $800 million was half the sum needed just to support vaccine development through Phase 3 trials.

"Call Debi," Yen suggested.

Debi was Dr. Deborah Birx, the U.S. global AIDS coordinator. The world of public health is an intimate network of alliances and friendships, mentors and protégés, but also jealousies and grievances that dog the reputations of so many of its major figures. In the mid-1980s, as a young Army doctor, Birx studied immunology and AIDS at Fauci's clinic. They walked the hallways together, watching their patients die. Birx then moved to Walter Reed Army Medical Center. Like so many immunologists, she broke her lance trying to create an HIV/AIDS vaccine. At Walter Reed, Birx worked with Robert Redfield. From 2005 to 2014, she headed CDC's Division of Global HIV/AIDS, making her Yen Pottinger's boss. In her role as global AIDS ambassador, Birx administered the President's Emergency Plan for AIDS Relief (PEPFAR), which started in the Bush administration and was then the largest financial commitment any nation has ever made to fighting a single disease. Birx was known to be effective and data-driven, but also autocratic. Yen described her as "super dedicated," adding, "She has stamina and she's demanding, and that pisses people off." That's exactly the person Matt was looking for.

Birx was in Johannesburg when Pottinger called. She quickly agreed that Covid posed a mortal threat to AIDS patients, and she found $200 million in her PEPFAR budget to advance the science. Then Pottinger moved to another subject. In January, when it was just getting started, he had tried unsuccessfully to persuade Birx to run the Coronavirus Task Force as its administrator. Now he was desperate.

Birx was ambivalent. When she started her job at CDC, some countries in Africa had HIV-infection rates as high as 40 percent. It wasn't just a health problem; the disease ravaged those countries' economies by wiping out much of the workforce. Through steady application of public health measures and the committed collaboration of governments, the virus's spread had been vastly reduced. Birx was just at the point where she felt the disease could be managed. What if she turned her attention elsewhere and the numbers skyrocketed? Then again, Covid-19 was likely going to run rampant through the same immune-compromised population she was devoted to protecting.

She had watched with alarm as the coronavirus took hold in China and then began its spread. She studied the graphs of its exponential growth. When victims of a disease are symptomatic, they tend to go to bed, which acts as a brake on the rate of transmission. Something else was happening with this coronavirus. It was moving too fast. The best explanation was that it was spreading asymptomatically.

Few people had as much experience as Birx in dealing with pandemics. They are disruptive, divisive, and always political. Science does not necessarily get the last word. Political leaders have to balance saving lives and saving the economy. Prejudice plays a role—so strikingly demonstrated with HIV—and the disparities in health outcomes prompt resentment and racial strife. Grief and fear generate irrational actions. There would be blame-shifting and bitter recriminations.

Birx flew back to Washington, expecting this would be the end of her career.

IN THE 2015 MERS outbreak in South Korea, 152 of the 186 patients infected no one else, but 5 patients infected 147 people. They came to be known as superspreaders. During the 2014–2015 Ebola outbreak, 3 percent of the patients were responsible for 61 percent of the infections. SARS-CoV-2 is even more insidious because most of the transmission occurs from people without symptoms. At the beginning of the pandemic, public health officials postulated that the disease spread through fomites—surfaces, such as a doorknob or a subway strap, that might become contaminated when touched by an infected person and would then pass along the contagion to people who came into contact with it. The other route was through the droplets of saliva or respiratory secretions emitted when a person coughed or sneezed, and even while speaking. Social distancing was based on the droplet theory: six feet should be ample distance to avoid the rain of infection. But neither of those means of transmission accounted for superspreaders.

There is a little-known study by Richard L. Riley, who was an expert on lung physiology at Johns Hopkins, and his mentor, William F. Wells, "an eccentric genius," as Riley called him, who first demonstrated that tuberculosis could be spread through respiratory droplets. In the late 1950s, Wells and Riley set out to prove that TB could also be spread through airborne transmission.

On the roof of the Veterans Administration hospital in Baltimore, they built a cage for guinea pigs that was connected to an air-tight ventilation system tied directly into the tuberculosis ward below. Guinea pigs are the only rodent that can cough and sneeze, which makes them ideal for respiratory experiments. The animals exposed to the contaminated air became ill, proving that a droplet from the nose or mouth of a patient could evaporate into a microscopic particle, float through the air, be inhaled by a guinea pig, and actually cause disease some distance away. The data were used to create a model that quantifies the risk of transmission in closed environments, such as hospitals, prisons, airplanes—and cruise ships.

On February 11, 2020, the *Grand Princess* departed San Francisco for Mexico. The ship docked again in San Francisco ten days later, and most of the passengers disembarked, except for 68 who joined the new cruise on the next leg to Hawaii, carrying 2,422 passengers and 1,111 crew members, from 54 different nations. Meantime, a sister ship, the *Diamond Princess*, was already quarantined in the port of Yokohama, Japan. It had journeyed to Hong Kong and Vietnam, but on its return a passenger who disembarked in Hong Kong tested positive for Covid-19.

With a common water supply, air conditioning, communal dining, and a semi-enclosed environment, cruise ships are exquisite laboratories for research on infectious disease. In the case of the *Diamond Princess*, a single infected passenger spread the disease to 687 of the 3,711 passengers and crew—at the time, the largest outbreak outside of China. Researchers were stunned that 18 percent of the passengers who were infected showed no symptoms at all. That percentage would prove to be far lower than in the general population because the passengers tended to be older and more likely to become extremely ill. Later studies determined that most of the spread of the infection was through aerosol droplets that could float through the air—down hallways, lingering in bathrooms, drifting through the dining halls. The infection rate of the disease on the *Diamond Princess* was eventually put at 19.2 percent; on some vessels, it reached 60 percent.

Marty Cetron was in charge of quarantine at CDC, and he was alarmed. "These cruise ships are the equivalent of mass gatherings of hundreds if not thousands of the most vulnerable populations," he warned director Redfield in an email. Despite the peril to passengers and crews, new cruises continued to get underway, spreading the virus to ports around the globe; other ships were on their way to dock in America. Cetron was furious at the government's inaction and the cruise industry's reluctance to police itself. "This is unconscionable," he told his colleagues. He was told to "go home and get some sleep."

As the *Grand Princess* continued on its way back from Hawaii, a seventy-five-year-old man who had disembarked after the Mexican leg of the trip died. He was declared to be the first Covid fatality in California. (Later tests found antibodies in a fifty-seven-year-old woman who died in Santa Clara County on February 6, making her the first known fatality in the U.S.) Those passengers who had been on that portion of the trip were asked to confine themselves to their cabins until they could be tested, but apparently that wasn't enforced. Gavin Newsom, the governor of California, ordered the ship to return, although it was unclear what health authorities would do with the passengers. Coast Guard helicopters dropped the few test kits they could spare onto the deck. Of the forty-five people tested, twenty-one tested positive, and about a hundred other passengers showed symptoms.

Thousands of passengers and crews were infected and hundreds died as cruise ships continued to sail and governments declined to stop them. Marty Cetron was finally allowed to issue a no-sail order in the middle of March, bringing the cruises to an abrupt halt.

NURSING HOMES ARE like cruise ships in their confinement. For several weeks firefighters had been summoned to Life Care, a skilled-nursing facility in Kirkland, Washington, to transport an unusual number of patients to hospitals with fever and respiratory distress—symptoms exactly like Covid-19—but they couldn't be tested because they had not traveled to China or been in close contact with someone known to be infected. Finally, on February 27, CDC relaxed its standards, and the next day doctors at EvergreenHealth hospital tested two patients from Life Care. Both were positive. On February 29, Washington governor Jay Inslee reported that a healthcare worker in his fifties had died of Covid. The governor immediately declared a state of emergency.

America's blindfold was finally coming off.

One of Senator Patty Murray's relatives had been in the Kirkland facility a few years before. "I knew how many people came in and out of it, visitors and staff and nursing assistants," Murray recalled, "and all I could think was, 'Wow, this contagious virus, it can't have just stayed in a nursing home.' It was within a short amount of time I began hearing from my family and friends, 'Oh my gosh, I've got the worst flu I ever had, I got this cold that won't go away, this cough that won't stop, my kids are sick.'" Some of her own family were extremely ill. Murray told them, "Go get a test," but they replied, "I can't get a test, I've asked my doctor, I've asked the public health people in the county, I've called the state health people—*nobody* has these tests." Her state was in turmoil. "I could just see this absolutely spiraling." But in the Senate hearings and briefings, she sensed a lack of coordination and urgency. Even during the impeachment hearings, as she sat with her colleagues, she noticed some of the senators coughing. Was it the flu? Just a cold? Allergies? Who could tell? In the meantime, thousands of Americans were returning from China. Cruise ships were angling back to port. Europe was about to get walloped.

At the end of February, the Senate Democratic caucus went on a retreat in Baltimore. Murray received a text from her daughter, whose children were in school in the same neighborhood as the initial nursing home outbreak. "They closed the schools," her daughter said. "Kids are sick, teachers are sick. This is really frightening." Murray called the school principal, who told her that 20 percent of the children in the school were ill.

Murray told her colleagues: "My granddaughter's school closed today. This is coming to you."

7

"Nothing Can Stop What's Coming"

WHILE THIS WAS happening, I was in Houston, in rehearsals for *Camp David*, a play I had written about the Jimmy Carter, Menachem Begin, and Anwar Sadat summit in 1978. Oskar Eustis, of New York's Public Theater, was directing. Oskar is a big man with a barking laugh, flowing brown hair, and a full, bristling beard I associate with Falstaff, which he strokes when he's cogitating. He directed the first production of *Angels in America*. Under his leadership, the Public has given birth to some of the most important works of the modern stage, notably including *Hamilton*. Few people in the theater world have made such an imprint as he.

We were presenting *Camp David* at the Alley Theatre with expectations that we would take it to New York. It was the third play Oskar and I had worked on together, and we had become good friends. So I was concerned when he seemed listless, especially at the end of rehearsal. We went for a walk along Buffalo Bayou and he was breathless. One could see the effort required to regain the heartiness that was always so natural to him.

I have a memory of that production that later came back to me charged with significance. The players were performing in the round, allowing the audience an intimacy one doesn't get with a conventional stage. Often, the actors would be only a few feet away. The slanted lighting created a dramatic portraiture, highlighting the faces of the cast against the shadowy figures of the audience in the seats across the way; and in that lighting, I noticed that, when one particular actor expostulated, bursts of saliva flew from his mouth. Some droplets arced and tumbled, but evanescent particles lingered, forming a dim cloud. At the time, I thought it was interestingly dramatic, adding to the forcefulness of the character. Later, I thought this is what a superspreader looks like.

As far as I know, none of my actors were ill or contagious. I have no idea how Oskar got sick. But on February 20, when he flew back to New York, missing opening night, I knew something was wrong.

Texas was thought to be out of the danger zone that month, but retrospective modeling showed that the disease likely had been infecting at least ten people a day since the middle of the month. That was also true for California, Washington, Illinois, New York, and Florida. By the end of February, there was probable local transmission in thirty-eight states.

ON THE NIGHT of February 26, Lawrence Garbuz, an attorney in New Rochelle, New York, awakened with a cough and a low-grade fever. He was an apparently healthy man with no underlying conditions. The next morning, he went to the doctor, who sent him immediately to the emergency room.

During the four days Garbuz was at NewYork-Presbyterian/Lawrence Hospital in Bronxville, he was attended by doctors and nurses; his room was crowded with friends and family; orderlies and janitorial staff freely came and went with no special precautions. An X-ray showed that Garbuz had pneumonia, but the severity was confounding; one person described his lungs as "full of cobwebs." A nurse in the intensive care unit ventured "I think this patient is Covid," but her concerns were considered alarmist. By the weekend, Garbuz was too weak to speak. He handed a note to a doctor, asking, "Am I going to die?"

On March 1, Garbuz was put on a ventilator. The next day, he was transferred to NewYork-Presbyterian/Columbia University Medical Center in Manhattan, where he was finally tested for Covid-19. He was positive. By that time, members of his family, nursing staff, healthcare workers and their families were beginning to show symptoms. So was the neighbor who drove him to the emergency room. Governor Andrew Cuomo tagged Garbuz "Patient Zero" in New York, but he was just one case of a cluster of more than ninety people in New Rochelle, where he had recently attended a funeral and a b'nai mitzvah. The synagogue was shut down, and the National Guard enforced a containment zone in a mile radius around it.

While Lawrence Garbuz lay unconscious, the coronavirus cast a kind of anesthesia over the entire country. It was a striking contrast to 2014, when there had been a small outbreak of Ebola in the U.S. Two people died, a Liberian national who brought the disease with him and a doctor who had contracted Ebola in Sierra Leone. Out of the eleven people treated, nine had contracted the disease in Africa and neither of the two people who were infected by the disease in the U.S. died. And yet the country was near hysteria. Governors in a number of states imposed mandatory twenty-one-day quarantines for anyone who had contact with an Ebola patient—mainly, healthcare workers—whether they had symptoms or not. Schools were closed even in districts where there had been no exposure. Donald Trump, then a private citizen, attacked the Obama administration's decision to send the U.S. military to West Africa to fight Ebola. "STOP THE FLIGHTS!" he tweeted. "NO VISAS FROM EBOLA STRICKEN COUNTRIES!" He wouldn't spare doctors, either. "People that go to far away places to help out are great—but must suffer the consequences!"

Where Ebola banged pans and tossed firecrackers in its path, the coronavirus slipped in on cat's paws. The virus hitchhiked on passengers coming from hotspots. Five million people had left Wuhan before Chinese authorities locked the city down. From December to March, there were 3,200 direct flights from China to the U.S., arriving mainly in Los Angeles, San Francisco, and New York. Sixty percent of flights from Italy to the U.S. landed in New York. They brought a new mutation of SARS-CoV-2 that would prove to be even more contagious than the Chinese original. Travel continued until Italy went into a nationwide lockdown on March 10. The next day, the WHO finally declared a pandemic. By that time there were more than 100,000 cases in 114 countries, and 4,291 had lost their lives. "It will go away," the president remarked. "Just stay calm. It will go away."

———

"WE ARE COORDINATED, we are fully mobilized, and we are fully prepared to deal with the situation as it develops," Governor Cuomo said. "This isn't our first rodeo." Mayor Bill de Blasio also sought to assure his constituents. "I'm encouraging New Yorkers to go on with your lives + get out on the town despite Coronavirus," he tweeted.

The New York City Health Department turned to Marc Lipsitch, a professor of epidemiology at Harvard University, to create a model that would give them some framework for how to respond. On February 24, Lipsitch and one of his students, Rebecca Kahn, presented the model, which allowed health authorities to plug in different factors, such as how many infected travelers had entered the city, what the rate of infection was, how many were asymptomatic. Lipsitch thought it might help the officials set guidelines despite the lack of political urgency, which he characterized as "if you don't see a problem, you don't have a problem."

The health authorities knew what an epidemic curve with exponential growth looked like. It measures the rate of doubling of the infections. Still, the graph was sobering. If there were five infections at the beginning of February, there could be more than 50,000 cases by the end of April.

The New York City Emergency Management Department was headed by Deanne Criswell, a former National Guard firefighter from Aurora, Colorado. Starting in January 2020, as soon as the new virus appeared on the horizon, Criswell conducted a series of tabletop exercises, involving the hospitals, schools, the police and fire departments, the health department, sanitation commissioner, the mayor's office, and other agencies. They were gaming worst-case scenarios. From the beginning, the main obstacle the city faced was the still-unknown nature of the virus. Added to that was the daunting responsibility of making decisions that would disrupt the lives of 8.6 million New Yorkers—decisions that would have cascading impacts across the region, the country, and the world—and what's more, they were being made before there were any known cases in the city. The nightmare scenarios included overwhelmed hospitals, staff reductions up to 40 percent, economic collapse, and mass fatalities. Reality would soon outstrip their worst imaginings.

The governor was giving mixed signals, demanding on the one hand that health departments in New York quarantine anyone who had been in contact with an infected person or had traveled to a country with an outbreak, which included much of the world. On the other hand, Cuomo was "a little perturbed" by the anxiety that was beginning to spread across his state. "The more people you test, the more positives you are going to find," he said, a complaint many politicians, not least the president, would echo.

All through February, the country remained unaware of the spread of the infection because of the faulty CDC test. Weeks had passed from the point when containment was possible. On February 25, Nancy Messonnier, a senior director at the CDC, warned that the situation was "rapidly evolving and expanding." She painted a sobering picture of the future: "Ultimately, we expect we will see community spread in this country. It's not so much a question of *if* this will happen anymore but rather more a question of exactly *when* this will happen and how many people in this country will have severe illness." Without a vaccine or treatment for the disease, communities would have to rely on nonpharmaceutical interventions, including school closures, social distancing, disinfecting surfaces, teleworking, canceling mass gatherings, and delaying elective surgeries. People should expect missed work and loss of income. Parents should consider what to do about childcare. "I understand this whole situation may seem overwhelming and that disruption to everyday life may be severe, but these are things that people need to start thinking about now."

Messonnier's straight talk crashed the stock market, the Dow Jones Industrial Average losing 12 percent of its value in one week. The president was enraged. He appointed Vice President Pence to head the White House Coronavirus Task Force, shoving aside Alex Azar, who remained on the force. But for the first time, America got an accurate diagnosis of its condition. The next time Messonnier spoke publicly, she was quick to praise the president, saying that the country had acted "incredibly quickly."

AMY KLOBUCHAR DROPPED out of the race for the Democratic nomination on March 2, hours before Super Tuesday voting began, and flew to Dallas to endorse Joe Biden. The stage was jammed with supporters, ranks of them, shoulder to shoulder, waving blue Texas for Biden signs.

"I believe, and it's the reason I'm up here, we are never going to out-divide the divider-in-chief," Klobuchar said to the crowd. "If we spend the next four months dividing our party and going at each other, we will spend the next four years watching Donald Trump tear apart this country." She embraced Biden as the crowd cried, "Let's go, Joe!" But as she did so, she was thinking, "Joe Biden shouldn't get Covid." She warned his advisers to begin taking greater precautions.

The following Friday she went to a Biden rally in Detroit. That night employees of the Wayne County sheriff's office gathered for an annual party at Bert's, a beloved soul food and jazz venue. They had been meeting there for twenty years. Most of them were Black, some were retired. Three weeks later, seven of the attendees had Covid and dozens more in the sheriff's office were ill. Three law-enforcement officials would be dead before the end of the month.

At the rally, Klobuchar noticed that people had become more careful. "I put on gloves," she said. "We didn't know about masks at the time."

The Democratic rallies soon came to a halt after Michigan, but people from all over the country flocked to New Orleans for Mardi Gras—some 1.4 million of them. So far, only fifteen cases had been confirmed in the U.S., but before the end of March, Orleans Parish would have the highest death rate per capita of any county in the country.

ON MARCH 6, on his way to play golf at his resort in Palm Beach, Mar-a-Lago, the president stopped off at CDC headquarters in Atlanta. There were no more dire warnings from this quarter; the CDC was now a captive agency.

The object of the president's visit was to publicize the fact that the revised CDC test was finally ready. The president claimed to feel right at home in the laboratory because of his innate understanding of medicine. "My uncle was a great person," he said. "He taught at MIT for, I think, like a record number of years. He was a great super genius. Dr. John Trump.* I like this stuff. I really get it. People are surprised that I understand it. Every one of these doctors said, 'How do you know so much about this?' Maybe I have a natural ability."

---

* John Trump was an electrical engineer who taught at MIT from 1936 to 1973. He won the National Medal of Science in 1983.

At Trump's side, gazing at him with a marveling expression, was Redfield. The president appointed him CDC director in March 2018, possibly at the suggestion of Redfield's friend and patron, W. Shepherd Smith Jr. An evangelical activist, Smith had started Americans for a Sound AIDS/HIV Policy, which advocated for sexual abstinence and mandatory AIDS testing, and opposed the use of condoms as a strategy for preventing the disease. Redfield, a devout Catholic, served on the advisory board of this organization. He also wrote the foreword for Smith's 1990 book, *Christians in the Age of AIDS*, which stated that AIDS was "God's judgment" against homosexuals.

Redfield spent many years as an Army physician at Walter Reed Army Institute of Research, where he led the AIDS division until 1994. He had a mixed record in that department. His research showed that HIV could be transmitted heterosexually, which did much to diminish the stigma of what was tagged a "gay disease." In July 1992, at an international AIDS conference in Amsterdam, he announced a breakthrough "vaccine," as he termed it, a treatment that he claimed lowered the viral load in patients already infected with the disease. Other scientists, including Anthony Fauci, challenged the results. Despite admitting that he had misrepresented the findings, he presented the same data at another conference a month later. In 1996, Redfield co-founded the Institute of Human Virology at the University of Maryland School of Medicine, with Dr. Robert C. Gallo, a well-known HIV researcher. Gallo characterized his partner as "a terrific, dedicated infectious disease doctor," but noted that he "can't do anything communication-wise . . . He's reticent, never wanting the front of anything—maybe it's extreme humility."

Director Redfield welcomed the president to the CDC and thanked him for "helping us put public health first." Trump toured the lab where the diagnostic tests were made. Alex Azar, the secretary of Health and Human Services, was there, boasting that four million tests would be available by the end of the next week, which was far from true.

Wearing a red "Keep America Great" cap and a presidential windbreaker, Trump was in a buoyant frame of mind, bouncing on the balls of his feet and jousting with reporters. "As of the time I left the plane," the president said, "we had 240 cases. That's at least what was on a very fine network known as Fox News." He turned to the reporter from that network. "And how was the show last night?" he asked, referring to his town hall appearance in Scranton, Pennsylvania. "Did it get good ratings, by the way?"

"I—I don't know, sir," the reporter said.

"Oh, really? I heard it broke all ratings records, but maybe that's wrong. That's what they told me." He returned to the point of his visit, which was to reassure Americans that there was nothing to worry about. "So we have 240 cases, 11 deaths," the president reiterated. "I don't want any deaths, right?" The case mortality rate for flu was under one percent, he pointed out. "But this could also be under one percent because many of the people that aren't that sick don't report. So they're not putting those people in there. And you're smiling when I say that," he said, noticing another reporter. "Who are you from, anyway?"

"I—I'm from CNN."

"You are? I don't watch CNN. That's why I don't recognize you."

"Oh, okay. Well, nice to meet you."

"I don't watch CNN because CNN is fake news."

One reporter, observing that the lack of testing made it impossible to know how many cases there actually were, asked Redfield, "Don't you think it's likely that there are a lot more people out there who are going to come and actually be sick?"

"No doubt we're going to see more community cases," Redfield conceded.

"In this great country of ours, we have 240 cases," the president reiterated, growing impatient. "Most of those people are going to be fine. A vast majority are going to be fine. We've had 11 deaths, and they've been largely old people who are—who were susceptible to what's happening."

A reporter asked if the coronavirus was contained in the U.S. "The overall risk to the American public does remain low," Redfield said. "It's not as if we have multiple, multiple—hundreds and hundreds of clusters around the United States." He added: "We're not blind where this virus is right now in the United States."

There was some confusion about how many tests would actually be available and when. "Anybody that wants a test can get a test. That's what the bottom line is," the president insisted, adding: "And the tests are beautiful." As for the *Diamond Princess*, which was still looking for a port as health authorities pondered how and whether to evacuate the passengers, the president made it clear that he didn't want the ship to dock at all. "I like the numbers where they are," he said. "I don't need to have the numbers double because of one ship that wasn't our fault."

The president flew on to Mar-a-Lago, where there was a birthday party for Donald Trump Jr.'s girlfriend, Kimberly Guilfoyle, and a visit from the Brazilian president. Several guests from the weekend later tested positive, including the Brazilian president. Trump refused to self-quarantine, but at a fundraiser that Sunday he remarked that he had shaken hands with a guest whose hands were annoyingly clammy. Some of the moisture clung to the president's palm. "You hear any bad things about the health of our president, there's the guy," Trump said. "Find out who the hell that guy was."

Tucker Carlson, the Fox News talk show host, walked in while the party was underway. He had arranged a private audience with the president, but he had no idea that there was a celebration underway for Guilfoyle, his former colleague at Fox. Carlson had come to warn Trump that the coronavirus was a genuine threat. The disease had sent a friend to an ICU, where he was now struggling for his life. "I think it'd be very hard to keep it from spreading given the nature of American life," he later said. "I could just feel a sense of real danger." Carlson's main concern, however, was the effect on the economy. "Millions of unemployed people makes your country volatile," he said. "You don't want to live in an unstable country, period."

The next day, the president retweeted a Photoshopped image of himself playing a fiddle. The meme sounded a QAnon slogan: "Nothing can stop what is coming!" Trump commented, "Who knows what this means, but it sounds good to me!"

THE NEW YORK CITY Health Department felt muzzled by the mayor. "Every message that we want to get to the public needs to go through him, and they end up getting nixed. City Hall continues to sideline and neuter the country's premier public health department," a health official complained in early March. "He doesn't get it," the official wrote in another memo. "Not convinced there's a volcano about to blow beneath us." Insurrection was afoot. There was talk of delivering an ultimatum to the mayor: "Either pivot to pandemic planning today or they start to deal with a health department that won't follow his orders." Mayor Bill de Blasio was under the spell of an email from Mitchell Katz, the CEO of New York's sprawling municipal healthcare system, who counseled the mayor to keep the city open. "Canceling large gatherings gives people the wrong impression of this illness," Katz wrote. "If it is not safe to go to a conference, why is it safe to go to the hospital or ride in the subway?" He argued, on the one hand, that the "terrible problem" in Italy was unlikely to happen in New York and, on the other, that many New Yorkers were going to get infected anyway. "Greater than 99 percent will recover without harm. Once people recover they will have immunity. The immunity will protect the herd." The mayor then went on *Morning Joe* and said a number of things he would soon regret, starting with his pledge to keep the schools open, even if students fell ill. "If you're under fifty and you're healthy, which is most New Yorkers, there's very little threat here."

Political leaders all over the world were facing a quandary. Was it wiser to let the disease roll through society, extracting its deadly toll, mainly of the elderly, the vulnerable, and a higher rate of minorities; or shutter the windows and try to keep the contagion at a manageable level? Mitchell Katz predicted that the case fatality rate in the city would work out to be about one percent—potentially 84,000 people—if nothing was done to flatten the curve.[*] But the idea of closing down the economy was chilling. Was it worth the sacrifice?

On March 10, the CDC announced there were more than five hundred reported cases in America, but they represented the meager population that conformed to the CDC's grudgingly evolving testing guidelines: someone who recently traveled to China, had contact with an infected person, was hospitalized with symptoms, or had fever, cough, and trouble breathing. The guidelines almost seemed designed to undercount the spread. Asymptomatic carriers and people with mild symptoms slipped through the nets.

That day, Oskar Eustis roused himself and walked a half mile from his home to an emergency clinic on Amity Street, in the Cobble Hill section of Brooklyn. He had been ill for nearly a month. His muscles ached.

---

[*] The infection fatality rate in the spring in New York City, despite the lockdown, was still 1.39 percent, and no doubt would have been much higher without the interventions. Wan Yang et al., "Estimating the Infection-Fatality Risk of SARS-CoV-2 in New York City during the Spring 2020 Pandemic Wave: A Model-Based Analysis," *The Lancet*, Oct. 19, 2020.

Twice he had to stop and catch his breath, sitting for a while on a fire hydrant. He was too exhausted to be afraid.

His vital signs showed dangerously low potassium levels and his heart kept skipping beats. An ambulance ferried him from the clinic to NYU Langone Hospital on 55th Street, in Brooklyn. Bloodwork showed worrisome heart abnormalities. The damage that Covid-19 can do to the heart wasn't yet known, and Oskar's symptoms weren't the ones normally associated with the disease; only later would an antibody test show that he was suffering from the coronavirus. A study in Germany scanned the hearts of 100 coronavirus patients and found abnormalities in 78 of them and myocardial inflammation in 60. Some patients have required heart transplants.

Despite his fragile condition, there was no room for Oskar. He was placed on a gurney with an IV potassium drip and left in a corridor overnight. He soiled himself, but nobody came to change him. He was given no food for thirty-six hours. The Covid surge had begun.

8

The Doom Loop

T HE FIRST REPORTED CASE of Covid in Washington, D.C., was on March 7. The virus was no longer "out there," it was in the capital, possibly in the same neighborhoods where the Coronavirus Task Force members and their families lived. The CDC's Robert Redfield observed that there were 3,656 new cases worldwide, and only 46 were in China. By now, the contagion had spread to 34 states, and the source of the disease was traced to Europe in 30 of them. The images from Italy on television were horrifying—overrun hospitals, people being treated in parking lots—and the data clearly showed that the U.S. was on the same dismal path. "The center of gravity is Europe," Redfield said, "and then it's the United States."

The vice president had taken over the chair and enlarged the group, so there were more voices in the room, but no direction. For days, the task force had been going round and round about what to do with the cruise ships without making any decisions. "We need to take steps that will cause people to say, 'You're crazy,'" Secretary Azar ventured at a task force meeting the next day. Up until then, Azar had resisted taking forceful action, but now he sensed that the virus was getting out of hand. "I know it's a scary proposition for the secretary of the Treasury and some of our other economic-minded officials, but we have to get a month ahead of it," he said.

Pottinger thought Azar's remark might serve to focus attention on what was really important, not on what was merely urgent. Pence seemed at least somewhat receptive. "Better safe than sorry" was his tepid endorsement.

Meetings were often full of acrimony. "I can't even begin to describe all these insane factions in the White House," Olivia Troye, a former homeland security adviser to Pence, said. Anthony Fauci was considered too "outspoken and blunt" with the media, which led Jared Kushner and Peter Navarro to describe him as "out of control." Troye summed up the administration's prevailing view of Deborah Birx crisply: "They hate her." At task force briefings, Birx typically presented a slide deck, and Troye noticed White House staff members rolling their eyes. She overheard Marc Short, Pence's chief of staff, remark, "How long is she going to instill fear in America?" Troye often thought, "If these people could focus more on doing what's right for the country rather than trying to take each other down, we'd be in a much different place."

The task force was awakening to the need to do something more than talk about the virus—but what? Thousands of travelers arrived daily in the U.S. from Europe and South Korea—another epicenter— possibly bringing new infections. Pottinger pushed for a more expansive travel ban. Birx agreed. "Every seed case you prevent is a cluster of cases you prevent," she said. Redfield, Birx, and Azar swung around to the idea that cutting off European travel might at least slow the rate of contagion and buy time. Fauci thought that was an illusion. He had supported the China ban, but once a pandemic has spread everywhere, he said, travel bans don't work. "There's no place in America where it's business as usual," he said. "By the time you mitigate today, we're three weeks late." The economists were dead set against any further restriction on travel.

On March 11, it was time to confront the president. At one in the afternoon, the task force crowded into the Oval Office, where they were joined by Kushner, Ivanka Trump, Secretary of State Mike Pompeo, and a dozen others. The discussion turned into a passionate argument. The immediate question was whether to close off all travel from Europe, but it led to a showdown over what was more urgent, saving lives or protecting the economy. The caseload in the U.S. had recently topped 1,000, which seemed ominous to the public health contingent but manageable to the economic team. Treasury Secretary Steven Mnuchin said a travel ban would cripple the U.S. economy and trigger a global depression. Every airline, every hotel, would be pounded. The markets would crater. "Forget about ballgames," he said, pointedly adding: "Forget about campaign rallies."

"It's the biggest decision of your presidency," Stephen Miller, Trump's senior policy adviser, said.

Matt Pottinger believed the president felt a need to witness such verbal brawls. There were two modes to Trump's decision-making process, Pottinger observed. When he was taking in new information, the president was receptive. He asked questions. He was open to hearing both sides. He didn't try to be the smartest guy in the room. Once he made a decision, though, God help you in trying to change his mind.

After an hour, the president had another obligation, and he asked Pence to keep the discussion going. The group adjourned to the Cabinet Room. The vice president remained standing as there was no place left to sit. Mnuchin argued that there must be ways to curb the spread of the virus without closing off all travel. The elderly were at high risk; why not sequester them and other vulnerable people, fence them off from their grandkids and likely sources of contagion?

"It's twenty-five percent of the population!" Robert O'Brien, the national security adviser, observed. "You're not going to be able to stick them all in hotels and think that's the end of it." Different generations have to interact. Caretakers will inevitably be exposed. People will continue to eat together. Even old people have lives to manage. It's just not realistic.

Everyone knew what was at stake. There were 1,272 reported cases in the U.S., but that was like believing the only stars in the sky were the ones you could see. Fauci declared it was just going to get worse and worse. Colleges were sending their students home. Yet another skeptical member of the task force observed that, in a bad flu season, there might be 60,000 deaths. So what's the difference?

"This is *twenty times* that," Pottinger argued. "This is two percent dead guys, where the flu is point-one percent." In Italy, the case fatality rate had reached 6.64 percent. "You're looking at twenty to forty times the deaths."

"If we just let this thing ride there could be two million dead," Birx added, "but if we take action, we can keep the death toll at a hundred and fifty to two hundred and fifty thousand." It was surreal hearing such numbers of dead Americans being laid out so nakedly.

Mnuchin demanded data. The U.S. was just going to have to live with the virus, he believed. It wasn't worth sacrificing the airlines, the cruise ships, the hotels, the entire travel and leisure industry. The effectiveness of a travel ban was unproven. Speculative health gains shouldn't outweigh the certain economic costs. "This is going to bankrupt everyone," he said. "Boeing won't sell a single jet."

"You keep asking me for my data," Birx said sharply. "What data do you have? Does it take into account hundreds of thousands of dead Americans?"

"OH, FUCK," the president said from the Oval Office that evening. On the C-SPAN screen there was a title page saying "Presidential Address," but the audio started broadcasting a few minutes early. "Oh, oh, I got a pen mark," the president's distinctive voice was saying. "Anybody got any white stuff?" he asked, presumably meaning correction fluid.

When the camera finally rolled, it found the president at the Resolute Desk, which had been used in the Oval Office by John F. Kennedy, Jimmy Carter, Ronald Reagan, George W. Bush, and Barack Obama. On the credenza behind him were the flags of the United States and the Presidency, along with photos of his parents and a display of tokens, called "challenge coins," from the many federal agencies under his command, as well as commemorative coins that Trump had printed for his club, Mar-a-Lago, and his visit with the pope. "We are marshaling the full power of the federal government and the private sector to protect the American people," the president promised, reading haltingly from a teleprompter. There were typos in the text because of the last-minute changes, as well as factual errors. "This is the most aggressive and comprehensive effort to confront a foreign virus in modern history," the president continued, emphasizing that it came from China. He said he was suspending all travel from Europe for the next thirty days, although he hadn't consulted the Europeans and the restrictions didn't apply to American citizens or legal permanent residents. He claimed that insurance companies had agreed to "waive all co-payments for coronavirus treatments," but in fact they had only agreed not to charge for testing. For the vast majority of Americans, he said, "the risk is very, very low. Young and healthy people can expect to recover fully and quickly." He pointed to the danger the elderly faced and urged nursing homes to suspend unnecessary visits. He had also signed a bill providing $8.3 billion to help the CDC and other government agencies fight the virus. "Our banks and financial institutions are fully capitalized and incredibly strong. Our unemployment is at a historic low . . . This is not a financial crisis," he said, even as futures on the Dow were plummeting during the speech, "this is just a temporary moment of time that we will overcome together." He advised social distancing and reducing large gatherings— practices that he hadn't yet adopted himself. He concluded: "We must put politics aside, stop the partisanship and unify together as one nation and one family."

Up until this moment, one could still grant that the missteps by the Trump administration were errors of inexperience. He had certainly been distracted by impeachment. In this speech, stilted as it was, Trump repackaged himself as a take-charge president, a unifier, a consoler-in-chief. If he had actually followed the course he outlined in the speech that night, the nation would have had a different experience with the contagion.

GLENN HUBBARD IS a conservative economist who served as chairman of President George W. Bush's Council of Economic Advisers. He decided to entertain his students at Columbia University's graduate school of business, in his course "Highlights of Modern Political Economy," with a lecture about how John Maynard Keynes and Friedrich von Hayek might have approached the economic consequences of Covid-19. Keynes and Hayek were among the most influential economists of the twentieth century. Their work continues to magnetize the thinking of the progressive left and the libertarian right.

Keynes, the avatar of liberal economists, had been puzzled by the persistence of the Great Depression. Classic economic theory held that savings and investment were like a seesaw; too much saving caused too little investment, and vice versa. But as long as government didn't meddle, markets would naturally settle into balance and trend toward full employment. "When Keynes saw how long the depression was lasting in the early 1930s, he came to the conclusion that the image of a seesaw wasn't quite right," Hubbard said. "It could be more like an elevator that could stall on any floor." In that case an outside force—government stimulus—was required to get the elevator back into service.

Keynes's great work, *The General Theory of Employment, Interest and Money*, published in 1936, changed the role of government in capitalist societies, leading to increased regulation and the creation of global institutions, such as the World Bank and the International Monetary Fund. It became accepted wisdom that, in times of recession, substantial government spending would kick-start consumption and cause businesses to expand, thereby reducing unemployment. The governmental bailouts during the 2007–2008 financial crisis in the U.S. were an example of Keynesian interventions.

Hayek's book *The Road to Serfdom* had been the bible of conservative economists since its publication in 1944, in the midst of the civilizational struggle between democracy and fascism. His thesis is that government control of the economy inevitably crushes individual freedom and leads to tyranny. Hayek's political influence reached its peak with the rise of Ronald Reagan and Margaret Thatcher and the neoliberals. When Reagan said in his first inaugural address, "Government is not the solution to our problem, government is the problem," he carved on the hearts of generations of conservative lawmakers a maxim that is the basis of Hayek's economics. In Hubbard's class at Columbia, the students discussed Hayek's 1945 article "The Use of Knowledge in Society," which argues that central planning can never replace market forces, which reflect the sum total of the "decentralized knowledge" available to a society. Jimmy Wales has said that he read Hayek's article as an undergraduate and it was central to his decision to create Wikipedia.

Hubbard observed that, in the face of this pandemic, Keynes would have proposed vigorous government intervention and deficit spending. He believed that the creation of jobs, even digging holes and filling them in again, is fundamental to getting people back into the economic system, putting money in their pockets, awakening demand, and lifting the "animal spirits" of businesspeople to open their doors and start hiring.

In a major recession, only government has the resources to prod society back on its feet. Hayek, on the other hand, would have argued that trying to return to the status quo would block the opportunity to create the economy of the future, leading to long-term stagnation. "The more we try to protect particular jobs and firms today, we may be slowing down an adaptation to a world that may be," Hubbard suggested. He nudged his students "to see paths forward in the middle." He added: "While I suspect members of Congress don't have *The Road to Serfdom* or *The General Theory* on their bedside table, those ideas about centralization and decentralization are probably front and center in their minds."

HUBBARD WAS INVOLVED in that discussion in Washington. As policymakers addressed the greatest economic crisis in nearly a century, Hubbard warned them that it was more dire than they imagined. "I and other economists had been worried about a doom loop since the beginning of the pandemic," Hubbard recalled. A doom loop is a term in modern economics that means a cycle of negative feedback. When the pandemic hit, the world suffered a supply shock: trade was disrupted, factories closed, stores shuttered. If workers didn't start earning again soon, the supply shock could turn into a demand shock, which would further weaken supply, which would increase unemployment and further diminish demand. The doom loop.

In mid-March Hubbard spoke with Republican senators Marco Rubio, Susan Collins, and Roy Blunt. They were in a state of shock. Economic forecasts were terrifying. The NBA had just suspended its season. States were closing schools. One day there were more than three hundred new cases; the very next day, more than five hundred. The historic scale of the damage was beginning to reveal itself. The senators were getting panicked reports from hospital administrators, local officials, business owners, and their frightened constituents, all demanding action.

Only Collins had been in office in 2008, during the Great Recession, when Congress reached into its purse and authorized $700 billion to bail out troubled assets—the outer limit of what these conservative politicians ever imagined spending. Now they were talking about trillions. Racking up debt, enlarging the deficit, and expanding the reach of the federal government were anathema to the Republican caucus, and to some members smacked of socialism or economic witchcraft. They were stymied.

"You need to do *something*," Hubbard told them. The doom loop might have sounded like a ride at Disneyland, but it now loomed as a possible future. He foresaw endless business failures and mass unemployment. And it wasn't just an economic question. Career-ending political consequences would be waiting to pounce on senators who made the wrong choice.

Hubbard tried to change the paradigm in the senators' minds. "We've been having a debate for decades now about the *size* of government," he told them. "The more interesting debate is the *scope* of government." He used the example of the first Republican president, Abraham Lincoln. "He decided to do the Homestead Act, land grant colleges, and to lay the foundation for the transcontinental railroad. If Lincoln, in the middle of the Civil War, had the idea of using government as a battering ram for opportunity, why can't we do that today? Instead of focusing on how big government is, think about what you want it to do."

Rubio, who was chair of the Small Business Committee in the Senate, could envision the economic damage already being done and what was likely to follow. He thought about the restaurants, the travel companies, gyms, hotels, hair salons, all of them service businesses—"the ones with the least ability to survive." The actions that Congress was contemplating were ruinous, from a Hayek perspective. But the alternative was a national calamity.

Rubio swung over to the side of action, but there was a surprising logistical problem: nobody knew how to give assistance to small businesses. The Treasury Department had previously bailed out corporations and given checks to individuals, but small business existed in a blind spot. There was no mechanism for providing assistance. Collins was considering a loan-forgiveness program, and Rubio was trying to figure out a way to create a new loan program through the Small Business Administration's existing network of lenders. "That's when the Paycheck Protection Program arose as an idea," Rubio said. Loans made to keep people on the payroll could be forgiven, offering employees assurance that their jobs would still be there when the clouds cleared.

For Rubio, the pandemic not only exposed many different fractures of society, it also revealed certain things about himself. "I would never vote to support the payroll of small businesses in normal times," he admitted. He was facing a handicapped economy, burdened by the massive debt that Congress was considering; at the same time, he foresaw communities hollowed out by the loss of industrial capacity, shocking unemployment, and declining opportunities. "I believe in free enterprise, it's the best way to generate growth," he said. "But the purpose of the economy is to serve people, not people to serve the economy." In the face of a national emergency, Marco Rubio became a Keynesian.

With the Democrats fully on board, Congress soon approved the Coronavirus Aid, Relief, and Economic Security (CARES) Act. It included $260 billion in increased unemployment benefits, $300 billion in one-time cash payments to citizens, and $350 billion in forgivable loans to small business, a figure that would be substantially increased in subsequent legislation. "We went from 'We don't know what to do,' to nine hundred pages and $2.2 trillion in about ten days," Delaware senator Chris Coons marveled. "I've never seen anything like it. This will be the biggest bill in our lifetime." It passed the Senate on March 25, with a vote of 96–0. The president signed it into law two days later.

"Nothing like a big shock to help people become more bipartisan," Glenn Hubbard observed.

FROM THE BEGINNING, the president was confronted with demands to take control and issue a federal plan, but his administration was reluctant to shoulder the responsibility—or the blame. The situation was fluid and confusing. "Should the federal government apply the same policy in states with different levels of contagion?" asked Kevin Hassett. He was Trump's first chairman of the Council on Economic Advisers and had been drafted to work with the White House Coronavirus Task Force. He related his experience to Glenn Hubbard's class at Columbia University. "If we told Alaska to shut down and they said no, what would we do? They could very well ignore us and there isn't very much federal authority to overrule them." The task force had looked into social distancing data in every zip code in the country and had been daunted by the fact that what Americans were told to do had little effect on their actual behavior. Hassett figured that was expectable. "Hayek would have told you that what government tells people to do is not so relevant because they're smart and they're going to figure it out."

The Trump administration was captivated by the promise—conveyed by the medical community, said Hassett—that the infection would die out in the summer. "Policymakers thought we would have to build a bridge to June, because by then it would be calmed down."

A student asked if the current recession offered an opportunity to rebalance the income inequality that has plagued American society. Hassett responded testily: "If you look at the period from when President Trump started to this January, wage growth was highest for the bottom ten percent, and income inequality declined sharply." He pointed out that wage growth was higher for African Americans than for whites. Then he ventured an attack on liberal economists who failed to recognize the achievements of the Trump administration. "By any metric of a just society, we had moved in a positive direction through January. And yet there was no remark about that from Thomas Piketty or Austan Goolsbee or Jason Furman. Left-wing intellectuals who complain about an unequal society weren't saying here's this guy I don't like very much but we just had the two best years for reduction of the increase in inequality we've had since the end of the world war."

But Hassett also noted that the pandemic had vividly exposed the painful inequalities in American society. "It's the bottom ten percent that loses their jobs," he said. "The folks who can't telecommute and have to go to work and expose themselves to Covid risk are minorities." He added: "I'm not so optimistic about inequality over the next year or so, because it's definitely the case that it's the bottom half of the income tier that suffers the most in a recession."

Another student asked if the future economic environment would resemble the low-growth, low-interest trap that has stymied growth in Japan since the mid-1990s. Hassett conceded that was the most likely outcome. "If it hadn't been for Covid, we would be close to escaping the low-interest environment. Now, it looks like we're stuck for another five or six years." Within the White House, there had been tempestuous arguments about the cost of the stimulus. "I was advocating big, long-term entitlement reform at the same time as we are spending all this money," Hassett confided. "We didn't do that." The economic future looked bleak to him. "There's a serious risk we are heading into a double-dip recession or maybe even something that has a worse name than that."

9

"Let It Be March"

O N THE AFTERNOON of March 11, Dr. Barron Lerner, a professor of population and health at the New York University Langone School of Medicine, was at his office in Bellevue Hospital, where he maintains a practice in internal medicine. The hospital had just begun implementing triage at the front desk for patients with respiratory problems. Masks were not encouraged among the staff unless they were seeing patients with fever and a cough. The only test available was the one from the CDC, which had to be sent to Atlanta, and the results wouldn't come back for four or five days; even then, the tests were only 70 to 80 percent accurate. Not useless, but not trustworthy.

Earlier that very morning at the staff conference, the policy for treating Covid patients was announced: "If you're talking to a patient you think might have Covid, you excuse yourself from the room; you say, 'Okay, I need to leave now. A nurse is going to come in and give you a mask.'"

Lerner met one of his regular patients who didn't speak English. Bellevue maintains a staff of a hundred translators for the many indigent immigrants that the hospital serves, and this patient spoke an obscure Asian language. They waited for the translator to connect to the dual telephone system. Time passed. Lerner was impatient. It was a Wednesday, his busiest day, with fifteen appointments. Eventually, the translator called. "About ten days ago, she had a fever," the translator said, "and then she was coughing, and she's been really short of breath since then"—exactly the symptoms described in the meeting that morning.

"I thought: I can't believe this just happened," Lerner recalled. "I was probably the first staff member to be exposed." He was sent home and told to take his temperature every twelve hours. The patient tested negative, which no one believed. Lerner and his wife began sleeping in separate bedrooms.

For many, March 12 was a moment of dismal clarity. The stock market suffered its biggest drop since the Black Monday crash of 1987. The Federal Reserve Bank of New York announced that it would generate $1.5 trillion in short-term loans to calm the financial markets. In Washington, Speaker Nancy Pelosi and Treasury Secretary Steven Mnuchin were about to conclude their negotiation of the $2.2 trillion CARES Act. It wouldn't be nearly enough.

Barron Lerner joined his friend Tom Frieden that day for lunch. They had been classmates at Columbia University's medical school in the 1980s. Frieden was the New York City health commissioner before President Obama appointed him director of the CDC. In that office, he oversaw the U.S. response to the 2014 Ebola outbreak. The CDC deployed 200 people to West Africa and committed another 400 staff in Atlanta. While coordinating an international response to confront the disease, CDC also trained thousands of health workers in Africa, set up laboratories for testing, and provided support for contact tracing, surveillance, and data management—all the things that had burnished CDC's reputation as the leading public health institution in the world. Ebola had been projected to infect 1.4 million people within four months; in the end, there were only 28,616 reported cases and 11,310 deaths in that outbreak; hundreds of thousands of lives were saved.

Lerner and Frieden met at Grand Central Oyster Bar, one of New York's treasures, with its elegant tiled arches and mischievous acoustics that sometimes volley intimate conversations into unexpected ears. Instead of shaking hands, Lerner offered to bump elbows, but Frieden responded with a namaste gesture. They discussed Lerner's probable exposure the day before. Even if he were infected, they agreed, the chances he was contagious were close to zero. "One more day, and I would have canceled," Frieden remarked. That very morning, he had closed his office and sent his staff to work remotely.

Usually the lunch crowd at the Oyster Bar was jammed with commuters and tourists and shoppers, buzzing with the nervous energy so characteristic of the city, but the bustle was gone. A third of the restaurant was roped off. It would turn out to be Lerner's last meal out for a long time. Frieden noticed that none of the waiters were wearing masks, nor did they make any effort to distance themselves. He was uncomfortable so they made it quick. Frieden had the clam chowder and Lerner the smoked trout.

Frieden handed Lerner a draft of a paper he had written for the CDC about superspreader events. He had been thinking about this poorly understood phenomenon for years. "We oversimplify, as if the average person is infecting 1.1 other persons, when in fact one out of twenty people is infecting twenty or thirty people and the other people are infecting zero to one people." There was no way to identify who the superspreaders are. "You gotta pounce on cases quickly," Frieden said, "and with that you can find superspreading events early and stop them."

Frieden had a full round of interviews that afternoon, capped by an appearance on *Tucker Carlson Tonight* on Fox. "He says that the death toll over one million is not an implausible figure," Carlson said by way of introduction. "That's a horrifying number."

Frieden allowed that no one really knows what's going to happen, but after watching the progress of the disease in Italy, he was sure it was going to get a lot worse in the U.S. He advised people to wash their hands, cover their coughs, and not go out if they're sick. "We may want to stop shaking hands for a while." Hospitals should stock up on supplies and prepare for a surge. He envisioned not having spectators at sporting events. Carlson looked appalled.

Barron Lerner and his wife watched the interview and went to bed in separate rooms. Five days later, the fever struck.

ON MARCH 12, Amy Klobuchar was back in Minnesota, while her husband, John Bessler, a law professor at the University of Baltimore, remained in Washington. He awoke that morning feeling ill. "He was going to take my place at my constituent breakfast in D.C.," Klobuchar recalled. "It was when he would have been most contagious, as we now know. There would have been around fifty people, in a small room. And then he was going to a faculty meeting—about sixty people, in a small room. Then he was going to get on an airplane and fly to Minnesota, with a bunch of people packed in. I was having some minor surgery at Mayo, and he was going to come there! He really would have had quite a day of infecting people." They had no idea how he'd caught the virus. He was fifty-two and, until then, in excellent health.

Bessler stayed home, self-quarantining, growing steadily worse. For more than a week, Klobuchar anxiously kept calling, asking what his temperature was. Their only thermometer was in centigrade, so Klobuchar had to Google the conversion. It was always over a hundred degrees. She could hear that he was short of breath. She urged him again and again to go to the doctor, worrying that "it was one of those cases where people are underestimating how sick they are, and then they die the next day. Those kind of stories." After Bessler coughed up blood, he finally agreed to go to the hospital to get tested. He had severe pneumonia. Doctors kept telling Klobuchar, "The oxygen is getting worse." She couldn't visit him, making the ordeal even more frightening.

Bessler spent five days in the hospital. He recuperated and was back in the couple's D.C. apartment when his test finally came back positive.

THE METROPOLITAN MUSEUM OF ART closed down, as well as the New York Philharmonic and the Metropolitan Opera. As the audience emerged from a matinee of *The Phantom of the Opera*, they encountered a notice pasted on the door to the ticket office: "Under the direction of Governor Andrew Cuomo, all Broadway shows in New York City have suspended performances." The sign promised that shows would resume a month later, but that fantasy wouldn't last long.

Phantom had run for thirty-two years in the Majestic Theatre, the longest run in Broadway history. Directly across 44th Street is the St. James, one of the largest of the Broadway stages. Musical theater is an especially American art form, and much of it was born in these two venues. In 1943, *Oklahoma!* opened at the St. James. Rodgers and Hammerstein's songs, along with the play's dramatic realism and bold portrait of America, created the modern musical. *South Pacific*, *The Music Man*, and *Funny Girl* followed at the Majestic; while the St. James hosted *The King and I*, *Hello, Dolly!*, *A Funny Thing Happened on the Way to the Forum*, *Hair*, and *The Producers*—each of these shows timeless but also a chronicle of the exuberant country they were born into.

Covid came on the heels of the highest-grossing season in Broadway history, as 14,768,254 audience members contributed a total box office gross of $1.8 billion. Then it hit a wall. The shows remained on the marquees but the forty-one great, opulent houses that make up Broadway were dark. "The theater is an inherently communal act. It doesn't exist without its audience," Jordan Roth, the president and owner of the Jujamcyn Theaters, one of the three Broadway chains, said. "So to be faced with this moment—when the very thing that makes the theater the theater is also the thing we must avoid at all costs—is an existential challenge." At the time of closing, his five theaters were showing *Hadestown* at the Walter Kerr, *The Book of Mormon* at the Eugene O'Neill, *Moulin Rouge!* at the Al Hirschfield, *Mean Girls* at the August Wilson, and *Frozen* at the St. James.

Roth has his office above the St. James, "this storied house," as he calls it. The shutdown caused by Covid-19 reminded him of the 1980s, the last time Broadway's future was threatened. Times Square was dirty and dangerous; tourists shunned it. Theaters were boarded up or turned into movie houses. Enlightened civic planning and the revitalization of Times Square, along with a jolt of energy from Britain in the form of mega-musicals by impresarios Andrew Lloyd Webber and Cameron Mackintosh, brought Broadway back from the grave. This time it was different. It was society that needed to be healed, not Broadway.

Another epidemic disease had devastated Broadway in the eighties, AIDS. When I asked Roth if he thought about the comparison with Covid, he began to weep. "Constantly," he said. "Constantly." After he composed himself, he said, "An entire generation of artists and storytellers is gone, and our community is still grappling with that. There's a huge, gaping hole where there should be lives."

Roth saw the shutdown as a period of introspection for the theater. "Everything is on the table for reinvention," he said, but he had no idea what might emerge. "It's a fascinating experience to be presented with the unfathomable, and you resist it—because it's unfathomable. And then you wrap your head around that, you take it in your hands, you say, 'Okay, I'm there—but only there.' And then the unfathomable moves.

And you do it again. And it keeps moving and moving and moving farther and farther into more unfathomable. Which seems impossible because unfathomable is like infinity. March was like five unfathomables from where we began. I now feel myself thinking, 'Oh, please let it be March.'"

OSKAR EUSTIS WAS RELEASED from the hospital after four days, still shaky. Upon returning home, he immediately went to bed. He turned out to have "long-haul" Covid symptoms, which persist in about 30 percent of people shown to have the disease. "It comes in waves," he told me. "I'm struggling with extreme fatigue and continued muscle pain." There was no going back to the office; every theater in New York was closed, including the Public. *Coal Country*, with Steve Earle, had recently opened to rave reviews. *The Visitor*, with David Hyde Pierce, was about to go into tech. *The Vagrant Trilogy*, a set of plays about a Palestinian Wordsworth scholar, with a Middle Eastern cast, was also shut down. Many shows would never get another chance.

Camp David had closed in Houston three days before. I wondered when theater would ever return. So much of a writer's life is solitary; the work can't be done unless one is comfortable being alone, mentally scratching the air for a thought, a word, parsing the use of a semicolon while pondering the human condition. Working in the theater was a vacation from myself. There, I became a member of a creative hive, involving costumes and electricians and wigs and music and actors who inhabit imaginary characters who no longer belong to me. Even when the subject is as weighty as the effort to make peace, there's something childish about the whole theatrical enterprise; and the reverse is true as well, the comedy of awkward situations being a route to enlightenment.

Social scientists have pointed out the decline of membership in clubs, unions, civic organizations, scouting, and churches; the bonds of community have been fraying for decades as people retreat into their virtual lives and politics becomes the main source of identity. Theater still brings us together. The experience can't be digitized. Being together, hearing a laugh or a sob caught in the throat, is solidifying. And when the house lights come on and we stand and look into each other's faces, there's acknowledgment that our feelings are shared and we've melded, at least for that moment, into a community.

My actors found work selling real estate or cleaning gutters, waiting for the chance to be themselves again. Real life was on pause, but would it ever be as real as it was?

10

"It's Like a Wind"

GREAT CRISES SUMMON profound social changes, for good or ill. The consequences of wars and economic depressions have been amply studied; those of pandemics, less so. I thought to look at the past through the eyes of Gianna Pomata, a retired professor at Johns Hopkins University. After retiring, Pomata returned to her hometown, the old city of Bologna. When we first spoke, on March 27, 2020, she and her husband had been locked down for seventeen days. Italy was in the teeth of the contagion.

"You know Bologna, right?" she asked.

Decades ago, I was the best man at a wedding there. I recalled the giant churches, the red-tiled roofs, the marble walkways under arched porticoes; a stately city, low-slung, amber-hued, full of students and indomitable old couples. During the Middle Ages, Bologna was home to more than a hundred towers, the skyscrapers of their era, which served as showplaces of wealth and ambition for powerful oligarchs. Two of the remaining ones have become symbols of Bologna: one slightly out of plumb, the other as cockeyed as its cousin in Pisa. "You remember the Piazza Maggiore, the very heart of the city near the two towers?" Pomata said. "That's where I live."

The day we spoke, confirmed cases in Italy reached 86,498, surging past China's total. Only the United States had a higher number, having just eclipsed China the day before. "In Italy, the streets are always crowded, night and day," Pomata said, as we spoke on Zoom. "Our cities are medieval, made for a different way of life. Not for cars but for people. Right now, to see them empty of people is so sad."

Pomata was sixty-nine, with brown hair and a long, open face. Her tortoiseshell glasses rested at half-mast on her nose, beneath upward-pointing, quizzical eyebrows. Since she had spent much of her adult life in the United States, her English had little accent, but she retained an Italian lilt, lingering on the broad vowels. Like me, she was beginning to show the pallor of confinement. The governor of Texas, Greg Abbott, had closed the restaurants, schools, bars, and gyms one week before; and although we hadn't gone into full lockdown yet, Austin, where I live, was already hibernating. But what world would we wake up to?

When I asked Pomata to compare Covid-19 to the pandemics of the past, she pointed to the bubonic plague that struck Europe in the fourteenth century—"not in the number of dead but in terms of shaking up the way people think." She explained: "The Black Death really marks the end of the Middle Ages and the beginning of something else." That something else became the Renaissance.

I asked Pomata if she were able to walk out of her apartment 672 years ago, during the Black Death, how would Bologna appear different? "If you try to imagine a plague-stricken city in the Middle Ages, the first thing you'd see would be dead people on the streets," she said. "Just as we have to send the army to take coffins to crematories in other cities, as in Bergamo right now, in the Middle Ages they couldn't cope with so many dead. The bodies just piled up on the streets." She paused and added, "I don't have an idyllic vision of the Middle Ages."

IN THE FOURTEENTH CENTURY, Tatar warriors in Crimea laid siege to the Black Sea port city of Caffa, which was owned by a group of wealthy Genoese traders. Like so many armies in history, the Tatars were also fighting an unseen enemy: they carried with them a ghastly disease, which killed some victims in a few days, and left others to die in indolent agony. Before retreating from Caffa, the Tatar general, Khan Jani Beg, ordered the diseased bodies of dead warriors catapulted over the city walls, perhaps the first instance of biological warfare. Terrified citizens took to boats, navigating through the Dardanelles into the Aegean Sea and the Mediterranean. A dozen ships made it to Sicily, in October 1347. The plague traveled with them.

Sicilians were appalled to find dead men still at their oars. Other sailors, dead or barely alive, were in their bunks, riddled with foul-smelling sores. The horrified Sicilians drove the ships back to sea, but it was too late. Rats and fleas, the carriers of *Yersina pestis*, the bacterium that causes the plague, quickly infested the port of Messina. By January, Italy was engulfed. Incoming ships were required to sit at anchor for *quaranta giorni*—forty days, which is where the term "quarantine" comes from.

Medieval mortality figures are a matter of speculation, but Bologna is believed to have lost half its population in 1348; Florence, as much as three quarters. Cities all over Europe were emptied. That first outbreak, between 1347 and 1351, is estimated to have killed at least seventy-five million people worldwide, and maybe as many as two hundred million.

"Child abandoned the father, husband the wife, wife the husband, one brother the other, one sister the other," a contemporary chronicler, Marchionne di Coppo Stefani, observed. Deep trenches were dug in the churchyards. "Those who were responsible for the dead carried them on their backs in the night in which they died and threw them into the ditch," Stefani continued. The next morning, dirt was thrown on the bodies as new corpses were piled on, "layer by layer just like one puts layers of cheese in a lasagna."

"Chroniclers of the plague describe the crumbling of the family," Pomata said. "At the same time, human beings are creative. They react to this perceived moral decay by creating new institutions; for instance, they create boards of health, which are in charge of quarantine." For the first time, hospitals split up patients into specific wards, so that broken bones and wounds, say, were treated separately from diseases. There was also a rise in trade associations, to take care of medical costs and funeral expenses. "So you can see both trends," Pomata said. "On the one hand, the plague works as a kind of acid; on the other hand, people try to recreate ties and perhaps better ties."

ITALY AT THE BEGINNING of the fourteenth century was a conglomeration of prosperous city-states that had broken free of the feudal system. Some of them, such as Venice, formed merchant republics, which became seedbeds for capitalism. Venice and other coastal cities, including Genoa, Pisa, and Amalfi, set up trading networks and established outposts throughout the Mediterranean and as far away as the Black Sea. Other Italian cities, such as Bologna, became free communes, which meant that peasants fleeing feudal estates were granted freedom once they entered the city walls. Serfs became artisans. A middle class began to form. The early fourteenth century was robust and ambitious. Then, suddenly, people began to die.

Bologna's famous university, established in 1088, the oldest in the world, was a stronghold of medical teaching. "What they had we call scholastic medicine," Pomata told me. "When we say 'scholastic,' we mean something that is very abstract, not concrete, not empirical." European scholars at the time studied a number of classical physicians—including Hippocrates, the Greek philosopher of the fifth century BC, who is considered the father of medicine, and Galen, the second-century Roman who was the most influential medical figure in antiquity—but scholastic medicine was confounded with astrological notions. When the king of France sought to understand the cause of the plague, the medical faculty at the University of Paris blamed a triple conjunction of Saturn, Jupiter, and Mars in the fortieth degree of Aquarius, which had occurred on March 20, 1345.

"Whether it descended on us mortals through the influence of the heavenly bodies or was sent down by God in His righteous anger to chastise us because of our wickedness, it had begun some years before in the East," Giovanni Boccaccio wrote in the *Decameron*, which was completed by 1353 and is set during the plague in Florence. "At its onset, in men and women alike, certain swellings would develop in the groin or under the armpits, some of which would grow like an ordinary apple and others like an egg." These pus-filled swellings, called buboes, were inflammations of the lymph nodes. They eventually erupted. Internal organs broke down in a bloody froth, and bodies darkened with gangrene, which is why the plague came to be called the Black Death.

Before arriving in Italy, the pestilence had already killed millions of people as it burned through China, Russia, India, Persia, Syria, and Asia Minor. It was said that there were entire territories where nobody was left alive. The source of the disease was sometimes thought to be "miasma"—air that was considered to be unhealthy, such as sea breezes. Paradoxically, there was also a folk belief that attendants who cleaned latrines were immune, which led some people to confine themselves for hours absorbing the presumed medicinal odors. "The advice of doctors and the power of medicine appeared useless and unavailing," Boccaccio wrote. Some people maintained that "the surest medicine for such an evil disease was to drink heavily, enjoy life's pleasures, and go about singing and having fun, satisfying their appetites by any means available, while laughing at everything." Others, he observed, "formed themselves into companies and lived in isolation from everyone else."

The *Decameron* tells the story of ten friends who shelter in place, trading tales while the plague rampages through the city. These ribald tales give little thought to medieval notions of sacredness or piety; indeed, the society the young, sequestered people describe is hypocritical and cheerfully amoral. Priests are portrayed as stupid, lustful, greedy connivers. Illicit sex is exalted. The earthy realism of the *Decameron*, written in Italian vernacular rather than classical Latin verse, sounded a fanfare for the approaching Renaissance.

I asked Pomata about Italy's economic experience after the Black Death. "It was a great time to be an artisan," she said. "Suddenly, labor was scarce, and because of that, market wages had to go up. The bourgeoisie, the artisans, and the workers started to have a stronger voice. When you don't have people, you have to pay them better." The relative standing of capital and labor reversed: landed gentry were battered by plunging food prices and rising wages, while former serfs, who had been too impoverished to leave anything but a portion of land to their eldest sons, increasingly found themselves able to spread their wealth among all their children, including their daughters. Women, many of them widows, entered depopulated professions, such as weaving and brewing. "What happens after the Black Death, it's like a wind, fresh air coming in, the fresh air of common sense," Pomata said. The intellectual overthrow of the medieval medical establishment was caused by doctors who set aside the classical texts and gradually turned to empirical evidence. It was the revival of medical science, which had been dismissed following the fall of ancient Rome, a thousand years earlier. "After the Black Death, nothing was the same," said Pomata. "What I expect now is something as dramatic is going to happen, not so much in medicine but in economy and culture. Because of danger, there's this wonderful human response, which is to think in a new way."

11

Bellevue

A S EACH DAY TRIGGERED a new cascade of consequences, Governor Cuomo and Mayor de Blasio quarreled over who had the authority to act, although neither did. By March 17, de Blasio opined that he was edging closer to deciding to order the citizens of his city to shelter in place. Maybe he would make a decision in the next two days, he said. Cuomo jeered at the suggestion. "I'm a New York City boy, born and raised if you can't tell," he said on CNN. "We're very good at getting around the rules." It simply wasn't practical to try to shut down the city, the governor said. "I don't even think you can do a state-wide policy." In his opinion, the mayor didn't have the authority to make such a decision, either. "No city in the state can quarantine itself without state approval," Cuomo asserted, adding that he had "no plan whatsoever to quarantine any city."

Three days later, the governor pivoted, ordering non-essential businesses in the state to shut their doors and workers to stay home. He was suddenly ablaze. "If you are in this line of work, we need masks," he pleaded. "If you're making clothing, figure out if you can make masks. I'll fund it." He compared the need for ventilators to the armaments required to wage the Second World War. "It's ventilators, ventilators, ventilators, that is the greatest need."

It was a crucial pivot, but it came woefully late. About a third of all the cases in the U.S. were in New York City. For once, de Blasio agreed with the governor. "I hate to say this, but it's true: We are now the epi-center of this crisis, right here in the nation's largest city."

On First Avenue in Manhattan, with its back to FDR Drive and the East River, stands Bellevue Hospital, "the grande dame of America's public hospitals," as historian David Oshinsky termed it, "the oldest pub-lic hospital and in many ways the most important." Since it opened as an almshouse in the eighteenth century, Bellevue has endured epidem-ics of cholera and yellow fever, which sent untold thousands to their graves in the potters' fields that are now Washington Square and Bryant Park. Bellevue also hosted an insane asylum, which added to its reputa-tion as a place where the marginalized and desperately poor mixed with disoriented immigrants, convicts, and drug addicts. It was a destination people spoke about in whispers.

And yet, Bellevue was also the vanguard of public health in America, providing the first maternity ward in the U.S., the first emergency pavil-ion, the first ambulance corps, and the first nursing school. The mission of Bellevue is that no one is turned away, whether they can afford treat-ment or not. "If a cop is shot, they send him to Bellevue. If a firefighter is overcome by smoke, or there's a terrorist attack, anyone who is injured goes to Bellevue," Oshinsky said.

By the mid-eighties, half the patients in Bellevue's medical wards had AIDS. It was a terrifying disease. Ambulance drivers would refuse to pick up patients in gay neighborhoods; morticians declined to embalm victims; and healthcare workers were naturally frightened of a disease that had no cure and whose progress to death was as grotesque as any-thing they had witnessed. Treating the disease was essentially hopeless and harrowing. Bellevue saw more AIDS patients than any other Ameri-can hospital.

Dr. Nate Link came to Bellevue from St. Louis in 1983 to do his internship. From the moment he first walked into the hospital, "I felt like I was in the epicenter of the universe. It was such an exciting environ-ment, just full of wonder." He had actually never heard of AIDS when he arrived; and then, in his first month of internship, Link accidentally pricked himself with a needle contaminated by HIV. He thought it was a death sentence, but he survived to become Bellevue's chief medical officer. The hospital finally shut its AIDS unit in 2012.

When the 2014 Ebola outbreak was raging in Africa, Link and his coworkers knew that if the disease spread to New York, the patients would end up at Bellevue. The hospital spent ten weeks building an Ebola unit and a dedicated laboratory, training hundreds of staff, and storing additional personal protection equipment. The instant they finished their preparations, a patient appeared: Dr. Craig Spencer, who had contracted the disease while working with Doctors Without Borders in Guinea. He survived. Bellevue then sent emissaries across the country to help hospitals prepare their facilities, develop protocols, and train their staff for future novel infections. Had it not been for the foresight of Link and his colleagues, America would have been much less prepared for the onslaught of Covid-19.

Once the coronavirus emerged, Bellevue's special pathogens team began preparing a protocol. "We thought we'd get one or two cases, just like Ebola," Link said. "We'll be totally ready for this." By early March, the hospital was admitting a number of patients with fever and unexplained respiratory problems who were labeled PUI—patients under investigation. There were zero tests available. Bellevue was flying blind, as was every hospital in the city. "We had this sense that there was this invisible force out there," Link recalled. He believed the city already had tens of thousands of cases, but "without testing, there was just no way to know—it was a sneak attack." When the city reported its first positive case, on March 1, only thirty-two tests had been conducted.

On March 18, Lawrence Garbuz, Governor Cuomo's "Patient Zero," finally awakened from his medically induced coma. It had been twenty days. As he was coming to, the city was going into a coma of its own.

BARRON LERNER'S COVID CASE was mild; he returned to work at Bellevue after twelve days. The city was eerily vacant. He noted the absence of pedestrians, of traffic, of street vendors. First Avenue resembled an abandoned set on a studio back lot. In the time that he had been gone, the hospital was transformed. A tent had been erected in the hospital courtyard, for screening patients. The lobby was weirdly empty. Everyone was masked.

Non-Covid patients in intensive care were shuttled to the post-operative surgical unit, which was available because elective surgeries were canceled. That freed up fifty-six ICU beds. Carpenters and plumbers moved in, redesigning the units, installing HEPA filters and creating negative pressure in each room, so that infected air would not escape into the hospital. Within a week and a half every cubicle on the ICU floor became a Covid-safe room, while the endoscopy suite and ambulatory surgery unit were converted into ICUs. Offices were turned into more patient units; as soon as the carpenters walked out of a room, a patient was wheeled in. Twenty-five more spaces for ventilator patients were added in the ER. When all the beds were filled, the ICU cubicles were doubled up. Lerner tended to his patients through televisits and assigned himself administrative duties. Still recovering, he would take hour-long naps while Bellevue whirled around him.

IN MID-MARCH, the first positive case in Bellevue was a middle-aged man with shortness of breath and low oxygen levels. He had no preexisting conditions, but an X-ray revealed widespread pneumonia. "It was an unexplainable syndrome," Dr. Amit Uppal, chief of critical care, said. That first patient would be dead in two weeks. "Among our staff, we just looked at each other and said, 'Okay, here we go.' And from there, it just exponentially ramped up."

Uppal, the son of Indian immigrants, was raised in a small town in Northern California. He did his medical training at Ohio State and his residency at the University of California, Irvine. He was drawn to Bellevue because he wanted to serve the disadvantaged segments of society—the poor, the homeless, the undocumented, those without adequate access to healthcare—but he was also impressed by the high caliber of the staff, "people that could work anywhere in the country and chose to defend this population." He elected to go into critical care specifically to deal with the most extreme diseases. He was prepared to face the knotty ethical dilemmas that reside at the limits of medical knowledge.

Part of the mission at Bellevue is helping patients die well. "It provides you a rare perspective on your own life," Uppal said. "I think many laypeople who don't do medicine and aren't exposed to end-of-life issues may not have the opportunity to reflect on what's really important to them until the end of their own life." But Covid-19 seemed cruelly designed to frustrate the rituals of death.

In the first two weeks of the surge, just as the early patients began dying, the hospital was flooded with new admissions. The typical mortality rate in the ICU was far lower than for Covid, so even critical-care staff, like Uppal, who see death all the time, were taken aback by the pace. Such doctors knew instinctively how to click into emergency mode. Before Covid, that might last thirty or forty minutes—say, with a patient who has a heart attack. If there is a bus wreck or a mass casualty event, emergency mode could last all day. But with Covid, it was day after day for weeks on end. Emotions were deferred, but they clawed deep scars.

During rounds, Uppal passed each of the ICU's fifty-six cubicles. The patients were all on ventilators, and the distinctive gasping sound was unvaried, room to room. The IV lines extended outside each cubicle so the attendants didn't have to enter to administer medication. Each patient was on an infusion pump, receiving seven or eight medications. They looked identical, shadowy figures in the antiseptic gloom. It was too easy to overlook their humanity. Uppal would force himself to examine their charts to recapture "what made them unique."

Patients were isolated from their families because of state-mandated restrictions on all visitations. Social workers and the palliative care team kept relatives updated, setting up video conferences on their personal phones so that family members could say goodbye. As he walked around the ICU, caring for one patient after another, Uppal would often see his colleagues holding up an iPhone to the tiny glass window for family members to go through the motions of talking to their relative. He was moved to see that they continued to speak to the patient, who was sedated and completely unresponsive. It helped the family to direct their final words into those isolated chambers where their loved ones were passing away.

Like everyone else, Uppal worried about getting ill and perhaps infecting his own family. His wife, Anjana, worked as an emergency room physician at the Jacobi Medical Center in the Bronx. They have two children, seven and four, and during most of that first wave they had no childcare. They rotated attending the kids, trading shifts so that one could be home while the other was at work. Amit was usually in the hospital from early morning until early evening, but sometimes he would go in extra early so he could finish up and get home in time for

Anjana to make it to her afternoon shift. On Sundays, when Amit did his overnight at Bellevue, he'd rush home by 7:30 in the morning so Anjana could make an 8:00 a.m. Monday shift at Jacobi. At the same time, they were having to homeschool their children. Quality time was subtracted from the children's lives, replaced by stress. The kids weren't themselves; they became irritable. They hadn't seen their friends for weeks, and they wanted to play, but Amit and Anjana had purposely instilled in them a fear of going outside. "They were grieving," Uppal said. "At times when we did have to go outside, you could see them flinch when someone came too close. It's heartbreaking."

OVERWHELMED HOSPITALS IN the outer boroughs began transferring patients to Bellevue, knowing that no one would be turned away. Over 600 patients came from other hospitals. The center of the crisis was Bellevue's emergency department, a hot zone where many people came in from the street flagrantly symptomatic and needing to be intubated immediately. Before Covid-19, the emergency department was always jammed; there would be twenty or thirty patients waiting for beds and stretchers strewn about everywhere. "When Covid hit, we made a promise to ourselves that we would not let the emergency rooms back up, and that we would keep them pristine," Nate Link told me. The hospital actually improved the flow. Healthcare workers had to be totally swathed in personal protective equipment. "And they wore that all day long," said Link. "In the end, only fifteen percent of the staff in the emergency department tested positive. That's lower than the hospital in general. It's even a bit less than the city average. The message is that PPE works."

The pace quickly wore down the staff, physically and emotionally. Every hour, day and night, the hallways resounded with emergency codes—*Airway team to ICU!*—summons after summons to the bedside of yet another doomed patient. Nurses had twice as many ICU patients to care for. Some departments, like emergency, were constantly on the verge of being swamped; others were looking for a role to play. Ophthalmologists were helping in the ICU; general surgeons treated non-Covid patients; and orthopedic surgeons began devoting their entire shifts to turning patients—"proning"—to facilitate breathing. "Everybody found a niche," said Link. "We were a completely different hospital for three months."

Running on adrenaline, the staff sometimes had to be ordered to go home, and when they did go home, they couldn't sleep. The disease was relentless, and for those, like Link, who had been at Bellevue during the AIDS era, it seemed frightfully familiar. "People come into the hospital short of breath; next thing you know, you're upping their oxygen, and then you've maxed out oxygen. Next thing you know, you've intubated them. Then you're upping the oxygen on the ventilator. The organs start to fail, the kidneys, the heart, the liver; and then they develop low blood pressure, and you have them on pressure agents. And that's the harbinger of death. Their blood pressure's dropping, their organs are failing. And then they die." This dismal progression can last weeks or move with startling rapidity. Doctors were finding Covid pneumonia even in patients they didn't suspect were ill—a gunshot victim, an old person who had fallen—some of whom had never reported feeling shortness of breath, but X-rays revealed lungs stuffed with fluid or pus. It is called "silent hypoxia." They were dying, many of them, in imperceptible increments. Typically, before patients are put on ventilators, they are gasping for breath, in shock or unconscious. Many Covid patients were using their phones even as they were being hooked up to monitors.

More than twenty thousand New Yorkers died from Covid in the spring. As the numbers mounted, Link noticed that the hospital staff were practicing what he called "psychological distancing." "Our staff had never seen so much death," he said. "Normally, a patient dying would be such a big deal, but when you start having a dozen patients die in a day, you have to get numb to that, or you can't really cope." That sense of psychological distance was shattered when the first staff member died: a popular nurse, Ernesto (Audie) De Leon, who had worked at Bellevue for thirty-three years. "He died in our own ICU," Link said. "His death was followed by a Covid-style 'wake,' as many of his colleagues approached his ICU cubicle in full PPE, put their hands on the glass door, and read Scripture, prayed, and wept. Because of the infection control restrictions, staff consoled each other without touching or hugging. It was very unnatural."

In the middle of the surge, when Bellevue's doctors were at their lowest ebb, reinforcements arrived. Hospital workers from other states flooded into New York to help shoulder the load. According to Governor Cuomo, 30,000 people responded to the city's call for aid. It was a rare glimpse of national unity. "Half the people in the ICU had southern accents," Link said. "That's what saved us."

ON A NORMAL DAY in New York, an average of twenty-five people die outside of the healthcare system. At the peak of the contagion, in April, ten times that many were dying at home or elsewhere. Their bodies were picked up by soldiers and members of the National Guard. They were added to the death toll of nearly eight hundred people a day. One funeral home was caught storing bodies in U-Haul trucks. Morgues and crematoriums were also overwhelmed. The emergency management system supplied 135 refrigerated trailers to the hospitals across the city, and ads were posted for "body handlers" to load the dead. A temporary morgue was set up at the South Brooklyn Marine Terminal, where the dead were stored in forty freezer units, each the size of a tractor trailer. Unclaimed or unidentified dead were laid to rest in hundred-yard trenches in a potters' field on Hart Island, just off the Bronx coast, beside anonymous victims of pandemics of the past, the 1918 flu and AIDS.

Outside of the hospitals, there was quiet. The streets were motionless. But somehow, the city knew. There were more than sixty hospitals in New York City, and they were all under siege. At 7:00 p.m., when the afternoon shifts ended, the city erupted in applause, cheers, banging pans. People cracked open their windows or stood on their balconies and sang "New York, New York." Healthcare workers felt gratified, but many didn't feel like heroes. Doug Bails, the chief of internal medicine, felt "leader guilt" because he wasn't on the front lines taking care of people. Some workers were dealing every day with the feeling that too many people had died on their watch. They headed home full of self-reproach. But the people who were cheering understood that. They knew a moral cost was exacted, along with the physical and emotional toll. The people in the blue cotton scrubs were carrying the city's guilt along with its grief. That's part of what made them heroic.

12

The No Plan Plan

O N MARCH 15, members of the Coronavirus Task Force presented recommendations on how to shut down the country. All Americans would work from home. Education would be virtual; travel and shopping would stop; restaurants and bars would close their doors. The goal was to break the transmission of the virus for fifteen days and "flatten the curve" so that hospitals would not be overwhelmed. Schools were already closed in twenty-nine states.

Trump's impatience flared. At a press briefing, he said of the virus, "It's something we have tremendous control over." Dr. Fauci corrected him, observing that the worst days lay ahead, noting, "It is how we respond to that challenge that's going to determine what the ultimate endpoint is going to be." Trump reluctantly issued the guidelines.

The following day he had a conference call with governors around the country, reporting progress on the creation of a vaccine and therapeutics. "We're marshalling the full power of the federal government," he said. "We're backing you one hundred percent." Then he explained what he actually meant. "We're backing you in terms of equipment and getting what you need. Also, though, respirators, ventilators, all the equipment—try getting it yourselves. We will be backing you but try getting it yourselves. . . . Much more direct."

It took a moment for this to sink in. Most governors had assumed that, just as in the event of a natural disaster—a hurricane or a forest fire—the federal government would rush to help. Federal agencies would be enlisted. FEMA would swing into action. The doors of the national stockpile would be thrown open and emergency equipment would be quickly dispersed. The governors had become aware of the shortages that might endanger the lives of their citizens—not enough ventilators, N95 masks, nasal swabs—vital weapons in the war against this virus. They expected the president to invoke the Defense Production Act, forcing private industry to produce whatever was needed. Surely, there was a national plan.

Jay Inslee, the Democratic governor of Washington State, was flabbergasted when he realized that the president did not intend to mobilize the forces of the federal government. Inslee told the president, "That would be equivalent to Franklin Delano Roosevelt on December 8, 1941, saying 'Good luck, Connecticut, *you* go build the battleships.'"

Trump responded, "Well, we're just the backup."

"Mr. President, I don't want you to be the backup quarterback here," Inslee said. "We need you to be Tom Brady. We need leadership. We need mobilization. We need to bring all the forces of government to bear on this existential crisis."

Larry Hogan, the Republican governor of Maryland, was incensed. "You're actively setting us up!" he told the president.

Gretchen Whitmer, the Democratic governor of Michigan, was stunned by how quickly the cases had exploded in her state since the first two were reported only five days earlier. Detroit hospitals were quickly at full capacity. When she hung up the phone from talking with Trump, she realized that, not only would there be no help coming from the federal government, Michigan was already practically out of masks for healthcare workers, not just for a day or a weekend—some healthcare workers didn't have enough PPE for their next shift.

Trump later defended his stance to reporters. "The federal government is not supposed to be out there buying vast amounts of items and then shipping," he said. "You know, we're not a shipping clerk."

It was now mid-March. In Washington State, medical workers and volunteers were making their own protective gear out of office supplies and materials from craft stores and Home Depot. Industrial tape, foam, elastic, and marine-grade vinyl were turned into face shields. Garbage bags became surgical gowns. Volunteers across the country began sewing masks. Doctors washed their now precious N95 masks in bleach in order to reuse them. There were still far too few tests to measure the extent of the contagion, and the particular nasal swab used for the test was also in short supply. It was too late to control the spread through contact tracing. The Strategic National Stockpile had been created to bridge such emergencies, but Secretary Azar had recently testified to the Senate that there were only twelve million N95 masks in reserve, a fraction of what was needed. There had been more than a hundred million in the stockpile, but many were used during the 2009 H1N1 flu pandemic, and the supply was never replenished.

It was a national problem, but there would be no national plan. The pandemic was broken into fifty separate epidemics and dumped into the reluctant embrace of the surprised and unprepared governors.

NED LAMONT IS a gregarious businessman who happens to be governor of Connecticut. He made a fortune in cable television and then went into politics, as a Democrat, losing a race for U.S. Senate in 2006 and his next race, for governor, in 2010. He finally won the governor's office in 2018, on a platform that included raising the minimum wage to $15 an hour and legalizing marijuana. He was one of the least popular governors in the country almost from the day he entered office. But Covid would reverse the fortunes of many politicians all over the world, for better or worse.

Much of Connecticut serves as a bedroom community for New York City. The Metro-North Railroad's New Haven Line, which connects southern Connecticut suburbs to New York's Grand Central Station, handled nearly forty million passengers a year, but the tracks were shaky and couldn't support faster trains that might shave thirty minutes off the two-hour commute. That could be economic salvation for the state, in Lamont's opinion. It wasn't entirely Connecticut's decision to make, so in 2019 Lamont called another governor who was lagging in popularity, Andrew Cuomo, and they made a date to meet. They spent an August afternoon on Lake Ontario fishing for steelhead trout. They each caught one, about the same size. "Twins," Cuomo declared.

Lamont paid court to other governors in the region—Phil Murphy, of New Jersey; Charlie Baker, of Massachusetts; and Gina Raimondo, of Rhode Island—so when the president made it clear that the states were on their own, Lamont picked up the phone. We need to act as a region, he said to his fellow governors, to speak with one voice. "If I close down bars and Andrew keeps them open in New York, that doesn't solve any problems," Lamont said. "Everybody's going to go down there to drink and bring back the infection."

The governors were daunted by the task facing them. Lamont imagined the furious reaction of his constituents. "You're going to close down the schools? My God!" But acting in concert with other states provided political cover and a sense of solidarity. "We weren't getting much guidance, to put it mildly, from the CDC and the White House," Lamont observed, "so we were on our own."

The governors closed gyms, restaurants, and bars at the same time. Lamont, Murphy, and Cuomo prohibited gatherings exceeding fifty people. Baker and Raimondo limited them to twenty-five. Casinos and racetracks were shut down. Cuomo announced, "If you were hoping to have a graduation party, you can't do it in the state of New York, you can't go do it in the state of New Jersey, and you can't do it in the state of Connecticut."

Was it necessary or prudent to lock down the country? An influential model from the Imperial College in London predicted that, without social distancing, 81 percent of the population in Britain and the U.S. would be infected, and that more than half a million people in Britain and two million in the U.S. would die. The figures were astounding and possibly overestimated, but neither country succeeded in getting the widespread cooperation found in Asian countries, such as Vietnam and Taiwan, which never let the contagion get out of control. Sweden, which more or less let it rage, was losing 574 people per million, but the U.K., which got off to a slow start, was even higher, at 623. The U.S. death toll was midway between them, at almost 600 people per million. In all of 2020, Taiwan reported fewer than 800 cases in total, and only seven deaths.

Unlike Taiwan, the U.S. lost the option of containing the disease through conventional public health measures because of the CDC's fumbled test, so the governors faced the dire choice of massive illness and death or a calamitous blow to their economies. Most of the governors steered a wavering course between competing disasters.

Governor Hogan of Maryland was head of the National Governors Association. In February, at the annual meeting in Washington, he convened a panel of health experts, including Fauci and Redfield, to brief the governors privately. Their message was harrowing, Hogan noted: "This could be catastrophic. . . . The death toll could be significant. . . . Much more contagious than SARS. . . . Testing will be crucial. . . . You have to follow the science—that's where the answers lie."

Hogan had been unnerved by the disparity between the president's dismissals and the blunt warnings of the experts. He and most of the other governors accepted the challenge that Fauci and Redfield put before them. And yet, when the governors acted, they discovered that the Trump administration was actively sabotaging their efforts.

Washington State and the Northeast were hit hardest at the beginning. Healthcare workers in Massachusetts were desperate for PPE. Nurses in Milford held up cardboard signs on street corners begging for protective gear. Charlie Baker, the state's Republican governor, arranged to buy three million N95 masks from China, but federal authorities seized them at the Port of New York, paying the supplier a premium and keeping the equipment. In another governors call with Trump, Baker complained, "We took seriously the push you made . . . that we should not just rely on the stockpile, and that we should go out and buy stuff and put in orders. . . . I got to tell you that, on three big orders, we lost to the feds. . . . I've got a feeling that if somebody has to sell to you or has a chance to [sell to] me, I'm going to lose every one of those."

"Price is always a component," Trump said unsympathetically.

Baker quietly secured another 1.2 million masks from China, but this time he enlisted the help of Robert Kraft, the owner of the New England Patriots, who used the team plane, "AirKraft," to fly the shipment directly to Boston's Logan Airport. The Kraft family also paid $2 million to defray about half the cost of the masks. As the governor stood on the tarmac beside the plane, he was overcome with emotion. "For the many, many dedicated frontline workers across this state who are battling Covid-19 on behalf of the people of Massachusetts every single day, this gear will make an enormous difference," Baker said. Then the masks were spirited away by the Massachusetts National Guard and hidden from federal authorities.

Governor J. B. Pritzker of Illinois also disguised his plans for securing masks and gloves. He said on PBS *NewsHour*: "I hate the idea that I'm competing against other people in the United States—other governors, even—to get what we need, but this is what President Trump has done to the country."

Governor Hogan's wife, Yumi, used her influence to secure half a million test kits from a laboratory in her native South Korea. They were taken to a refrigerated warehouse in a secret location. "We weren't going to let Washington stop us from helping Marylanders," the governor remarked. The president was disdainful. "The governor of Maryland could've called Mike Pence, could've saved a lot of money," he remarked.

Some Democratic governors, including Laura Kelly of Kansas and Gretchen Whitmer of Michigan, complained that their supply orders were purposely blocked by the White House. "Vendors with whom we had contracts are now being told not to send stuff to Michigan," Whitmer said. "We've been told they're going first to the federal government." After Whitmer voiced her complaint on a Detroit radio station, Trump said at a press conference that he had instructed Vice President Pence, "Don't call the woman in Michigan."

"Look at the bizarre situation we wind up in," Governor Cuomo fumed at a briefing. "Every state does its own purchasing. . . . So you have fifty states competing to buy the same item. We all wind up bidding up each other." Medical devices and protective equipment were essentially being auctioned. "You now literally will have a company call you up and say, 'California just outbid you.' It's like being on eBay with fifty other states bidding on a ventilator. And then FEMA gets involved, and FEMA starts bidding!" Cuomo threw up his hands. "What sense does this make? The federal government—FEMA—should have been the purchasing agent. Buy everything, and then allocate it by need back to the states."

"It's a struggle to get the supplies we need," Colorado governor Jared Polis, a Democrat, complained on CNN, as his state topped four thousand cases. "We had a good lead with a manufacturer on vents . . . and they got swept up by FEMA, so we're not getting them." His message to the federal government: "Either work with us, or don't do anything at all. This middle ground where they're buying things out from under us and not telling us what we're going to get—that's really challenging to match our hospital surge." South Florida firefighters were about to start coronavirus testing for housebound residents, until a million masks they had ordered were seized. An order of thermometers for Florida hospitals was commandeered with no explanation. Testing supplies bound for hospitals in the Northwest and Alaska disappeared.

Rhode Island was wedged between two epicenters, New York and Boston. "I spent hours and hours of my days and nights scouring the earth to find PPE for my state," Governor Gina Raimondo said. "I'd call FEMA and say, 'Uh, can we tap into our national stockpile?' And I'd just constantly get the runaround." Finally, the federal agency promised that a truck full of PPE was on its way. "Tell me the time, I'll check on it myself," she said. She was told 7:00 p.m. Finally at 9:00 p.m., she got a text from FEMA saying the truck had arrived. "Hallelujah! I called my director of health. 'Great news, the truck is finally here!' She says, 'Governor, it's an empty truck. They sent an empty truck.'"

Some of the governors turned to Vice President Pence, a former governor of Indiana. They say he did what he could to help. California governor Gavin Newsom sought assistance from Jared Kushner, the president's son-in-law and all-purpose fixer, who had taken on the task of managing supply-chain issues. Kushner reportedly told the governor to call the president and personally ask for swabs, which Newsom did, and fulsomely praised the president after being promised a shipment.

"You've suggested that some of these governors are not doing everything they need to do," a reporter asked Trump at a news briefing. "What more, in this time of a national emergency, should these governors be doing?"

"Simple," said Trump. "I want them to be *appreciative*."

JARED KUSHNER INSERTED himself into the discombobulated White House response, but he only added to the chaos. It was characteristic of the Trump administration to go around the very government it controlled. Kushner set up an "impact team" composed of about a dozen young volunteers, mostly from the financial sector. The mission of this group of amateur bureaucrats was to break down the governmental barriers and streamline the process of getting assistance to the states and healthcare institutions. The volunteers, all in their twenties, were eager, patriotic, and ready to go, but they had little to no experience in healthcare or governmental procurement procedures. One of the volunteers was Max Kennedy Jr., the twenty-six-year-old grandson of Robert F. Kennedy, the former attorney general and presidential candidate. He and the others expected to help out the professionals, but they were surprised to learn that wasn't their job. "We *were* the team," Kennedy said. "We were the entire frontline team for the federal government."

They were given a conference room at FEMA headquarters, but no phones or computers. Using their personal laptops and email accounts, they reached out to suppliers and manufacturers all over the world, claiming to represent the U.S. government. They were told to call contacts from a spreadsheet called "VIP Update," which listed many of the president's friends, including Fox News stars and a former contestant on *The Apprentice*, seeking tips about where to purchase PPE. Jeanine Pirro, a Fox News host, repeatedly pressured the impact team to send PPE to a particular hospital, which eventually happened.

"We would call factories and say, 'We think the federal government can send you a check in sixty days,' and they would say, 'There's someone with a briefcase of cash, and they're offering to pay me right now,'" Kennedy recalled. "And we would run around the FEMA building looking for someone who could tell us what payment terms the government was allowed to offer, and no one ever told us." In the end, he said, "Our team did not directly purchase a single mask."

Governor Cuomo was desperate for ventilators, and the impact team had a lead. An electrical engineer in Silicon Valley, Yaron Oren-Pines, had no experience in healthcare but he had recently posted a tweet claiming he could supply them. New York took the bait and paid $69 million for 1,450 ventilators, which was at least three times the market price. There were no ventilators. The federal government awarded another contract, for $55.5 million, to purchase N95 masks from a tactical training company in Virginia, one of the largest orders for masks by the federal government. Not only did the company have no experience in making masks, or anything, it was also bankrupt and had no employees.

"The bottom line is that this program sourced tens of millions of masks and essential PPE in record time and Americans who needed ventilators received ventilators," Kushner claimed. "These volunteers are true patriots."

Mike Bowen at Prestige Ameritech, who had been pestering the federal government to purchase PPE before the country ran out, finally got a yearlong contract for a million masks a month, but he was never asked to open up his spare production capacity, which could have done much to ease the shortage.

Some officials received favorable treatment going through Kushner. Mayor de Blasio credited Kushner with supplying one million N95 masks and over 500,000 Tyvek gowns to the city hospitals. Governor Hogan credited Kushner with helping Maryland get 138 ventilators.

Kushner promised a nationwide network of thousands of testing sites, but only seventy-eight were ever set up. A proposed screening website never happened. He redirected purchasing orders that had already been promised to certain states, telling FEMA to send them to other states whose governors had called him personally. The White House had turned aid to states and hospitals into a form of patronage.

Cuomo, the governor of Kushner's own state, was his biggest defender. "I saw him as the key to New York getting anything from the federal government," he later recalled. "He was attentive and he delivered. Jared was the person who eventually produced the PPE, ventilators, and military personnel for New Yorkers, and I am grateful on their behalf."

"WE NOW HAVE five days of gowns and surgical masks," Dr. Paul Pottinger wrote his brother Matt at the White House on March 20. "We are buying lab coats, if we can get them, in desperation. . . . We are in a bad way." Paul included pleas from other doctors in the Seattle area: "The PPE situation is dire. We have received 655 requests from healthcare partners and have been able to fill only 52 of them. Please help. . . . There are people in the community NOW that do not have any or about to run out of masks and/or N95. We are currently drafting up guidelines for how to make homemade masks from cloth . . . if we can do ANYTHING that would be better than nothing."

Matt responded: "I'm doing all I can, and help is on the way, but it probably won't be in time—so start tearing up bedsheets and turning them into lab coats, raid the Salvation Army for garments, wrap bras around your faces in place of face masks if you have to. Just stay clear-headed and remember to get some rest."

Pottinger and Robert Kadlec, an assistant secretary at Health and Human Services, came up with an idea to put masks in every mailbox in America. Hanes, the underwear company, offered to make antimicrobial masks that were machine washable. "We couldn't get it through the task force," Pottinger told his brother. "We got machine-gunned down before we could even move on it." Masks were still seen as useless or even harmful by the administration and even public health officials.

"WHAT IF THERE'S already a cheap and widely available medication that's on the market to treat the virus?" Laura Ingraham said on her March 16 show on Fox News, *The Ingraham Angle*. She introduced Gregory Rigano, whom she identified as the co-author of a new study showing the benefits of two drugs widely used to treat malaria. "Gregory, how big a game changer could chloroquine and its sister drug hydrochloroquine [sic] be if, say, we began using it fairly promptly to treat Americans who are highly at risk?"

Rigano, who was not otherwise identified on the show except as the author of the paper, was a thirty-four-year-old lawyer from Long Island. He had recently started several blockchain funds that aimed to "cheat death" and "end Alzheimer's." What brought him to Ingraham's attention was a document he self-published on Google Docs with his co-author, James Todaro, a medical school graduate who is also a cryptocurrency investor. Ingraham quoted from the document, which claimed that the drugs were "effective in treating Covid-19," and could be used as a prophylactic to prevent contracting the disease. Rigano spoke about a study, yet to be published, of thirty patients, half of whom received hydroxychloroquine and the other half a placebo. "Within a matter of six days, the patients taking hydroxychloroquine tested negative for coronavirus . . . the patients that took the control tested positive."

"That's a game changer," Ingraham declared.

Apparently, Rigano and Todaro got the inspiration to write about choloroquine and hydroxychloroquine from a Twitter conversation with Adrian Bye, who describes himself as a philosopher living in the Wudang Mountains in China, where he tweets white supremacist musings. "My hobby is researching Jews," he has said. He also prophesied that the coronavirus would "destroy feminism." Bye developed his ideas about chloroquine through "philosophy." He was upset that Rigano and Todaro left his name off their paper.

On March 18, Rigano was on *Tucker Carlson Tonight* on Fox. Carlson identified him as an adviser at the Stanford University School of Medicine. (Rigano is not affiliated with Stanford Medical School.) Rigano referenced a different paper by "the most eminent infectious disease specialist in the world, Didier Raoult"—a microbiologist at the Institut Hospitalo-Universitaire Méditerranée Infection in Marseille. Raoult, a famous contrarian, had boasted, "We know how to cure the disease," using hydroxychloroquine in combination with the antibiotic azithromycin. On the Carlson show, Rigano said that Raoult's study showed a "hundred-percent cure rate against coronavirus."

"It's very unusual for a study of anything to produce results of a hundred percent," Carlson observed. "It's our job to be skeptical of all and any claims. However, I very much want to believe this."

The next day, at a press conference, President Trump said he had ordered the FDA to fast-track approval of chloroquine and hydroxychloroquine. "It's been around for a long time, so we know that if it—if things don't go as planned, it's not going to kill anybody." It was Trump's first mention of the drugs, which would become an obsession for him. Echoing Ingraham, Trump labeled them "a game changer."

Fox News drove the story relentlessly. During the two weeks between March 23 and April 6, Fox hosts and their guests promoted hydroxychloroquine nearly three hundred times.

"We have to be careful, Laura, that we don't assume something works based on an anecdotal report that's not controlled," Dr. Fauci said on *The Ingraham Angle* on March 17. "And I refer specifically to hydroxychloroquine. There's a lot of buzz out there on the internet, on the social media about that."

"Oh, there have been studies published though, right?" Ingraham asked.

"Those studies, some of them were not controlled," Fauci responded.

He promised, "We're going to look at that data very seriously." But at a task force briefing at the White House on March 20, Fauci was asked if he thought hydroxychloroquine was a promising treatment for coronavirus. "The answer is no," he said.

The president glowered and stepped toward the mic. "I'm a big fan, and we'll see what happens," he said. "I feel good about it. That's all it is, just a feeling, you know."

On March 24, a man in Arizona died after eating a form of chloroquine used to clean fish tanks. "I used to have koi fish," his widow told NBC News. "I saw it sitting on the back shelf and thought, 'Hey, isn't that the stuff they're talking about on TV?'" Four days later, under immense pressure, the FDA approved the emergency use of chloroquine and hydroxychloroquine, only to withdraw it three months later. The FDA found it ineffective in treating Covid-19 and reported "serious cardiac adverse events" and other side effects, including blood disorders, kidney injury, liver problems, and death. When hydroxychloroquine was paired with azithromycin—a combination that Trump publicly championed—patients were twice as likely to suffer cardiac arrest as those who took neither drug.

Fox News eventually stopped talking about hydroxychloroquine, but the president, who said he had been taking hydroxychloroquine himself, continued to defend the drug. "It certainly didn't hurt me," he said when the damning report came out. "I feel good."

The president said he wanted America "opened up and raring to go" by Easter. "You can destroy a country this way, by closing it down," he observed in a Fox News town hall in the White House Rose Garden on March 24. This was while caseloads in New York were doubling every three days. By the end of the week, refrigerated trailers were serving as emergency morgues and the East Meadow of Central Park was covered with field hospital tents, as it had been before—during the Civil War.

EIGHTY PERCENT OF the Covid deaths are over the age of sixty-five—my demographic. The disparity in vulnerability means that each generation experiences a different pandemic. The case fatality rate overall is 2 percent, but for people eighteen and under it is .02 percent, and for people over seventy, it's 18.8 percent. Why be surprised by the anger—compounded with envy—that the elderly feel when they see younger people mingling, freely breathing disease into the air. The coronavirus was like a plexiglass prison, one from which we could view life, but we were cautioned not to escape into it because the air itself might carry our destruction.

The devaluation of elderly lives was evident in the low standards of care in so many nursing homes, where 40 percent of all the U.S. deaths occurred, despite accounting for only 8 percent of the cases. Yes, the elderly are more vulnerable and more likely to have underlying conditions, but one of the risk factors was incompetent management and insufficient staffing.

In March, there were 235 military veterans living at the Soldiers' Home in Holyoke, Massachusetts. Some had served in the Second World War. They were once brave young men who survived America's greatest conflict in the twentieth century. Now they were old and helpless, captive to a system that they fought to protect but which was failing to protect them in turn.

Before the contagion came, the facility was operating with only 80 percent of its staff, in part because of a hiring freeze. On March 17, a veteran who had been showing symptoms for weeks was tested for Covid. He lived in one of two dementia units; he wasn't isolated, not even after his test came back positive four days later. Contagion took hold. Before the end of March a quarter of the staff were not reporting to work. Remaining nurses and orderlies floated from one ward to another, possibly carrying the contagion with them. Overburdened medical officers made the fateful decision to combine the two dementia units, crowding together the infected and uninfected veterans, instead of isolating those who showed symptoms. Many disoriented veterans climbed into the wrong beds, accelerating the spread. A recreational therapist told a state investigator she felt like she was "walking [the patients] to their death." The veterans were "terrified," another staffer said. It was "total pandemonium." Another staff member asked, "Where is the respect and dignity for these men?" A nurse was heard to say, "All in this room will be dead by tomorrow."

A social worker described the scene: "I was sitting with a veteran holding his hand, rubbing his chest a little bit. Across from him is a veteran moaning and actively dying. Next to me is another veteran who is alert and oriented, even though he is on a locked dementia unit. There is not a curtain to shield him from the man across from him actively dying and moaning, or a curtain to divide me and the veteran I am with at the time . . . I don't know . . . how many of us will ever recover from those images."

On Friday, March 20, Michael Miller, who is retired from the Army National Guard, got a call from his two sisters, Linda McKee and Susan Perez. "They're not thinking Dad's gonna make it through the night," they said. Their father, James L. Miller, was ninety-six, and had been at the Soldiers' Home since 2015. The siblings drove to the facility. Only one family member was allowed to enter. Mike went in while his sisters waited in the car. His father "looked like a corpse," he said. "He had been in that state of decay for a week, and nobody called us."

Jim Miller had landed at Normandy Beach on D-Day. After mustering out, he became a postal worker and a firefighter. He was a taciturn man who had rarely discussed his military service with his children. Mike almost never saw his father get angry, but one day he had exploded when someone denied that the Holocaust had happened. "He was irate," Mike recalled. His father dug around in the closet and found a shoebox full of photographs—pictures of a concentration camp near Nordhausen, Germany, that Jim had helped liberate. He donated them to a local Jewish museum in West Springfield, Massachusetts; they eventually wound up in the Holocaust Museum in Washington, D.C. "He wanted to make sure that never happened again," Mike said.

Now this stoic veteran was dying in the midst of bedlam. "Men were just wandering around," Mike said. "They were in various states of dress. There was a curtain drawn for my dad—other veterans would open the curtain and stand there. And these gentlemen I knew. They meant no disrespect."

The room was full of death and the groans of others soon to die. Staffers couldn't offer the residents anything but "comfort measures"—morphine under the tongue. Jim was so dehydrated that he couldn't swallow. "Give him an IV!" Mike pleaded. But the staff wasn't authorized to do that, nor could they transport patients to a hospital. Administrators were nowhere to be seen. There was nothing for Mike to do but moisten his father's mouth with a foam swab. Nurses broke down. Mike recalled: "They loved my dad. But they couldn't do anything."

Mike returned each day as his sisters kept vigil in the parking lot. On Saturday, they witnessed the arrival of a refrigerated truck that had been sent to store the bodies. On Monday, Jim Miller passed away. Before it was all over, at least seventy-five other veterans had died.

13

Little Africa

I N COVID WORLD, everyone is in disguise. When Dr. Ebony Hilton enters the room, the patient sees wide-set, lively eyes above her surgical mask. Her hair and body are hidden by a bonnet and a gown. Her accent marks her as a southerner. She calls herself a "country girl," which is at odds with her assured manner. When the call comes to intubate a patient, "it's already a situation where somebody is dying," Hilton says. "The only reason I'm placing this breathing tube is because your body is shutting down, your heart has stopped, you're not breathing at all at this point, so if I don't touch you, you're dead." She adds: "If I do touch you, *I* could die."

Hilton is a professor and anesthesiologist at the University of Virginia Medical School, in Charlottesville. The university's hospital has some six hundred beds, but at night, Hilton often works alone. "I'm literally the only anesthesiologist attending for the entire hospital. At that moment I can't shut down, I can't go to my room and let this fear stop me. I don't think any of us have slowed down to think that this could be the one that gets me sick. You don't have time to consider Options A, B, C, and D. You've got to gown up and go."

The lungs of Covid patients often display an unusual pneumonia. Fluid fills the air sacs to fight the infection, limiting the oxygen intake and causing the shortness of breath so characteristic of the disease. What makes the pneumonia unusual is that the blood vessels in the lungs also start leaking fluid, which leads to respiratory distress. At that stage, without a ventilator, the patient is confronting a terrible death.

One day in early March, Hilton got a page. A patient was septic, meaning that an infection had entered her bloodstream and was rampaging through her body, damaging major organs. Her kidneys were beginning to fail. Under ordinary circumstances, doctors would suspect bacteria as the cause, but the infection's spread had been alarmingly rapid, and the symptoms matched what the doctors were learning about Covid patients from China and Italy. Many healthcare workers noted the speed with which the infection killed when it made its move.

Hilton entered the room wearing an N95 mask but no goggles or face shield, as would soon be mandatory. The patient had no blood pressure; without intervention, her oxygen-starved brain would start dying within seconds. The procedure for intubation requires a pillow to be placed under the patient's shoulder blades, so that the head is tilted back in the "sniffing position." Hilton made sure the patient was oxygenated and given a sedative and a muscle relaxant; then she pried her mouth open, pushed her tongue aside, and inserted a laryngoscope—a thin curved metal blade attached to a handle, which looks like the head of a walking cane. The device lifts the epiglottis. If the vocal cords don't readily appear, pressure on the larynx can bring them into view. Hilton carefully snaked a plastic tube through the narrow portal between the vocal cords, down into the trachea. Once the tube was secured, the patient was connected to a ventilator.

That was probably Hilton's first Covid patient, but there was no way to know. Like many states, Virginia had barely any tests in early March. There was, however, a sharp rise in pneumonias—doubling in some states, tripling in others—that were suspicious but not yet ascribed to Covid. It will never be clear how many people perished of the disease before widespread testing began to take hold.

EBONY JADE HILTON COMES from a community near Spartanburg, South Carolina, called Little Africa. After the Civil War, Simpson Foster, a former slave, and a Cherokee named Emanuel Waddell founded the community as an agrarian refuge. "It's tiny," said Hilton. "We don't have a red light. We only have my great-uncle Hobbs's store."

Little Africa sits on high ground in the foothills of the Blue Ridge Mountains. "When you're sitting on the porch, you can see the skyline of the peaks," Ebony's mother, Mary Hilton, told me. "We have doctors, lawyers, judges—we have so many professions coming out of the Little Africa community, because we put so much emphasis on education, taking care of each other, reaching back, lifting up," she said. "Eb is coming from a very powerful place."

When Ebony was eight, her little sister asked Mary if they could have a brother. The question caught Mary by surprise, but she replied that her first child had been a boy. "I was seventeen," she recalled. "I had never heard of an ob/gyn. We always went to the clinic." She went alone; her mother was in the fields picking cotton. Mary suspects that, during a pregnancy exam, a technician punctured her amniotic sac. The boy was born prematurely and died after three days. "I told Eb that story, not knowing it would change her life," Mary said. The moment she heard it, eight-year-old Ebony announced that she was going into medicine. Her resolve must have been evident; right then, Mary began calling her Doctor Hilton. There was never any question about what Ebony was going to do with her life.

Not long ago, Ebony and her sisters, Brandi and Kyndran, placed a tombstone for the older brother they never knew in the churchyard of the New Bedford Baptist Church, in Little Africa. It says:

INFANT SON OF
TYRONE AND MARY HILTON
FEB. 8, 1978
FEB. 11, 1978

"He was a fighter," Ebony told me. "He tried to beat the odds. So I try to finish out that mission for him."

EBONY'S IMAGE OF her future was formed by watching *Dr. Quinn, Medicine Woman*, a television series about a physician on the western frontier. She attended the Medical University of South Carolina intending to be an obstetrician-gynecologist. "One night when I was on my OB rotation, there was a lady having a seizure—she actually had eclampsia—and this guy ran into the room and started shouting orders, like: 'I'm going to do the A-line. You start a magnesium, you do this, and you do that.' I leaned over and asked, 'Who is *that* guy?' One of the OBs said, 'Oh, that's the anesthesia resident.'" Hilton resolved: "I want to be the person that, when there's utter chaos, you know what to do."

In 2013, Ebony Hilton became the first Black female anesthesiologist to be hired by the Medical University of South Carolina, which opened in 1824. U.Va. hired her five years later. "Growing up in medicine, what I've come to realize is that, should I have a child, it would actually be at more risk of dying than my mom's child was," she said. She cited a Duke University study that correlated race and education levels. "If you look at white women with my same level of degrees, my child is five to seven times more likely to die before his first birthday than theirs. It's been that way historically for Black women. Our numbers haven't really changed, as far as health outcomes, since slavery times."

Many minorities suffer from comorbidities. "That's where the social determinants of health kick in," said Hilton. Asthma and chronic respiratory diseases can be the result of air pollution—for instance, from an industrial plant in a low-income neighborhood. "If you're in a gated community, you don't see smoke bellowing out of these industries, because you have the money and power to influence the policymakers to say you can't put that here." Heart failure, obesity, and diabetes are tied to whether or not there are restaurants and grocery stores with healthy food options instead of fast-food restaurants or the gas station that might be the only source of groceries in the neighborhood. Minorities are wildly overrepresented in prisons, "because we have the school-to-prison pipeline. We know their chances of going to prison are based on their third-grade reading exam. And then you have to go back and ask, why is it this third-grader can't read? Is it possibly the fact that he was born prematurely, because the mother did not have access to prenatal care?" She pointed out that in South Carolina, one in every five counties doesn't have a hospital; eleven counties don't have a single ob/gyn. "The net has a big hole in it."

The moment the first American Covid death was announced in February, Hilton said, she "started doing a tweet storm to CDC and WHO saying, 'We know racial health disparities exist, and they existed before Covid-19. And we know where this will end up.'" She demanded: "Tell us who you're testing and who you're not." The CDC didn't release that information until July, after the *New York Times* sued for it, and then it was sketchy, missing race and ethnicity data from more than half the cases. The information portrayed a country that was experiencing wildly different pandemics. For every 10,000 Americans, there were 38 coronavirus cases; however, for whites, the number was 23; for Blacks, it was 62; and for Hispanics, it was 73.

Hilton and her colleagues went to minority communities in and around Charlottesville to provide testing at churches and shopping centers. "Minorities are less likely to be tested, which means they might go back home, where they have the capability to infect their entire community." People of color were also more likely to be exposed because so many are essential workers. "Only one in five African-Americans can work remotely," she said. "Only one in six Hispanics can work from home. So they were having to go out into the community, face-to-face with the virus."

Nationwide, Blacks and Latinos contracted the virus at a rate three times greater than whites. Virginia senator Mark Warner told me that Hispanics in his state accounted for 45 percent of the Covid cases, although they make up only 8 percent of the population. Dr. Hilton pointed to an article in a Richmond paper, on April 26, which stated that by that date every single person who had died of Covid in the city was Black. At Hilton's hospital, seven of the first ten Covid fatalities were people of color. In the first half of 2020, life expectancy for Black Americans fell by 2.7 years, erasing two decades of gains.

Staffers at U.Va.'s hospital prepared their wills. Hilton's neighbor, a nurse in the Covid unit, has two children. Fearing that she might expose them, the woman moved into her basement. Hilton realized that she would be spending long hours away from her dog, Barkley, so she bought a puppy—"a dog for my dog"—that she named Bentley. "They barely get along," she admitted.

ONE OF THE HARDEST MOMENTS at Hilton's hospital came when Lorna Breen, a forty-nine-year-old doctor, was admitted to the psych unit. Her father, Philip Breen, is a retired trauma surgeon; her mother, Rosemary Breen, had been a nurse on the ward where Lorna was admitted. Lorna had been living in Manhattan, overseeing the ER at New York-Presbyterian Allen Hospital.

When Covid inundated New York, Breen worked twelve-hour shifts that often blurred into eighteen. Within a week, she caught Covid herself, sweating it out in her apartment while managing her department remotely. After her fever broke, she returned to work, on April 1.

Breen was defined by her zest for life. She was a salsa dancer; she played the cello in an amateur orchestra; she ran marathons; she drove a Porsche convertible; in her spare time, she was pursuing an MBA. "She never left the party," her sister, Jennifer Feist, said.

During the surge, Breen told Feist that a trauma nurse was walking through the ER triaging patients based on how blue their faces were. So many doctors fell ill that, at one point, Breen supervised the ERs in two hospitals simultaneously. It became too much, even for this immensely vigorous woman. As her father put it later, Lorna was "like a horse that had pulled too heavy a load and couldn't go a step further and just went down."

Breen called her sister one morning and said she couldn't get out of a chair. "She was catatonic," Feist said. "Covid broke her brain."

Feist and her husband, Corey, decided that Lorna needed to come home to Virginia. A friend in Connecticut drove her to Philadelphia; another friend took her to Baltimore, where Feist was waiting on the side of the road to drive her to Charlottesville.

During the eleven days that Breen spent in U.Va.'s hospital, she was terrified that her career was over. Licensing boards, she knew, might flag evidence of mental illness, although before Covid, Breen never had a trace of instability. Jennifer and Corey, both attorneys, assured Lorna that she wouldn't lose her license. She seemed to improve; she even tried to do her MBA homework on her phone. Jennifer took Lorna home with her on the last Saturday of April. The next day, Lorna killed herself.

The pandemic has added immeasurable stress to a public health workforce already suffering from burnout. "She got crushed because she was trying to help other people," Feist said. "She got crushed by a nation that was not ready for this. We should have been prepared. We should have had some sort of plan."

14

The Mission of Wall Street

GOLDMAN SACHS IS a resonant and controversial name in the world of high finance. Its influence pervades American economic policy. Trump's secretary of the Treasury, Steven Mnuchin, was a Goldman alum, as was Gary Cohn, Trump's first director of the National Economic Council, as have been a number of presidents of the Federal Reserve. For many Americans, Goldman represents the pinnacle of avarice. They hold it responsible in part for the vast income disparities in America and the manipulation of government policy to further enrich the already wealthy. But in the upper chambers of power, Goldman is revered because it has created a culture of success. Winning is what matters, in Washington as well as on Wall Street.

In the first quarter of 2020, the Goldman view of the economy was near ecstatic. "We had come fully out of the deep downturn post-2008," Jan Hatzius, Goldman's chief economist, said. Unemployment was near historically low levels, and wages were creeping up; the Federal Reserve seemed willing to let interest rates stay low, so cheap money lubricated investments, consumer spending, and increased employment. Yes, there were longer-term issues. Median incomes hadn't risen substantially since the 1970s. The gap between the rich and the poor appeared unbridgeable. But at the end of 2019, Goldman looked forward to continued robust growth.

At first, when the Wuhan outbreak began, the risk to the American economy seemed low. Previous pandemic scares, such as H1N1 and SARS, had negligible economic impact in the U.S. On February 12, with Covid already rooted in America and beginning to spread in Italy, the Dow Jones closed at 29,551, a record perch at the time, from which the economy would take one of the steepest dives in history.

"For the next four weeks, until the end of March, we made the biggest downward revisions to our growth forecasts that we've ever made," said Hatzius. "We began the deepest contraction in the global economy on record." Normally, when Hatzius is compiling data for the quarterly Goldman forecasts, he breaks down the GDP into different industries. "You estimate the ups and downs of a business cycle by, say, relating people's propensity to spend on consumer goods to their labor income or tax changes, or the effect of interest-rate changes on the willingness or ability to buy homes." This situation was different. "It wasn't the case that people didn't have the money to go to restaurants—they *couldn't* go to restaurants. Restaurants were shut." Airlines stopped flying. Automobile production ceased. Entire sectors were subtracted from the economy. "It was more arithmetic than econometrics." As he did the math, Hatzius said, "the numbers were mind-blowing once we got into double digits for the second quarter GDP decline." He pegged the drop at 24 percent of the GDP, which turned out to be less than the actual figure. "We thought, 'Wow, this is like four times larger than anything we've ever seen before.' But it seemed to be coming out of these relatively simple calculations."

On March 27, the front page of the *New York Times* posted an extraordinary graph, illustrating the 3,300,000 unemployment claims filed in the past week. The graph stretches across the bottom of the page, starting in the year 2000, with a weekly average below 345,000 claims. It rises in 2008 during the financial crisis, cresting in the first quarter of 2009 with 665,000 claims; it then shows a steady downward trend. At the beginning of March 2020, only 200,000 workers had applied for relief, a historic low. Then the graph shoots up like a telephone pole, climbing the righthand margin of the front page, peaking just below the headline: JOB LOSSES SOAR; U.S. VIRUS CASES TOP WORLD. At that same moment, the Dow Jones Industrial Average had reversed its sharp plunge and begun a long climb that was strikingly at odds with the actual economy.

STEVE STRONGIN IS a senior adviser at Goldman Sachs. He describes himself as "a systems analyst of the old school. I focus on how things connect." He retired in January 2020 after twenty-five years, twelve of them as head of research. Before that, he spent a dozen years at the Federal Reserve in Chicago.

As a kind of farewell, he was invited to Hong Kong to give a lecture to some of his Goldman colleagues stationed there. When he arrived, on January 20, he saw about ten people in the city wearing face masks; a week later, as he departed, nearly everyone was wearing one. Had he waited one more day to return to the U.S., he would have been quarantined. Then he traveled to Europe, and Covid was there to greet him. In February, he taught a course at the RAND Corporation in Los Angeles, and by early March the restaurants were empty and it was getting hard to find a place to eat. He flew back to New York on March 14, six days before the city shut down. All along he was one step behind the virus, "a lagging indicator," he said.

Strongin was sixty-two, thin, tousled, with rimless glasses that gave him a kind of nineteenth-century European intellectual look—Henrik Ibsen without the sideburns. He spent his career at the summit of the financial world. "It was my job for thirty years to foresee the future," he said. The markets were his crystal ball. "Markets very often get talked about as though they're some kind of giant casino. But they actually have a deep economic function, which is to move capital, both equity and debt, from businesses that no longer serve a purpose to businesses we need *today*."

In 2019, Strongin wrote a paper titled "A Survivor's Guide to Disruption," in which he analyzed what he termed an "Everything-as-a-Service economy." Businesses fare better when they organize around what they do well and outsource everything else, he argued. He gave the example of Apple, which does not actually manufacture any part of the iPhone. "Apple has so little to do with the actual production chain that when a customer purchases an iPhone it is quite possible no Apple employee has touched any part of that phone," he wrote. That makes for faster, easier competition, which is good for the economy, but it means that established companies face potential rivals that can scale up quickly and cheaply—a near-constant threat of disruption. In such an environment, the key to survival is resilience.

The market's reaction to the pandemic passed through a series of revelations, Strongin observed. "First are the classic crisis ones. How to keep operating. How to keep our people safe. How to connect to our clients." This was not a time to rethink the world. The mentality at the beginning was "Somehow we are going to freeze in place, the virus will pass, and then we'll unfreeze and go back to normal." During that phase, the function of Wall Street was to provide liquidity as clients turned to preservation strategies—raising cash, drawing on lines of credit—while they waited out the contagion. But the pandemic settled in like a dinner guest who wouldn't leave and was eating everything in the pantry.

Strongin had run research at Goldman through bird flu and SARS. Those diseases left not a scratch on financial markets, having been successfully contained by contact tracing and by health officials in airports with fever-detecting infrared guns. But how do you control a contagion that can be spread by people who show no signs of disease? "The moment when everybody was forced to reassess the severity and longevity of the crisis is when people realized that asymptomatic carriers were important," Strongin said. "That meant that all the prior controls were going to fail."

His crystal ball told him that thousands of businesses would be lost. There would be paralyzing gaps in production. Government would wade in with historic levels of assistance, but it was unclear that would suffice. No one alive had seen a catastrophe of such scale. The rules were going to change. The pandemic was a historic disrupter, forcing a shift from short-term to long-term thinking. "Once that realization came into place," Strongin said, "you saw the rush to opportunity."

Investors pivoted to the consolidation phase—going with the winners. Facebook, Apple, Microsoft, Google, and Amazon: the market recovery was led by these five stocks, which accounted for more than 20 percent of the S&P, each of them setting a new record high. "But the Darwinian reality of capitalism is not about this brilliant insight into the five winners," said Strongin, "it's about taking money *away* from the fifty thousand losers. It's a blinding revelation that the past is dead and it's time to figure out what the future will be."

———

PART OF THE CULTURE of Goldman Sachs, Strongin believes, is the freedom it awards its associates to wander intellectually, searching for interesting questions. One such question is why government policy has failed to narrow the jobs gap—the gap between the jobs people want and those that are actually available.

Globalization and technological change have led to higher standards of living, but that is of little comfort for people whose jobs have been displaced. "Part of the political failure around globalization was an inability to understand how badly some people were being hurt even as society as a whole did better," Strongin said. "Dealing with that pain should have been a major focus of policy; instead, policy tried to pretend it could make the pain go away with a few training courses."

From the Hayek perspective, new jobs should arise from the crisis and labor will simply adjust. But in fact, labor is not so easy to move around. Workers may lack the resources or the knowledge to fit into the new paradigm. "If you think about the decision of a forty-five-year-old steelworker in the seventies deciding to learn a new trade and move to the Southwest, it is virtually impossible to construct a policy that makes that decision rational," Strongin pointed out. "They are giving up all their social networks to make a highly concentrated, risky investment decision about which they know little and which requires a huge part of their financial reserves and a great deal of time and energy. The Keynesian answer of ramping the economy until steel jobs return is just as unworkable. The only real answer is recognizing the financial losses from change and mitigating the community damage."

After years of studying markets, Strongin has learned that "the secret for success is to stop doing things that are not working. Everything you do that doesn't work prevents you from doing something that might. It's the core of the capitalist economic system: we don't prop up failures." He added: "The U.S. will come out of this notably stronger as long as we learn this lesson instead of trying to reinforce the past."

That's Hayek talking, but Strongin drew a distinction. "My own view is that the policy should follow Keynes, but the outcome will follow Hayek." He explained in an email: "The current split between the stock market and the employment numbers is a flashing warning that the economy and the people are not the same. The markets and most large companies are having an easy time moving on to the new post-

Covid economy (Hayek). Many workers will have a much harder time making that transition (Keynes). If we don't spend real money the pain will be very real and the political consequences dangerous at best."

LONG BEFORE THE Covid contagion, the American economy was suffering from severe structural problems. Raj Chetty, a professor of economics at Harvard, founded an institute called Opportunity Insights, with the goal of restoring the American dream. Evidence that the dream is fading is starkly depicted in a graph showing the steadily diminishing number of Americans who earn as much as their parents did in the year of their birth. Ninety percent of Americans born in 1940 earned more than their parents, but by 1980, that ratio had fallen to 50 percent. The legacy of the coronavirus will likely make the American dream even more difficult to achieve.

Chetty and his colleagues have constructed an economic map of the United States by zip codes, examining income and employment to see which areas are hit hardest by the virus. Classic recessions, such as in 2001 and 2009, begin with a reduction in consumer spending. Low- and middle-income workers decide they can't afford a new car, the effect is felt in Detroit; autoworkers are laid off; secondary industries and services feel the contraction as spending slows, and the downward spiral begins. In 2020, however, the fundamental concern was about health, so the reduction has been with in-person services rather than durable goods.

Initially, the economists expected that, as with previous recessions, the impacts would be concentrated on less-affluent areas, but the data surprised them. Workers were more likely to have lost their jobs in places like Manhattan's Upper East Side, which lost nearly 90 percent of small business revenue—the restaurants and shoe stores and boutiques that had flourished in the wealthy ecosystem—than in the Bronx, where businesses lost only about 30 percent of their revenue. Chetty concluded that the decline in consumer spending wasn't driven by the absence of money, it was driven by affluent Americans who didn't want to take the risk of leaving their homes because of the contagion. The result was massive unemployment among lower-income workers who once served drinks at the Caledonia Bar or sold sweaters and jeans at J. Crew. Similar effects were shown in other affluent neighborhoods. Low-income workers in Silicon Valley, for instance, were among the most likely to have lost their jobs, a regional impact counter to what would normally be expected. Repairing the damage would require different economic remedies, but the policymakers were still looking at the crisis through the paradigms of the past.

By April 14, the stimulus checks of up to $1,200 for more than eighty million Americans were deposited; the 21 percent surge in spending that followed was spent on durable goods, like microwaves ordered from Walmart, but spending on in-person services only rose 7 percent, doing little to repair the holes in the economy. Small businesses had lost 40 percent of their jobs. The $500 billion Paycheck Protection Program was meant to plug the employment drain, but when Chetty and his colleagues calculated the increase in employment, it was only 2 percent. They figured that each job saved cost taxpayers about $375,000. In part, this was because checks went to companies that weren't planning to lay off many workers anyway. But according to the Small Business Administration, there were also indications of widespread fraud, including businesses that suddenly popped up after the pandemic started. The FBI opened hundreds of investigations. Among the ironies was the fact that more than $850,000 went to five anti-vaccine groups.

In Chetty's study, government-ordered shutdowns and reopenings showed little effect on economic activity. Traditional economic tools, such as stimulus spending or providing liquidity to businesses, would have limited effect as long as health concerns were not assuaged. The best that government can offer, Chetty suggested, was extended unemployment benefits.

"To be clear, if the government had done nothing, and had no stimulus, no monetary policy, and no unemployment benefit extension, we would be looking at possibly a Great Depression here," Chetty said.

CHETTY'S STORY IS shaped by the immigrant experience. He was born in New Delhi in 1979 to a family of scholars. Both of his parents were professors, his father, Veerappa Chetty, of economics, and his mother, Anbu, of pediatrics. The family moved to the U.S. when he was nine. Veerappa taught at Columbia University and consulted with the U.N. and the World Bank. Anbu is a pediatric pulmonologist at

Tufts Medical Center. Raj's two older sisters both became biomedical researchers.

Chetty wondered why there are so many more opportunities to succeed in America than in India. His own life was an example. He whizzed through Harvard in three years, becoming a tenured professor at the age of twenty-eight, one of the earliest in Harvard's history, picking up a MacArthur genius grant along the way. His work has reflected his concern that the dynamism that marked America, and which opened up so many opportunities to his own family, has faltered.

Government alone cannot restore the economy to health. Innovation is a primary driver of economic growth. One way of measuring inventive creativeness is through patent applications. Chetty, along with Alex Bell, Xavier Jaravel, Neviana Petkova, and John Van Reenen, studied the childhoods of more than a million patent holders, linking family income with elementary test scores and other key factors. Children at the top of their third-grade math class were the most likely to become inventors—but only if they also came from a high-income family. High-scoring children who were from low-income or minority families were no more likely to become inventors than affluent children with mediocre scores. Successful inventors were also less likely to be women, Black, Latino, or from the Southeast. Chetty called these failed inventors the "lost Einsteins." "If women, minorities, and children from low-income families were to invent at the same rate as white men from high-income (top 20%) families, the rate of innovation in America would quadruple," the authors said.

The most ominous finding by Chetty and his colleagues was the effect of Covid-19 on educational progress. Using a popular math program called Zearn, the economists plotted the achievement of children from upper-income families versus those from lower incomes. When schools shut down and instruction switched to remote learning, children in the upper-income tier suffered a small drop in the lessons completed, but low-income children fell in a hole—a 60 percent drop in the rate of progress in learning math. The long-term economic prospects for those children are dire. "We're likely to see further erosion of social mobility the longer this lasts," Chetty said. The American dream was drifting farther out of reach for another generation.

————

WHEN I CALLED Gianna Pomata again, in April, she had set up an avatar on her Zoom page: a bouquet of plumbago. "There was a big bush of plumbago next to the door of my grandmother's little country house when I was a child," she explained. The house was in Sardinia, where Pomata grew up. "I loved my grandmother, and I loved that house. So I just love that plant. It's a color I remember from when I was very, very little." Plumbago blossoms are a delicate blue, like a summer afternoon in Texas, when the color has almost been bleached out of the sky. Plumbago grows well in the heat.

Gianna's sister, Daniela, was an emergency room doctor, in Sant'Orsola-Malpighi Polyclinic, the largest hospital in Italy. The two sisters lived in the same building. "We used to be together constantly, and now I can't see her," Gianna said. From the start of the outbreak, her sister had emphasized that the coronavirus was not an ordinary flu. She told Gianna, "I've never seen such pneumonias, they're devastating."

The crisis in Italy had begun to ease just as it was making itself felt in Texas. The state's governor ordered a lockdown on April 2, although he refused to call it that. Austin was about to have the experience Bologna had had the month before.

I asked Pomata if Italians who recovered will be allowed to return to work. "There is no work for them," she said. Even before the economic crisis caused by the coronavirus, unemployment for young Italians was 30 percent. "What you need is exactly what the Fed is doing in the United States—you inject money into the system."

Pomata's daughter, Catherine, lived in New York, where she worked in the film industry. "I don't like the situation there at all," Pomata said. "She is with her husband, she's not by herself, so that's good." They lived in a tiny apartment near Columbia University, on the Upper West Side. "Catherine loves New York," said Pomata. "Living in New York was a dream. But now I think she's very scared."

There was another feature of the pandemic that reminded her of the Black Death. "We cannot go and visit the dying, we cannot celebrate funerals. I think, what if something happens to my daughter, and I couldn't even see her body? It just feels intolerable."

———

MICHIGAN GOVERNOR GRETCHEN WHITMER issued a statewide stay-at-home order in March and extended it on April 9, by which time there were more than 20,000 confirmed cases in the state and nearly a thousand deaths, the third-highest in the nation at the time. The auto industry closed shop and the economy went into deep freeze. Through all this, Whitmer's lockdown order was broadly popular. And then Trump began to tweet. "LIBERATE MICHIGAN!" he wrote on April 17. Two weeks later, he tweeted, "The Governor of Michigan should give a little, and put out the fire. These are very good people, but they are angry. They want their lives back again, safely! See them, talk to them, make a deal."

On April 30, thousands of protesters, spurred on by Trump's tweets and Fox News commentators, participated in "Operation Gridlock," surrounding the state capitol in Lansing and demanding that restrictions be lifted. They carried Trump 2020 campaign signs and chanted "Lock Her Up," meaning Whitmer, not Hillary Clinton. "They had a Trump float and they were waving the Confederate flag, which in the state of Michigan is not something you see very often," Whitmer said. She was called "Hitler" and hanged in effigy. A number of the protesters armed with assault weapons stormed into the Capitol building, menacing state police who barred them from entering legislative chambers. This went on week after week.

"The whole political reality on the ground changed when Trump singled me out," Whitmer said. "Up until that point I had pretty good support out of my legislature, which is totally Republican controlled. And when that happened, they stopped extending the state of emergency, they started suing me, they threatened to impeach me." Protesters not only continued to besiege the Capitol, they showed up at the Governor's Mansion with assault weapons, wearing tactical gear.

Whitmer was inside with her husband and two teenage daughters. "I called the leader of the Michigan senate," Whitmer said, referring to Mike Shirkey, who represents Jackson, Michigan, one of the spots that lays claim to being the birthplace of the Republican Party. She left a message on his cell phone. "We need to bring the heat down," she said. "I need your help." She told him that there had been death threats against her and her family. "He didn't even return my phone call," she said.

15

The Man Without a Mask

T HE THIRD AND FINAL chance to contain the infection—masks—was the easiest, the cheapest, and perhaps the most effective. But the administration, and the country, failed to meet the challenge.

In the early morning of March 4, as Matt Pottinger was driving to the White House, he was on the phone with a source in China, a doctor. Taking notes on the back of an envelope while holding the phone to his ear and navigating the city traffic, Pottinger was excited by all the valuable new information about how the virus was being contained in China. The doctor specifically mentioned the antiviral drug remdesivir—which was just emerging as a possible therapy in the U.S. Then he talked about masks, which he said were extremely effective with Covid, more so than with influenza. "It's great to carry around your own hand sanitizer," the doctor explained, "but masks are going to win the day."

Still on the phone when he parked his car, a stick-shift Audi, on West Executive Avenue next to the West Wing, Pottinger left the car in neutral and neglected to apply the parking brake. As he rushed toward his office, the Audi took a journey of its own, rolling backward into the street in a long, wide arc, narrowly missing a collision with the vice president's limo, then hopping the curb and coming to rest against a tree.

While the Secret Service was examining the errant Audi, Pottinger kept thinking about masks. America's pandemic response had already been handicapped by China's withholding of information about human-to-human and asymptomatic transmission. The testing imbroglio would set the country back for months. But masks offered a ready solution for a desperate situation.

Deborah Birx had told Pottinger that, whereas mask-wearing was part of Asian culture, Americans couldn't be counted on to comply. It wasn't just a cultural failing, however; Pottinger began to see America's public health establishment as an impediment. In those early days, the U.S. health officials looked at SARS-CoV-2 and flatly applied the algorithm for SARS and flu: sick people should wear masks, but for others they weren't necessary. Redfield admitted: "We didn't understand until mid-March that many people with Covid weren't symptomatic but were highly infectious."

Pottinger felt sure he had the data on his side. He argued that whenever a large majority of people wore masks, it stopped contagion "dead in its tracks." He pointed to the success in Taiwan, which was manufacturing ten million masks per day for a population of twenty-three million. It was almost untouched. Hong Kong was one of the most densely populated cities in the world, but there was no community spread of virus because nearly everyone wore masks. Pottinger's arguments stirred up surprisingly rigid responses from the public health contingent; in his opinion, when Redfield, Fauci, Birx, and Hahn spoke, it could sound like groupthink, echoing the way that their public messaging was strictly coordinated.

No one in the White House wore a mask until Pottinger donned one, in the middle of March. Entering the West Wing, he felt as if he were wearing a clown nose. People gawked. The president asked if he was ill. Pottinger replied, "I don't want to be a footnote in history—the guy who knocked off a president with Covid."

NSC staffers worked in close quarters in the Situation Room, monitoring news and global developments. They had heard over and over again that masks were useless and maybe dangerous. Pottinger asked the staff virologist to teach them how to mask up. Some people were annoyed. Masks had become a political litmus test, with many conservatives condemning mask mandates as infringements on liberty, and wearing one in Trump's White House seemed borderline treasonous, as well as a risky career move. Pottinger was shocked to learn that, in any case, the White House had no ready supply of masks.

He called an official in Taiwan and asked for guidance about controlling the virus. Masks, he was told again. Prompted by the call, Taiwan's president donated half a million masks to the U.S., via diplomatic pouch. Pottinger took 3,600, for the NSC staff and the White House medical unit, and sent the rest to the national stockpile.

In early April, new studies showed dramatic reductions in transmission when masks were worn. Pottinger put copies of the studies into binders for key task force members. One anecdotal study out of China reported on an infected traveler who took two long bus rides. He began coughing on the first ride, then purchased a face mask before boarding a minibus. Five passengers on the first ride were infected, and no one on the second. Another study failed to detect any viral particles in aerosol or droplets from subjects wearing surgical masks. The president remarked, "It turns out Pottinger was right."

On April 3, the CDC finally concluded that masks were vital in slowing the spread of infection. It was the last opportunity to do something meaningful to curb the pandemic.

Redfield admitted that the sudden reversal by the CDC was awkward and confusing. "When you have to change the message, the second message doesn't always stick." The president made things worse when he announced the new mask advisory in a Coronavirus Task Force briefing. "This is voluntary," he stressed, adding, "I don't think I'm going to be doing it."

In that task force meeting in April when the CDC reversed its guidance, Pottinger was still the only one wearing a mask. Not a single member of the public health contingent was masked. Vice President Pence congratulated Pottinger for his foresight. That same afternoon, Pottinger was notified by Pence's chief of staff that at the next task force meeting "No masks will be worn."

That was a signal. Pottinger stopped attending the task force.

TRUMP WAS A notorious germophobe. He recoiled when anyone near him sneezed and once chastised his acting chief of staff, Mick Mulvaney, on camera when Mulvaney coughed in the Oval Office. "If you're going to cough, please leave the room," Trump told him. He hated shaking hands and suggested to visitors that they wash up before they entered the office. He once told talk show host Howard Stern that he had a hand-washing obsession, which "could be a psychological problem," and later admitted he avoided his son Barron when he had a cold.

"I had a man come up to me a week ago," the president recalled in a task force briefing. "I hadn't seen him in a long time, and I said, 'How you doing?' He said, 'Fine, fine.' And he—he hugs me, kiss. I said, 'Are you well?' He says, 'No.' He said, 'I have the worst fever and the worst flu.' And he's hugging and kissing me. So I said, 'Excuse me.' I went and started washing my hands." Trump recounted this story as an amusing insight into his personality, the only frailty he admits to. He seems intrigued by his horror of contamination.

By rejecting the CDC guidance and refusing to wear a mask, the president was making a powerful statement, far more dangerous than his idle speculation about injecting disinfectant. He demanded a reporter take off a mask at a press conference, then mocked him for being "politically correct" when the reporter refused. Immune to irony, he even toured a mask-making factory in Arizona without a mask.

What was going on with this man who shrank from personal contact, who tried to "bail out" whenever someone sneezed, but refused to wear a face mask in the middle of a pandemic? It was not just Trump, of course; the people around him submitted to the example he set. Vice President Pence visited the Mayo Clinic without a mask, violating hospital policy. Many Republican legislators shunned masks even after members of their caucus became infected. It was not just Republicans, but Democrats were twice as likely to say that masks should always be worn. It was not just men, but women were more in favor of masks than men. It was not just white people, but they were much more averse to mask-wearing than Blacks and Latinos. If you sorted each group into those least likely to wear a mask, the result would roughly coincide with the average Trump voter.

Some anti-maskers called the coronavirus a hoax; others believed it wasn't all that dangerous. But the image of the maskless president animated his base. Maskless, he appeared defiant, masculine, invulnerable, whereas to wear a mask would be caving in, being weak; it might "send the wrong message" and hurt his chances for reelection. Eventually, he would come to believe that people wore masks to show their disapproval of him. And yet, from his perspective, exposing himself to microbes that could readily kill him must have seemed heroic.

He knew the virus was dangerous—"deadly stuff," he admitted to journalist Bob Woodward in a February interview that surfaced months later, "more deadly than even your strenuous flus." Yes, there was testing in the White House, but the tests were fallible and not a shield against infection. He dared the virus to touch him, like Lear raging against the storm, the full Shakespearean drama unfolding with the uncloaked emotions Trump and his family and his entire entourage invariably displayed. The absence of complexity in their characters made them all the more theatrical, as we instantly sensed what drove them—vanity, avarice, and ambition being the most obvious.

In part because of the president's courtship of the virus, millions of people followed his example, giving the pandemic access to new communities, infecting new families, endangering healthcare workers, prolonging unemployment, sabotaging efforts to open the economy, and causing untold numbers of people to die.

MASKS HAVE BEEN a part of public health for over a century, but until April, the WHO and other health agencies actively discouraged their use among healthy people, speculating that masks might cause people to take risks, and if worn incorrectly could put them at greater risk. In the U.S., health experts also advised against wearing masks. "If it's not fitted right you're going to fumble with it," Secretary Azar advised a House of Representatives subcommittee. "Seriously people—STOP BUYING MASKS!" Jerome Adams, the surgeon general, tweeted on February 29. He claimed he was concerned about the shortage of masks for frontline workers, but he had added, "They are NOT effective in preventing general public from catching #Coronavirus." In March, he went further, asserting on *Fox & Friends*, "You can increase your risk of getting it by wearing a mask if you are not a healthcare provider."

"Right now in the United States, people should not be walking around with masks," Dr. Fauci said on March 8. "When you're in the middle of an outbreak, wearing a mask might make people feel a little bit better and it might even block a droplet, but it's not providing the perfect protection that people think that it is." And yet, the CDC recommended that all healthcare workers in contact with Covid patients wear hospital-grade N95 masks, so from the beginning there was a sense among many people that the government, and even the highest medical authorities, couldn't be trusted.

One turning point in scientific perception concerning the importance of masks was a paper in the CDC publication *Morbidity and Mortality Weekly Report*. The *MMWR* is the central repository of information from state health departments and the CDC's Epidemic Intelligence Service. The investigators described a choir practice in Skagit County, Washington, north of Seattle. On March 10, 61 singers were at practice, half of the total membership. Their median age was 69. One of them had cold-like symptoms—what turned out to be Covid-19. In less than two weeks, 53 positive cases were identified among the singers, three were hospitalized, two of whom died. Only seven people (not counting the index case) failed to be infected in the two and a half hours of practice.

Much was learned from this event. Loud singing generates aerosols, the most likely way the infection spread. "Certain persons, known as superemitters, who release more aerosol particles during speech than do their peers, might have contributed to this," the authors state. They recommended that people avoid face-to-face encounters, maintain a social distance of at least six feet, and "[wear] cloth face coverings in public settings." When the CDC recommended that congregations consider ending or at least decreasing the use of choirs, the president's aides demanded that the guidance be dropped. Jay Butler, the infectious disease specialist who had made the recommendation, wrote an email to his colleagues: "There will be people who will get sick and perhaps die because of what we were forced to do."

It is dispiriting to think that employing the simple precaution of wearing a mask could have avoided much suffering, death, impoverishment, and grief, had it been widely implemented from the start. Asian countries where mask-wearing was common reported sharply lower rates of transmission. As of March 17, when U.S. officials were still weighing in strongly against masks, Hong Kong, Singapore, and Taiwan had fewer than a thousand cases of Covid-19 altogether. The WHO changed its stance after commissioning a meta-analysis of 172 observational studies across sixteen countries of the effectiveness of social distancing and face masks, finding they made a significant difference.

An enlightening natural experiment occurred in Kansas, when the governor issued an executive order in July to wear masks in public but allowed counties to opt out. It was as if Kansas were performing a clinical trial on itself. Within two months, infections in mask-wearing counties had fallen by 6 percent; elsewhere, infections rose 100 percent.

Plague doctors in seventeenth-century Europe wore beaked masks stuffed with aromatic herbs that were thought to fend off contagion. When plague returned in the early twentieth century, in Manchuria, Wu Lien-teh, a Chinese doctor from British Malaya, tried to convince his colleagues that the disease—what we now call pneumonic plague—was spreading through the air from human to human and not just through flea bites, the source of bubonic plague. Like Matt Pottinger, Wu Lien-teh advocated wearing masks to halt the contagion, which was contrary to conventional public health wisdom at the time. A prominent French doctor ridiculed the idea and then visited a hospital without covering his face; he died days later, and masks were suddenly in demand. It's a lesson that apparently needs to be relearned again and again.

Jan Hatzius, Goldman's chief economist, decided to examine the effect of mask-wearing on the gross domestic product. He noted that most of East Asia and many European countries had imposed mandatory mask-wearing or normally wore masks in time of illness. The U.S. scored surprisingly well in terms of the number of people saying they were wearing masks in public—just below 70 percent, compared to 90 percent in East Asia and 80 percent in southern Europe. The rate in the U.K. was only 30 percent. There were broad differences within the United States, with about 40 percent of respondents in Arizona saying they "always" wear a mask in public compared with nearly 80 percent in Massachusetts. Drawing on data from state-mandated mask-wearing, Hatzius estimated that a national mandate would increase the average number of people who "always" or "frequently" wear masks by 15 percent. But would that actually lower transmission?

Based on the data from states, Hatzius observed that, once a mandate was issued, "the growth rate of infections is cut by 25%." Fatalities also showed a dramatic decline. "Our numerical estimates are that cumulative cases grow 17.3% per week without a mask mandate but only 7.3% with a mask mandate, and that cumulative fatalities grow 29% per week without a mask mandate but only 16% with a mask mandate." A national mandate would cut the average growth rate in Covid cases to between 0.6 to 0.7%—below the rate at which a virus is considered under control. "The upshot of our analysis is that a national face mask mandate could potentially substitute for renewed lockdowns that would otherwise subtract nearly 5% from GDP."

BY COINCIDENCE my pandemic novel, *The End of October*, was published on April 28, in the first wave of the pandemic, and although it received good notices, I heard whispers that I was exploiting a worldwide catastrophe. "I suppose if it weren't for the pandemic, no one would pay attention to this book at all," a late-night talk show host in Britain said to me, as if publishing a novel when the bookstores were shuttered and the airport newsstands empty was a sinister plot of mine.

The main reaction, however, was that I was clairvoyant, that I knew before anyone else that a pandemic awaited us, and that it would unfold in ways I had eerily foreseen. I don't have those powers. The reason the novel parallels reality is that I read the playbooks, I watched the tabletop exercises, I talked to the experts. They all knew what was going to happen. The knowledge of how the virus would disrupt society was always there. I just lifted the expert reports and turned them into fiction.

If a lowly novelist knew, my critics persisted, why didn't the government know? The president kept saying, "Nobody knew there would be a pandemic or an epidemic of this proportion. . . . There's never been anything like this in history," and "What a problem. Came out of nowhere." But of course lots of people knew. The administration simply didn't trust its own public health officials. Instead of framing policy around the advice they were giving, the administration decided to control the narrative, play down the threat—this was something I actually did predict.

The question the novel posed was: How could civilization collapse? I'm intrigued by fallen empires, the ruins, the once-great fortresses, the literature of bygone peoples, the failed cultural impulses that swelled into greatness and then collapsed. I'm not a pessimist about the durability of the American republic, but I did think we were drawing closer to the edge. What could push us over? A nuclear war, of course, but civilizations have ended long before humanity had hold of the tools of annihilation. Often the force that brings about the end is disease.

I set about to educate myself on viruses and I was immediately astonished by the fact that science still knew so little about them. Scientists were shocked to learn that there were viruses in seawater; a single liter can contain about 100 billion of them. I interviewed Curtis Suttle, a marine virologist at the University of British Columbia, who was trying to conduct a rough census of the viral world. Ninety percent of the viruses he found in seawater were totally unknown. In 2018, he and other researchers placed buckets on mountaintops in Spain, at the approximate height of jet travel; according to their calculations, more than 800 million viruses a day were raining down on every square meter of the earth's surface. They were apparently able to be swept up in the atmosphere and travel across oceans and continents. Ian Lipkin, the distinguished epidemiologist at Columbia University, surprised me by describing archaic viruses frozen in the tundra, which were being brought back to life by global warming.

I had thought of viruses as being harmful aliens, but I learned that they were a guiding force in human evolution. Portions of viral DNA from ancient infections have wedged themselves into our genome, accounting for as much as 8 percent of it, including genes that control memory formation, the immune system, and cognitive development. The more I learned, the more intrigued I became. I could certainly understand the spell that viruses cast over scientists like John Brooks and Yen Pottinger.

The moment that the idea of writing the novel occurred to me was on a trek with my wife in Britain, in 2014, from Winchester to Dover. The path was called Pilgrim's Way because it passes through Canterbury, where the great cathedral stands. Now the many churches along the path were mostly abandoned, testaments to the bygone era of faith. We often ate our picnic lunches in a picturesque churchyard among the gray granite tombstones. The death dates stretched back hundreds of years, but one year stood out: 1918.

Of course, many were soldiers. Britain paid a terrible price in that war, which overshadowed the flu, but the Spanish influenza killed far more people worldwide than the war. The year 1918 is carved into graveyards like the iridium layer that marks the date, sixty-six million years ago, when an asteroid struck Earth and extinguished the dinosaurs.

The war was remembered, chronicled, and memorialized, but recollections of the 1918 pandemic were boxed up and hidden away. My own father had been stricken, when he was three years old, living on a farm in central Kansas, and his father had a terrible round of it, but they survived. Daddy never spoke of it. Instead, his earliest memory was of the church bells and fireworks that marked Armistice Day, ending the First World War. In that conflict, 53,000 American soldiers died in combat, and 63,000 by disease. Howard Markel estimates that the total number of Americans who died of the 1918 pandemic was between 500,000 and 750,000; the average life expectancy in the U.S. fell by nearly twelve years. Of course, death by disease was far more common then. The great advances of medicine were over the horizon. With few effective treatments or vaccines to ward off contagion, people felt helpless and resigned to their fate. There was nothing heroic about getting sick and dying from the flu, and nothing unique. It was as arbitrary as it was deadly. No wonder people wanted to put the experience behind them. And yet it was the worst natural disaster in modern times.

I was asked what I got wrong in the novel. I underestimated the willingness of people to isolate themselves, at great cost—financially, emotionally, spiritually—and do this for months. Of course, much of the early sense of solidarity deteriorated into an upsurge of rebellion and conspiracy-mongering, looking more like what I imagined. I didn't expect the food chain to be so resilient, or banks to be able to keep the cash flowing. My fictional virus is deadlier, more like the one that may come one day.

On a sunny afternoon in April I went for a jog on a school track near my home in Austin. A group of young women were running time trials in the hundred-meter dash. They were the fastest people I had ever seen. Occasionally, as I came around a curve, I'd pull even with one of them just as she was taking off. It was like Wile E. Coyote eating Road Runner's dust. Their feet rarely touched the track. There was an element of flight.

"What school do you guys run for?" I asked one of them, who was cooling off.

"Oh, it's not a school," she said, and then added, "We're Olympians."

Instead of competing in Tokyo, here they were, on a middle-school track in Austin, trying to maintain peak condition as they waited for the games to be rescheduled. So many dreams had been deferred or abandoned—weddings canceled, funerals avoided, high school musicals called off, vacation plans dropped, and businesses closed. After seeing what happened to New Orleans following Mardi Gras, the mayor of Austin shut down South by Southwest, one of the biggest sources of revenue in the city. My niece Elizabeth Shapiro fronts a ten-piece jazz band in L.A., Lizzy & the Triggermen, and SXSW was going to be her big breakthrough. There might be other chances, but would the band even survive the shutdown? As the quarantine dragged on, my wife and I forced ourselves to take an occasional drive, partly to keep our car battery alive. We would prowl through downtown and along the University of Texas campus, taking note of the vacant streets and boarded-up businesses and wondering what our country would be when we emerged from the prison of Covid-19.

THE VIRUS PLAYED an April Fool's trick on the Trump White House. Mark Meadows, the chief of staff, essentially replaced the Coronavirus Task Force with his own small group of advisers, including Kevin Hassett and other economists who sought to open the country as quickly as possible. The data seemed to show that the contagion in the U.S. was following a similar downward slope as Italy. Of course, there was no way to see into the future, but that's what models were for. One, compiled by the University of Washington and followed closely in the White House painted an optimistic picture of an epidemic that was losing its grip on America. But the projections were illusory.

By the end of April, more than thirty million Americans had filed for unemployment over the previous six weeks, roughly one in five American workers. Over one million Americans had tested positive and more than 63,000 were dead. But a new wave of the virus was about to engulf the country, just as more than half of the states planned to be partially reopened by the end of the week.

In Texas, Governor Abbott decided to open certain sectors of the economy—retail, restaurants, theaters, and more. In his press conference, he sounded serious and considered, referencing the public health advisers he had consulted, the contact tracers that the state was hiring, the ramping up of tests, and so on. But it was all premised on the idea that the number of cases and the death toll were diminishing. The governor cited the declining rates of positive cases to tests conducted, and the decreased hospitalizations, but the very day he eased restrictions, fifty people died, the most in the state since the siege began and only a prelude to the hundreds of Texans who would die every day by the end of July. It was also the first day in weeks with over a thousand new cases, although it was impossible to even estimate how many people were actually infected—Texas was vying with Kansas to be dead last in the country in terms of tests per capita. The contact tracers the governor promised never materialized in sufficient numbers to make a difference. After offering local elected officials the authority to set stricter standards for their communities in March, in April the governor caved in to political pressure from the right flank of his party and ordered municipalities to stop enforcing mask orders, with predictable consequences.

But it still felt like there was reason to be optimistic. By the end of spring, the spread of the disease in the U.S. appeared to have stabilized. The average daily case rate dropped from 30,000 in April, to 25,000 in May, and 20,000 in June. "In recent days, the media has taken to sounding the alarm bells over a 'second wave' of coronavirus infections," Vice President Pence, the leader of the White House Coronavirus Task Force, opined in the *Wall Street Journal*. "Such panic is overblown. Thanks to the leadership of President Trump . . . we are winning the fight against the invisible enemy."

SAN QUENTIN STATE PRISON, on the north shore of San Francisco Bay, has perhaps the most beautiful setting of any operating penitentiary in the U.S.—not that the view was on the minds of the prisoners who built the facility, which opened in 1852. California's oldest state building, and first public work, is a dungeon that is still preserved on the property. Located in Marin County, San Quentin is just one of the 1,833 state prisons in the U.S., where the majority of the more than 2 million incarcerated people in the U.S. are housed, but its long history and reputation for hosting some of America's most notorious criminals has awarded it an outsized spot in the public imagination. Charles Manson was imprisoned here, as was Richard Ramirez, the "Night Stalker"; Sirhan Sirhan, the assassin of Robert F. Kennedy, spent time on San Quentin's death row until the California Supreme Court overturned the death penalty. Merle Haggard was a prisoner in San Quentin when Johnny Cash performed there, and he decided to dedicate his life to music.

On May 30, 122 prisoners from the California Institution for Men in Chino, which had experienced one of the first outbreaks of Covid-19 in the state prison system, were transferred to San Quentin, where, until then, there had been no positive cases. A healthcare executive in the system explicitly ordered that the transferees—among the most medically vulnerable prisoners in the system—not be tested. They were crowded onto buses and delivered to San Quentin. Some of them arrived obviously symptomatic. The next day, the first case in the prison was detected. By mid-summer, San Quentin was the site of one of the largest coronavirus outbreaks in the U.S.

Juan Moreno Haines was incarcerated in San Quentin when the transferees arrived. He was convicted of bank robbery in 1996 and was serving a sentence of fifty-five years to life. Despite its fearsome reputation, San Quentin had a number of educational and recreational programs, including a newspaper, the *San Quentin News,* where Haines became the senior editor. He noted that the day the transferees arrived, two of the cell blocks were at 188 percent of capacity. Prisoners were crowded into the gym, with cots spaced twelve inches apart, head to head.

Haines is a wiry African American with a moustache and wire-rimmed glasses. At San Quentin, he wrote, "prisoners are reluctant to report when they're sick—everyone knows they'll be sent to Carson, known as the Hole, where prisoners are kept in the punishing conditions of solitary confinement." Haines himself fell ill in July. He said that he received only cold meals and no medical attention while he was ill.

In Kansas, half of the prisoners were infected; in South Dakota, the figure was six out of ten. Overall, 20 percent of all state and federal prisoners tested positive for the virus, a rate four times as high as the general population. At San Quentin, by the end of August, 2,237 prisoners and 277 staff members were infected; 28 prisoners and one staff member died. It was history repeating itself: San Quentin suffered terribly during the Spanish flu pandemic, with over 76 percent of the prison population reporting sick at the height of the first wave. In April 1918, the public health officer at San Quentin recorded the first influenza infection, which he attributed to "the entrance into the institution of a prisoner who had come from the county jail in Los Angeles, where, he stated, a number of other inmates had been ill." "This assessment is strikingly similar to the recent mass outbreak of COVID-19 at San Quentin State Prison," the California inspector general concluded a century later.

16

Waves

AM REFLECTING on the idea of disease waves," I said, when Gianna
Pomata and I spoke again in May. Despite Vice President Pence's
assertion, scientists were talking about a second wave of Covid-19 in
the fall, or perhaps many waves. The 1918 Spanish flu began in the early
spring, disappeared in the summer, then returned in the fall. A third
wave came in the spring of the following year; after that, the disease
retreated, leaving tens of millions dead in the space of a year.

The bubonic plague came in three great pandemics. The first, known
as the Plague of Justinian, lasted from the sixth century till the eighth,
with few letups, ravaging the Byzantine Empire. The second pandemic,
the Black Death, arrived in Italy in December 1347, and spread quickly
across Europe. Pilgrims carried it to Mecca. The plague soon infested
Scandinavia. A third of the population of Egypt died. Subsidiary outbreaks continued to appear in Europe for three hundred years. The
Great Plague of London, which Daniel Defoe chronicled, hit in 1665.
After that, the plague mysteriously faded away.

"There was a much more circumscribed episode in Marseille in the
early eighteenth century," Pomata told me, "and that's it for Europe, but
not for Asia." The last plague pandemic began in the mid-nineteenth
century, in China, and spread to India, where it killed six million people. At the beginning of the twentieth century, the disease journeyed
to America, where a Chinese resident of San Francisco was the first to

die. Henry Gage, the governor of California at the time, tried to play down the outbreak, speculating that white people were immune to the disease; scores died. The plague has never been entirely eradicated, but it may have killed so efficiently that with each wave it starved itself of human hosts. Having persisted in flea and rat populations, the bacterium continues to infect humans from time to time. As many as two thousand cases are reported to the World Health Organization every year, often including a handful in the American Southwest.

AT ONE POINT in our conversations, while we were discussing the challenges facing our societies when we emerge from the Covid crisis, Pomata confessed, "I'm so upset and emotional, it's difficult to think clearly." I asked her what troubled her. "First of all, it is rediscovering the extreme fragility of life. So much of our way of life is insane. Right now, for instance, in Italy we don't have proper face masks." Such masks used to be manufactured there, but production had been outsourced to China. If the pandemic had struck in the early 1990s, she believed, Italy could have handled it better, and not just because masks would have been on hand. "Our national healthcare system was better funded, we had more hospitals, the hospitals were better equipped, they had more intensive care units, and all that has been cut, cut, cut for austerity policies dictated by Brussels"—that is, the European Union. Nevertheless, the talk about how the crisis could spell the end of the European Union frightened her. "I am a Europeanist. I have always believed in Europe as a culture and a political idea. But right now I see this. And I'm very angry."

Pomata mentioned an essay that Mario Draghi, the former president of the European Central Bank, had published in the *Financial Times* in March. Draghi, a neoliberal, has been at "the pinnacle of the European bureaucracy that has been enforcing the economic policy called austerity," Pomata explained. The southern tier of European countries—mainly Spain, Italy, Portugal, and Greece—were struggling with heavy debt loads; northern countries, including Germany and the Netherlands, which held the debt, insisted it must be repaid on a rigid schedule. Pomata described the E.U.'s reasoning as "spending more than we have is heresy and we should never do it." It was a classic Keynes-Hayek split.

Draghi had described the coronavirus as "a human tragedy of potentially biblical proportions." He added: "The challenge we face is how to act with sufficient strength and speed to prevent the recession from morphing into a prolonged depression, made deeper by a plethora of defaults leaving irreversible damage. It is already clear that the answer must involve a significant increase in public debt."

Pomata was astounded. "For a long time European bureaucrats and the European ruling class has been firmly anti-Keynesian," she explained. "And Draghi was part of that class—he was at the top of it! And suddenly he writes in the *Financial Times* saying the opposite of what he has been preaching all these years." In a softer voice she said, "I'm glad at least that Draghi spoke up. But that ruling class, the European elite, has to really rethink."

Pomata described the pandemic as "an accelerator of mental renewal. We listen more, perhaps. We're more ready to talk to each other. Once again, I give Draghi's example, because I'm so struck by it. An anthropologist should write about this kind of thing. Draghi's world was very stable. He had some beliefs about how the economy should be handled. And suddenly he's in a whirlwind, and he has to think anew."

IN 1345, shortly before the plague devastated Verona, the Italian poet and scholar Petrarch was rummaging through the library of the city's cathedral. Among the crumbling manuscripts, he found letters from Marcus Tullius Cicero, the Roman statesman and orator who is sometimes credited with making Latin a literary language. Until Petrarch's discovery, Cicero was almost totally forgotten, as were most of the great figures of the classical era. Reading Cicero's letters—or other abandoned works, like Livy's *History of Rome*—revealed to Petrarch how degraded civilization had become. He christened the period after the fall of Rome the Dark Ages. The beauty of Cicero's language, the rigor of his thought, inflamed Petrarch with an ambition to restore the glory of the past. And that meant opening the minds of his contemporaries to the possibility of change.

"For Petrarch, it was about disliking his time and his age and the condition of Italy," Pomata said. Petrarch expressed his frustration by writing letters to the ancients. "It could be like someone today disliking the present state of America and wanting to talk to Thomas Jefferson or Martin Luther King."

The Middle Ages didn't end definitively until the fall of Constantinople, in 1453, when scholars of the Byzantine Empire migrated to Europe, especially to Italy, bringing their libraries with them. But new thinking was already underway, spurred by Petrarch's discovery of old thinking, which is why he is often cited as the instigator of the Renaissance. Artists reclaimed ancient techniques for drawing and painting with perspective. Musicians rediscovered melody. Humanism displaced the stagnant rule of religion over people's minds. Michelangelo, da Vinci, Palladio, Brunelleschi, Boccaccio, Petrarch, Machiavelli, and Dante Alighieri became foundation stones of European thought. Italian explorers, including Christopher Columbus, Giovanni da Verrazano, and Amerigo Vespucci, changed the map of the world. Galileo established the scientific method. The Italian Renaissance was the greatest efflorescence of science and art in Western civilization.

I believe we are at another inflection point, when society will make a radical adjustment, for good or ill. History offers mixed lessons. The Plague of Athens, in 430 BC, led to a prolonged period of lawlessness and immorality. Citizens lost faith in Athenian democracy, which never regained its standing. The millions of deaths caused by the 1918 Spanish flu and the First World War brought about women's suffrage but also inaugurated the Roaring Twenties, which featured disparities of wealth unequaled until the present day. On the other hand, during the Great Depression, the United States remade itself into a stronger, more unified and compassionate society. The shock of the Second World War caused America to transform itself into the strongest economic power in history, largely through an expansive middle class. But after 9/11, the U.S. forged a dark path. Instead of taking advantage of surging patriotism and international goodwill, America invaded Iraq and tortured suspects in Guantánamo. At home, prosperous Americans barricaded themselves off from their fellow citizens, allowing racial and economic inequalities to fester.

Pomata and I began to speculate again on positive outcomes of the current pandemic. "People are noticing in Venice that the water is suddenly transparent," she said. "It's clean. And even I, here in Bologna, I open the window and usually it smells foul because of too many Moto-rini, and now it smells nice. It's like being in the countryside."

I also treasured the quiet, the absence of the traffic roar, the neigh-borhood streets given up to pedestrians and exhilarated children on bicy-cles. I was inspired by the photographs of Los Angeles, looking eerily pristine, and by newfound vistas of the Himalayas from Punjab, hidden for decades by smog. I wondered if these images will have a galvanizing effect, like *The Blue Marble*, that iconic 1972 photo of Earth from space taken by the crew of Apollo 17, which helped stir the environmental movement to life. The atmosphere felt scrubbed clean; the stars were sharper and more visible. The relationship between humanity and the natural world was more balanced and harmonious. This restoration came at an awful cost in terms of collapsed economies and punctured dreams.

Of course, traffic would resume, oil would be pumped, airplanes would take off, and astronauts might fly to the moon again, but I hope the glorious experience of living without pollution, however momen-tary it might be, will linger in our consciousness as an achievable destiny.

17

I Can't Breathe

T HE CORPSE ON the autopsy bench was a middle-aged Black man with Covid-19. Six feet four and a muscular 223 pounds, he had suffered many of the comorbidities Ebony Hilton had described. The Hennepin County medical examiner identified signs of heart disease and hypertension. Both are chronic problems among Black Americans, producing higher rates of strokes and heart attacks. The autopsy also noted the presence of fentanyl and methamphetamine, which could also be considered comorbidities, although they didn't really factor into this case. The cause of death was a police officer's knee on the neck. The man on the autopsy bench was George Floyd.

According to the charging documents, "The autopsy revealed no physical findings that support a diagnosis of traumatic asphyxia or strangulation." This was to explain the decision to charge one of the four officers at the scene of the killing with third-degree murder and second-degree manslaughter. "The combined effects of Mr. Floyd being restrained by the police, his underlying health conditions and any potential intoxicants in his system likely contributed to his death." The document read like an excuse for minimizing charges against the one officer.

The whole world knew what happened. Four Minneapolis policemen killed George Floyd as he was handcuffed and lying facedown in the street. It was May 25, 2020, Memorial Day. One cop stood watch as two knelt on Floyd's back and held his legs while the fourth, Derek

Michael Chauvin, the only one initially charged, pressed his knee into Floyd's neck for more than nine minutes,[*] long after this massive man had stopped crying for his mother and saying "I can't breathe" twenty times.

After the Floyd family commissioned an independent autopsy, which said that Floyd died of asphyxia, Hennepin County revised its findings, calling Floyd's death a homicide. On June 3, Chauvin's charge was upgraded to second-degree murder, and the other three men were charged with aiding and abetting.

This being America, in the year 2020, racial issues were both more complex and essentially unchanged. Cup Foods is a corner convenience store and deli in south Minneapolis, owned by Mahmoud "Mike" Abumayyaleh and his three brothers. The Abumayyaleh family are Palestinian Americans. Many such stores in minority neighborhoods in Minneapolis—and other cities across America—are owned by Muslim immigrants. Because they serve as a hub of commerce in places often stigmatized as high-crime districts, stores like Cup Foods often have been venues for encounters between the police and Black residents. Eric Garner was choked to death two doors down from Steve's Deli, owned by Steve Ali, in Staten Island, in July 2014. Alton Sterling was shot to death outside the Triple S Food Mart, owned by Abdullah Muflahi, in Baton Rouge, in July 2016.

Cup Foods had been in the neighborhood for more than three decades, offering stamps, keys, notary service, wire transfers, and utility payments, in addition to groceries. It was started by Mike's father, and Mike had worked there since the age of ten. He knew most of his customers by name. George Floyd was a regular for about a year; it's where he bought credits for his cell phone. Abumayyaleh later described him as "a big teddy bear."

Floyd had been a bouncer in a nightclub, but like so many Americans, the pandemic put him out of work. That may be why, at about eight in the evening, he alledgedly bought a pack of cigarettes with a counterfeit $20 bill. A teenage clerk examined the bill and called the police. He told the dispatcher that Floyd appeared drunk. Abumayyaleh said the clerks in the store are supposed to let one of the owners know

---

[*] Initial reports put the length of time Chauvin had his knee on Floyd's neck at 8:46 minutes, but according to court filings the figure is closer to nine and a half minutes.

if something like that happens, so it can be settled privately before the police get involved, but Abumayyaleh had taken the holiday off. Many states had chosen Memorial Day weekend to begin reopening the bars and restaurants. Americans were at the beach or enjoying themselves. It was the kickoff for a massive new surge.

At first, two rookie cops arrived. J. Alexander Kueng was the son of a white mother and an absent African father, like Barack Obama. He joined the police force in 2019, becoming one of about 80 black cops in a force of nearly 900. He said he hoped to reform the department from within. This was just his third shift. Thomas Lane was in the same rookie class with Kueng and they were paired together. Lane had wandered through a dozen jobs before joining the force at the age of thirty-six. He also had volunteered as a mentor to at-risk kids and was tutoring Somali children in math and science.

Lane and Kueng found Floyd sitting in a car nearby with two other people. Lane held a gun on Floyd and repeatedly asked him to show his hands. After Floyd put his hands on the steering wheel, the cops pulled him out of the car and handcuffed him. Floyd was cooperative until the cops tried to get him into the squad car. According to prosecutors, Floyd "stiffened up, fell to the ground, and told the officers he was claustrophobic."

Two more cops arrived.

Tou Thao's family was Hmong, a nomadic people from Southeast Asia who were U.S. allies during the Vietnam War. Thousands of them resettled in the Twin Cities, becoming the largest concentration of Hmong in the U.S. When Thao first joined the force in 2008, he was hired as a part-time community service officer, part of the department's efforts to diversify. In 2017, Thao was sued by a Black man who said that Thao and his partner beat him while he was being arrested. The case was settled out of court.

Derek Chauvin, a nineteen-year veteran of the force, was married to a Hmong immigrant, Kellie Xiong, whose family escaped from Laos in 1977; in 2018 she realized one of her dreams when she was crowned Mrs. Minnesota. Chauvin had a mixed record on the force; his file contained two medals for valor along with at least seventeen complaints of misconduct, only one of which resulted in a verbal reprimand. He was also involved in several previous cases of using excessive force while restraining people, none of which resulted in disciplinary action. It said a lot about the Minneapolis police department that it assigned Chauvin to train Kueng and Lane, apparently so they could learn to emulate his behavior. When off-duty, Chauvin sometimes worked at a club, El Nuevo Rodeo, the same place where Floyd did security work, but they don't seem to have known each other.

The cops who killed George Floyd were not stereotypical racists; they were complexly entangled in the net of interracial relationships that characterize modern America. But they did act as the face of established power in the city. Despite its progressive self-image, Minneapolis has a history of systemic oppression of its Black citizens. In 1999 alone, over half of all the Black males between eighteen and thirty in Hennepin County were arrested. Police in Minneapolis still used force against Black people at a rate seven times higher than against whites.

In the age of smartphones, the murder of George Floyd was a kind of performance, with the whole world serving as an audience. The police were well aware that they were being recorded by a crowd of witnesses screaming at them to let the man breathe. And yet, none of the four officers moved to stop the murder from progressing. While he held on to Floyd's legs, Lane twice asked Chauvin, "Should we roll him on his side?" The bystanders called for the police to check Floyd's pulse, and when Officer Kueng finally did that, he couldn't find one.

The performance suggests a presumption of impunity—they did this in full view, on the record, like a public execution. Even if they didn't believe that Floyd was dying, there's an absence of discretion about their flagrant abuse of a helpless, handcuffed man. One supposes that, in the minds of the four officers, they were doing their job, enforcing the social order.

MINNEAPOLIS UNDERSCORES a disturbing paradox in American society. Despite its reputation as one of the most progressive cities in the country, Minneapolis has stunning wealth disparities; and yet, for decades, tax income from well-off communities has been redistributed to poorer neighborhoods, providing more money for social services, improved schools, and affordable housing. The state income tax rate is 9.85 percent for individuals making over $150,000 per year, among the highest in the country. But the outcome of decades of progressive tax policies in Minneapolis is that whites are richer and Blacks are poorer than the national average. Blacks are five times as likely to live in poverty as whites.

A study by brightbeam, a left-leaning educational foundation, argues that schools in conservative cities have better outcomes for minority students than those in progressive cities.* In San Francisco, one of the wealthiest cities in the country, run for years by liberal Democrats, 70 percent of white students were proficient in math, but only 12 percent of Black students were—a gap of 58 points. In Washington, D.C., the gap was 62 points. Overall, the twelve most progressive cities in America had an average gap in math scores of 41 percent between whites and Blacks, and 34 percent between whites and Latinos. There were similar disparities with reading ability.

On the other hand, three of the twelve most conservative cities— Virginia Beach, Anaheim, and Fort Worth—had effectively closed the gap in at least one of the academic categories. In Oklahoma City, students of color actually graduated at a higher rate than whites. Overall, the Black-white proficiency gap in math was 41.3 percent for progressive cities and 26.2 in conservative cities; the gap for Latinos and whites was 34.4 percent versus 19.1. The researchers examined the size of cities, number of students in private schools, greater income inequality, and higher poverty rates, but only one factor could account for these disparities: "The biggest predictor for larger educational gaps was whether or not the city has a progressive population." The report was titled "The Secret Shame."

With all the wealth, political idealism, community effort, and apparent goodwill directed by the white progressive power structure of Minneapolis to the Black community, nothing changed, except for the fact that, year after year, things got worse for the Black citizens. Their anger grew. And it is not only in Minneapolis. America has been engaged in a vast effort to "level the playing field" for minorities by providing better education and job opportunities and access to housing, but that effort has fallen short because society has built in safeguards to protect itself from structural change. In Minneapolis, the police have served that function for many years.

---

* My son, Gordon Wright, serves as chief of digital content and platforms for brightbeam.

The Black community in Minneapolis saw a link between police mistreatment and the medical establishment. Hennepin Healthcare, which operates the county hospital, inaugurated a years-long study of the sedative ketamine, best known as a date-rape drug but one that paramedics sometimes administer to agitated or aggressive people who are suffering from a condition called "excited delirium." The police encouraged the use of the drug on crime suspects for purposes of the study, at times over the objection of the persons being drugged and sometimes when no crime had been committed. In some cases, the ketamine injections led to heart stoppage or lung problems that required intubation. African Americans account for a disproportionate number of the people enrolled in clinical trials without consent.

In Minnesota, African Americans make up only 6 percent of the population but 19 percent of confirmed cases of Covid-19; 5 percent of the population was Hispanic, but they made up 17 percent of the cases. Added to the list of comorbidities leading to racial disparities in health outcomes was the frustration of minority citizens with constant reforms that never led to meaningful improvements in their lives. Incrementally, there was progress. Minnesota attorney general Keith Ellison took over the George Floyd case. Ellison was the first Black person elected to the U.S. House of Representatives from Minnesota; when he was elected attorney general, he became the first Black person elected to statewide office in Minnesota, and the first Muslim elected to statewide office anywhere in America. Derek Chauvin became the first white officer in Minnesota to be charged with the death of a Black civilian.

DR. EBONY JADE HILTON JOINED a Black Lives Matter protest in Charlottesville on June 7. Hundreds of people marched from the Freedom of Speech Wall on the Downtown Mall to the Rotunda at the University of Virginia, carrying homemade placards saying "Let My People Breathe." Three years before, Charlottesville had been the site of a "Unite the Right" rally. Hundreds of torch-carrying white nationalists, Klansmen, neo-fascists, and right-wing militia members confronted counterprotesters, who had linked arms around a statue of Thomas Jefferson, a slave owner, the third president of the United States, and the founder of the university. The next day, a twenty-year-old white supremacist drove his Dodge Challenger into a crowd of anti-racist marchers, then backed up and ran over more of them. Many were hurt but one, Heather Heyer, was killed. President Trump had remarked on the occasion that there were "very fine people on both sides."

This day was different. There was no violence, but there was resolve. "I did not speak. I mainly wanted to listen," Hilton said. "I've often said that I grew up 'in the gap.' My parents and their parents lived during times of Jim Crow and slavery before that. When I was born in '82, racism was clearly still there but not as in your face with violence as it was with the lynchings of my grandparents' generation or the 'colored only' of my mother's. But now, the generation of my nieces and nephew, they are seeing this daily onslaught of Black men and women dying—murders, paraded on television to the point of normalcy. And that makes me incredibly sad. So I wanted to listen. I was protected from seeing those images as a child. They weren't. These students at U.Va. were ten to fourteen years old when Trayvon Martin was murdered. And it hasn't stopped for them." She added: "They also grew up with their first knowledge of a president being a Black man. How do you juggle those two positions of status—one of power, the other of being hunted?"

She acknowledged that she expected to see a rise in infections within the week following the march, but added: "For Black men, one in every thousand is at risk of dying in their lifetime from an encounter with a police officer. If you think about that number, that's what leads Black people to say it's worth me dying and going out to this protest and saying enough is enough. Police brutality is almost like a pandemic, a generational pandemic. It's a feeling—I'm going to die anyway, so I might as well risk this virus that I can't see, to speak about the virus of systemic racism that I can."

IN 2016, during a Black Lives Matter march, a sniper killed five Dallas police officers on downtown streets. Seven other officers and two civilians were injured by the shooter. He intended to kill as many white officers as he could in retaliation for police killings of Black men. The killer was a supporter of the New Black Panther Party, which has encouraged violence against whites and especially Jews. The cops finally killed the sniper with a robot bomb.

"Our profession is hurting," David Brown, the Dallas chief of police, said after the killings. "We are heartbroken. There are no words to describe the atrocity that occurred to our city." These words came from a Black man whose brother was slain by drug dealers and whose own son killed a police officer.

David Brown became a legend in Dallas. He reformed the department despite resistance from the rank and file. Under his leadership, crime dropped, as did police shootings. When asked what he had to say to the protesters, Brown replied, "We're hiring." He promised to assign new officers to their own neighborhoods so they could "resolve some of the problems you're protesting about." Applications tripled. The Dallas police force became almost evenly divided between whites and minorities, one of the few in the country to do so. Brown was lured to Chicago to take over the troubled police department there.

His successor, U. Reneé Hall, was the first woman to lead the Dallas force. In the aftermath of the George Floyd murder, Chief Hall, who is Black, struggled to deal with what many saw as the overreaction by the Dallas police to contain the protests, which took place at the end of May. More than a dozen officers were injured by bricks, fireworks, and frozen water bottles hurled at them. Six officers required medical attention; two protesters and a police horse were also badly hurt. The SWAT Unit arrived, along with armored personnel carriers. The cops fired tear gas and less-lethal rounds, including "Stingers" and "PepperBalls," injuring a number of protesters. Among them were members of the Boogaloo Movement and Antifa. Downtown stores were vandalized. Neiman Marcus was robbed. Cop cars were burned. The SWAT team gassed the crowd. It was a melee. This went on for four days. Nearly seven hundred people were detained. Fifty use-of-force complaints were filed. Chief Hall's job was in danger as city council members said they had lost confidence in her leadership.

She knew her time was short, but there was a historic wrong she felt called to address. The chain of history had led her to this moment.

On a hot July night in 1973, police took a twelve-year-old boy named Santos Rodriguez and his brother, David, a year older, from their home in Dallas's Little Mexico neighborhood. It was around 2:30 in the morning and the cops didn't even allow them to put on shoes. They were tall, handsome boys, Santos with curly hair and the beginnings of a wispy adolescent mustache.

There had been a break-in at a gas station. A vending machine had been burglarized, eight dollars in total. The boys were handcuffed and driven to the scene of the crime for a spur-of-the-moment interrogation, with no lawyer present. When the boys denied having anything to do with the robbery, one of the cops, Darrell Cain, said he would make them talk. He later claimed that he had removed all the bullets from his .357 Magnum revolver before playing Russian roulette with Santos. He put the gun to the head of the terrified child and pulled the trigger. Nothing happened. The boy said, "I am telling the truth." Cain pulled the trigger again and blew the boy's brains out. David remained in the back seat, his bare feet soaking in his brother's blood.

Officer Cain was convicted of murder, sentenced to five years, and served half of that time.

When Reneé Hall was six months old, her father, a police officer in Detroit, responded to a call at a gas station in the middle of the night. It was eerily similar to the event that led to the police killing of Santos Rodriguez, although that time it was the cop, Reneé's father, who was killed. The shooter was never caught.

For forty-seven years, Bessie Rodriguez had been holding a vigil at Oakland Cemetery in South Dallas to commemorate her son's murder. On July 25, 2020, the beleaguered chief came and laid a bouquet on Santos's grave. Then Chief Hall apologized to Santos's mother. "We were responsible then and we are responsible now," she said through her mask. "We are committed to being a different police department."

On September 8, Chief Hall announced her resignation.

History can be understood as the revenge of the dead on the living. Hall might never have been a cop if her father hadn't been killed. She might still be chief of police if she had been able to bring under control the clashes that took place after George Floyd's death. Floyd might still be alive if he hadn't passed a counterfeit bill, having lost his job because of the pandemic. So much death will have consequences we can never account for.

FIVE DAYS AFTER Floyd's murder, 1,300 public health officials signed a letter supporting the mass protests that arose in Minneapolis and spread across America and then to cities around the world. This was at a time when health officials had been begging people to stay at home and not assemble in groups. People took to the streets by the tens of thousands—not just in America but in cities around the world—to protest the death of an unemployed Black man with a criminal record and a drug problem. If George Floyd's life could matter, so might the lives of every minority citizen.

There were many elements contributing to this massive outpouring. Part of it was the simple fact that people were tired of confinement and they had time on their hands. The weather was nice. They were outdone with the mixed signals they had gotten from their political leaders. Some had lost their jobs and those who hadn't worried that day would soon come. But there was a deeper note sounded in these protests. Many of those who marched, of all races and ethnicities, realized that they were actually putting their lives at risk. They didn't doubt the danger. A moment had arrived, inconveniently, but there was no avoiding it.

The protests called to mind the Liberty Loan parades in 1918, which served as potent vectors for the killer flu. And yet, in 2020, the marches did not appear to be significant drivers of transmission. "We tested thousands of people," Michael Osterholm, the director of the Center for Infectious Disease Research and Policy at the University of Minnesota, told me. "We saw no appreciable impact." One study found lower rates of infection among marchers than in the surrounding community. Epidemiologists concluded that mask-wearing and being outdoors protected the marchers.

GIANNA POMATA UNDERSTOOD the reasons for the mass protests and political rallies, but, as a medical historian, she was uncomfortably reminded of the religious processions that had spread the plague in medieval Europe. And, as someone who had obediently remained indoors for months, she was affronted by the refusal of so many Americans to wear masks at the grocery store and maintain social distancing. "What I see right now in the United States is that the pandemic has not led to new creative thinking but, on the contrary, has strengthened all the worst, most stereotypical and irrational ways of thinking. I'm very sorry for the state of your country, which seems to be in the grip of a horrible attack of unreason." She continued: "I'm sorry because I love it and have received so much from it."

On the other hand, things were looking up in Italy. "Starting tomorrow, they're going to relax the rules a bit," Gianna Pomata told me when we spoke at the end of May. "You're supposed to be able to go and visit 'relatives,' but of course nobody knows what is meant by relatives. A fiancée? A lover? A mistress? We're making lots of jokes about the meaning of a relative in Italy at this moment."

Pomata's optimism was buoyed by the fact that her country's shutdown, cohesive and well managed, had worked: new infections were petering out there. Italy had six thousand new cases a day when spring started and only two hundred a day when the first wave subsided in early summer. Moreover, the leaders of Germany and France proposed creating grants, rather than loans, that would help prevent the poorer regions of Europe from falling into a prolonged recession. It could mark the moment when the European Union moved toward a truly federal system, like the United States.

I asked Gianna what she wanted to do when she finally ventured out. "I don't actually feel starved for human contact," she said with a bit of surprise. "I've never written so many letters as in this period of my life. Of course, I see my sister from the window, but we cannot hug each other. I cannot hug my mother—I cannot even visit my mother because she lives in Sardinia and I just cannot go there." She paused, then added, "So there's something about the joys of human contact, of hugging each other, and kissing each other, that I don't even dare to think about. It's like an impossible dream right now. And it would hurt too much to think about it."

She especially missed swimming. "Older people need exercise," she said. "I haven't yet given up on Sardinia and the sea and swimming. Sardinia fortunately has been spared from the contagion. They've had very few cases. If they open up, they're going to ask people to take the test. I'm going to take the test immediately!" She added: "I don't spend time at the beach gossiping with friends. I don't even take the sun. I just go immediately into the sea and spend an hour swimming in the water. And that's what I want to do. Wish me luck!"

18

Tulsa

MORE THAN TWO MONTHS after General Robert E. Lee surrendered at Appomattox Court House, Union Major General Gordon Granger disembarked at Galveston and brought the news that the war was over and slavery had been abolished in the former Confederate states. "All slaves are free," the general's order declared. "This involves an absolute equality of personal rights and rights of property between former masters and slaves." That day, June 19, 1865, "Juneteenth," became a day of celebration in Texas. It has since been designated as a holiday in forty-seven states and the District of Columbia. The president was unaware of the significance of the date until a Black Secret Service agent advised him. Trump had been planning to hold a rally in Tulsa on June 19, 2020. "I did something good: I made Juneteenth very famous," the president said, after postponing the rally for a day. "Nobody had ever heard of it."

As it happens, Tulsa was in the middle of a painful reexamination of its past. In 1921, a nineteen-year-old Black man, Dick Rowland, who worked at a shoeshine parlor, was suspected of raping a seventeen-year-old white girl, Sarah Page, an elevator operator in the nearby Drexel Building. A lynch mob went to the county courthouse. A group of about fifty to sixty African American men, some of them armed, many of them soldiers who had recently returned from fighting in the world war, told law enforcement officers at the courthouse they were there to help defend it. It was Memorial Day, the same holiday on which George Floyd would be killed a century later.

Many in the mob carried weapons. In this tense standoff, someone fired a pistol, perhaps a warning shot, but it set off a riot. Gunplay continued for two hours, moving into an all-Black district called Greenwood. At dawn, a force of white citizens, police, and National Guardsmen moved in. Airplanes circled the neighborhood, dropping firebombs and picking off fleeing residents with rifle shots. More than 6,000 Blacks were detained at the city's convention center and fairgrounds, and 800 people were hospitalized. The death toll has never been firmly established. Officially, the count was 26 African Americans and 10 whites, but modern historians estimate as many as 300 killed. No one knows. No one was ever charged with anything. Dick Rowland, the young suspect, was let go, the charges having been dropped at Sarah Page's request. What happened in the elevator has never been made clear; in 2001, a commission established to get to the truth decided that Rowland may have accidentally stepped on Page's foot as he got onto the elevator. She cried out; he fled; and hysteria took over from there.

Tulsa began a search to locate the mass graves described in contemporary reports. Whether or not the bodies are ever discovered, something else was buried by that bloody riot. Around 11,000 Black people had resided in Greenwood. Booker T. Washington, the author and educator, had termed it "Negro Wall Street" because of the neighborhood's flourishing business district. More than 60 of those businesses were burned, along with churches, schools, a hospital, doctors' offices, two newspapers, some 1,200 homes—virtually every structure in the thirty-five city blocks that once composed Greenwood.

THE PRESIDENT HAD big plans for the Tulsa rally. He had not gathered with supporters since March, and he was eager to plunge again into the pool of adulation. "It's going to be a hell of a night," he promised. He tweeted, "Almost One Million people request tickets for the Saturday Night Rally in Tulsa, Oklahoma!" A million people is more than twice the population of Tulsa.

Trump had chosen as his venue the BOK Center, which had only 19,000 seats, and clearly that wouldn't be enough. Spillover spaces were set aside at the nearby convention center and an outdoor stage was constructed. But when the president arrived, the BOK Center was glaringly empty. Only 6,200 people showed up; a group of TikTok pranksters had subverted the turnout by falsely requesting tickets. The outdoor stage was hastily taken down.

Trump was enraged by the dismal turnout but delivered his usual blustery speech. "We've tested now twenty-five million people," he said. "When you do testing to that extent, you're going to find more people, you're going to find more cases. So, I said to my people, 'Slow the testing down, please.'" However, everyone who entered the auditorium had to be fever-checked, as did anyone who came within sneezing range of the maskless president, and attendees were made to release the Trump campaign of responsibility for any exposure. Just before Trump went onstage, two Secret Service officers and six campaign staffers tested positive.

In the audience was Herman Cain, the former CEO of Godfather's Pizza and an erstwhile presidential candidate, who had become one of Trump's most prominent Black supporters. His test upon entering the Tulsa auditorium was negative. Like nearly everyone else, he hadn't worn a mask at the event, although Oklahoma had just seen a record increase in Covid cases. He flew home to Atlanta the next day, feeling exhausted—"from his travels," his daughter, Melanie Cain Gallo, believed. It was Father's Day, and she stopped by to give him a gift. They embraced. She had seen a photograph of him at the rally and wondered why he hadn't worn a mask. Cain had preached the virtue of social distancing and hand-washing on *The Herman Cain Show*, a web series that he hosted, and he regularly wore a mask in public.

Gallo worked with her dad all week on his show. By Friday, they were both feeling ill, but Cain filmed another episode. Flanked by the American flag and a painting of Ronald Reagan, he looked wan, his eyes rheumy. He quoted a newspaper headline: "U.S. DEATH RATE FALLS FOR THIRD DAY IN A ROW." Other newscasts had hyped rising case counts, he complained, adding, "They never get to the death rate is *falling*."

On Monday, both were sick enough to go to a clinic for a test. Cain was feeling weak, so he waited by the car while Gallo stood in a long line. Suddenly, he passed out. An EMS truck took him to the emergency room. "They checked him out and said he was fine," Gallo recalled. They returned to the testing site. Both were positive.

Her case was mild. On July 1, Cain was hospitalized. That day, he tweeted an article about a forthcoming Trump rally at Mount Rushmore. "Masks will not be mandatory," he tweeted, adding approvingly, "PEOPLE ARE FED UP!" It was a defiant nod to Trump's base. Cain died on July 30. He was seventy-four.

IT'S EASY TO BE blind to the geological layers of history that shape the surfaces of our lives. Lisa Cook, an economist at Michigan State University, dug into the effects of violent conflict and social instability on patents granted to Black inventors between 1870 and 1940. It required diligent and resourceful work to unearth the race of patent holders, which she did by examining correspondence, obituaries, archives, programs from "Negro Day" science exhibitions, and directories of African American scientists, doctors, and engineers. She was able to match 726 significant patents by Black inventors during that span. They included Alexander Miles, for a means of automatically opening and closing elevator doors; George F. Grant, for a tapered golf tee; Clarence Gregg, for a machine gun. One of the most successful Black inventors was Garrett Morgan, who invented a traffic light and hair-straightening products. He also came up with an early gas mask, which he sold to fire departments while disguised as an Indian chief assisting a white actor he hired to pose as the real inventor. Percy Julian, a relative of Professor Cook's, was the first African American to head a major corporate laboratory. He came up with treatments for glaucoma and rheumatoid arthritis, as well as a process for synthesizing cortisone. Eventually he would be awarded more than a hundred patents, but most of them were outside the time span Cook was studying.

Cook plotted the 726 patents—a rotary engine, a telephone system, a fruit press, a flying machine, a roller mechanism for player pianos, carbon filaments for electric incandescent lamps, and on and on—over the seventy-year span and compared them to white patents during the same period. Black patents were at a much lower rate per capita, but they run roughly parallel through the 1870s and early 1880s, a fertile period of invention for both races. Around 1884, the number of Black patents shoots up, reaching a peak in 1889, then plunges to negligible levels. Cook attributes that to the implementation of the Supreme Court's decision several years before in *Plessy v. Ferguson*, which established "separate but equal" as the law of the land. After that, patents for Black inventors follow a different course from that of whites. Something else was affecting the creative output of Black Americans.

Cook then added to the graph incidents of violent conflict against African Americans to see if that could account for the variation in patents. As lynchings climbed in the 1890s, patents steeply dropped but quickly recovered by 1899, when lynchings diminished. Starting in 1921, a new pattern takes hold: lynchings have sharply decreased, but so have Black patents. What could account for that?

The decline coincided with the Tulsa massacre. "Accounts of the Tulsa riot suggest that many at the time believed that government failed at all levels, and that this was a turning point in federal policy and national practice related to property-rights protection, and that the country was likely headed toward racial warfare," Cook wrote. After Tulsa, annual patenting by African Americans compared with whites was lower by a factor of 2.2, on average. It has never recovered. The peak year for patents for Black inventors, per capita, is still 1899.

The Tulsa riot changed America. Imagine the country that might have been. Tulsa is Indian Territory, located in the Creek Nation. Imagine Tulsa as a sanctuary of wealth for all races. One might believe there could have been an alternate future if Sarah Page had not cried out, but the destruction of that dream was already on the minds of the mob that went to lynch Dick Rowland.

19

Thelma and Louise

FOR SOME MEMBERS of the public health community, Deborah Birx had become an object of scorn. "She's been a disaster," a former head of CDC confided. The Yale epidemiologist Gregg Gonsalves tweeted, "Dr. Birx, what the hell are you doing? What happened to you? Your HIV colleagues are ashamed." Birx was accused of being an enabler of an incompetent and corrupt administration. The opprobrium reached a peak when, in the middle of another coronavirus briefing, in April, Birx sat beside the podium as the president offered his wisdom on coronavirus cures. "So, supposedly we hit the body with a tremendous, whether it's ultraviolet or just very powerful light. . . . Supposing you brought the light inside the body, which you can do either through the skin or in some other way," he mused. "Sounds interesting, right?" The awkward look on Birx's face as the president bumbled forth became a social media meme for how compromised the scientists were. She sat there, wearing one of her signature Hermès scarves, gaping, then looking down at the floor and straightening her back as the president went on to talk about using bleach: "And then I see the disinfectant"—Birx's head recoiled—"where it knocks it out in a minute, one minute. And is there a way we can do something like that, by injection inside, or almost a cleaning, because you see it gets in the lungs and it does a tremendous number on the lungs, so it'd be interesting to check that."

Birx took a deep breath. And yet, when Trump later turned to her and asked, "Have you ever heard of that, the heat and light, relative to this virus, safe to say as a cure?" she helpfully responded, "Not as a treatment. I mean, certainly fever is a good thing, when you have a fever, it helps your body respond." Such remarks made some public health workers cringe. They didn't know what she was saying in private.

Birx told colleagues that she had lost confidence in the CDC. She disparaged the agency's hospital reports on Covid, which relied on models, not hard data. A CDC staffer told *Science* that compiling precise totals daily in a pandemic was impossible. But hospitals quickly complied after Birx informed them that supplies of remdesivir could be portioned out only to hospitals that provided inpatient Covid data.

In August, Dr. Scott Atlas, a neuroradiologist, a fellow at Stanford University's Hoover Institution, and a frequent commentator on Fox News, joined the task force. He was adamant that children should return to school—as was the American Academy of Pediatrics, which urged a "safe return" to schools in the fall, warning of learning deficits, physical or sexual abuse at home, and depression. That was a debate worth having, but Atlas also proposed that only symptomatic people should be tested for Covid and claimed that masks did little to stop the spread of the virus. He advocated creating "herd immunity" by allowing the virus to spread among those who are at lower risk. Herd immunity could be gained when a major portion of the population had effective antibodies to the disease, either through infection or vaccination. Atlas pointed to the example of Sweden, which rejected lockdowns, allowing schools, bars, and restaurants to remain open. Sweden would experience more than ten times the number of Covid deaths per capita than neighboring Norway.

Once Atlas got to the White House, Trump stopped speaking to other health advisers. The great appeal of herd immunity was that it could be achieved by doing nothing at all, and that became the president's unspoken policy.* At the same time, Atlas was encouraging the president to believe that the contagion was waning. "His voice is really very welcome combating some of the nonsense that comes out of Fauci," Stephen Moore, a White House economic adviser, said. "He's a real asset for the president." This was at a time when Birx and other

---

* The Trump White House denied that "the President, the White House, or anyone in the Administration has pursued or advocated for a strategy of achieving herd immunity."

health officials were looking at projections for the fall and foreseeing a coming catastrophe.

Birx and Atlas had it out in the Oval Office, in front of the president. Birx accused him of costing American lives with his unfounded theories. Atlas cursed her. Birx, who spent twenty-eight years in the Army, gave it right back. Atlas said that young, asymptomatic people shouldn't be tested. "She just wants to lock them down and not let them live their lives," he asserted. The president calmly watched as they shouted at each other. "The president just let them go at it," one of Birx's colleagues said. "It's all reality TV to him."

Birx decided she had had enough. She would not sit through another meeting listening to Atlas's theories about the virus. She demanded that the vice president, who chairs the task force, remove Atlas, but Pence declined. The task force began to dissolve after Atlas took a seat.

WHEN BIRX WAS working in Africa, she and her chief epidemiologist, Irum Zaidi, had met with presidents and village elders across the continent, learning the value of personal diplomacy. Now the pair decided to take to the road in America. The contagion had moved from the coasts to the heartland. In June, when the virus suddenly gripped Texas, Birx and Zaidi traveled with the vice president to Dallas to meet with Governor Greg Abbott at the University of Texas Southwestern Medical Center. Abbott's dithering response to the pandemic had led to attacks by Democrats, who noted that the death rate soared when he lifted restrictions too soon, and by Republicans, who called him a tyrant for imposing any restrictions at all. At a press conference, Birx urged Texans to mask up, especially young people. "If they're interacting with their parents and grandparents, they should wear a mask," she said. "No one wants to pass the virus to others." She praised Abbott for closing the bars, knowing that he was being pressured to fling open the doors. The governor reluctantly issued a mask mandate. Then, Birx and Zaidi rented a car and hurried to New Mexico.

Zaidi grew up in Atlanta. Her father was a statistician for CDC, so public health has been a part of her entire life. For family vacations, they would take long car trips, a passion Zaidi inherited, only she likes to drive fast—really fast. When she lived in Atlanta, she would sometimes go to Little Talladega Gran Prix Raceway, outside Birmingham, or Road Atlanta, to work on her driving skills. Speeding through America was her ideal assignment. Right away, as they were leaving Dallas, a state trooper pulled her over. She had been doing 110.

"Little lady, what's the hurry?" he wanted to know.

Zaidi explained that they had just met with Governor Abbott in Dallas and were on their way to New Mexico to talk to Governor Michelle Lujan Grisham. "Surely you recognize Dr. Birx," Zaidi said.

In an act of clemency rare for the Texas Department of Public Safety, the trooper let them off. Birx chastised Zaidi for dropping names to avoid a ticket. "At least I didn't mention the vice president," Zaidi cheerfully replied.

Soon after their visit to New Mexico, the governor announced a hundred-dollar fine for going maskless in public. Birx and Zaidi headed to Arizona and met with Governor Doug Ducey as well as state and local health officials. Birx explained that even a small increase in the percentage of positivity—going from 3.5 to 5 percent—could spark an unmanageable crisis. "She gave me a tutorial," the governor said. "If you want to participate in *any* good or service in Arizona, you're going to wear a mask."

After that first swing through the west, Birx and Zaidi kept traveling, mostly by car. Sometimes they hitched a ride on Air Force Two if the vice president was going to a hot zone, but most of the time Zaidi was at the wheel, racking up 25,000 miles as they crossed the country eight times, visiting forty-three states, many more than once. They saw rural areas and the cities, red America and blue America. They drove past cotton farms, cattle ranches, soybean fields—a vast and fertile land—but they also saw derelict oil rigs and abandoned factories, remnants of a vanishing industrial age. There were gleaming cities, bold and glassy, with construction cranes crowning the skyline; and broken towns, tumbling in decay, with all the promise bled out of them.

The women, who got regular Covid tests, established their own protocols. They sanitized rental cars and motel rooms with Clorox Wipes. In the early morning, they'd pick up coffee and pastries at Starbucks. Lunch was often peanut butter spread on bread with a plastic knife. Dinner was served at a drive-through window. Baristas and gas station attendants were useful informants of community outbreaks and served as indicators of local mask compliance. They met mayors and community organizers; they visited hospitals and nursing homes; they turned HIV activists into Covid activists. In Atlanta, they urged officials to test migrant workers working on chicken farms. They visited more than thirty universities, talking to students and administrators. Schools that conducted mandatory weekly testing of students had positivity rates below 1 percent; but in those where only symptomatic people were tested, 12 to 15 percent of the student body were positive. Both Republican and Democratic governors privately had the same complaint: folks wouldn't listen as long as the president refused to set an example.

One of the most effective governors Birx and Zaidi encountered was Jim Justice of West Virginia. He issued a mask mandate, and in his press briefings he reviewed the daily toll of West Virginians who had succumbed to the disease. The demographics of the state placed it in special peril, the governor noted, describing it as "absolutely the oldest, the sickest, the most vulnerable." He urged residents to "be great, loving neighbors" by wearing a mask. The state developed a plan to safely reopen schools by constantly assessing the level of risk in every county, represented on a color-coded map—a data mine bound to delight Birx. "I think the reason why I like it is it's practical, it's something that every county and every state can do," she said. "West Virginia represents exactly what we want to see across the country—a common-sense approach based on the data." Oklahoma governor Kevin Stitt, who had tested positive in July, sat on Birx's report that recommended closing all the bars and issuing a statewide mask mandate. Six Oklahoma cities were listed as being in the red zone for increased case numbers, but local officials were kept in the dark until the report was leaked to the press.

Birx and Zaidi saw a country that was suffering from ill health even before Covid attacked, where 40 percent of the adults are obese, half have cardiovascular disease, and one in thirteen has asthma. According to the CDC, 94 percent of Covid fatalities would be among people with comorbidities. America was deathly ill before the pandemic hit.

Native Americans have been particularly ravaged by Covid. Birx received a mask with the Salt River tribe shield inscribed on it, which the leaders told her now represented the tribe's fight against the virus. When North Dakota recorded the nation's highest rate of infection, Governor Doug Burgum refused to issue a mask mandate. Birx met with him, along with local, state, and tribal officials. "We were in your grocery stores and in your restaurants, and frankly even in your hotels, and this is the least use of masks that we have seen in retail establishments of any place we have been," Birx scolded them. "It starts with the community deciding that it's important for their children to be in school, the community deciding that it's important not to infect the nursing home staff who are caring for their residents—for North Dakotans—every day." Burgum eventually agreed to a mask mandate. In South Dakota, Governor Kristi Noem couldn't find the time to meet with Birx.

By late summer, it was clear that Americans were exhausted by the restrictions. "I've been so struck by the number of Americans across the country that have just had it," Birx said in Arkansas. She admitted, "When you're asking people to change behavior, you have to meet them where they are."

For more than six months, Birx corralled politicians, hospital executives, and public health officials, often bringing such leaders together for the first time. She took charts and slides from state to state, promoting a simple message about masks, social distancing, transparency, and responsible leadership. And she was the only federal official doing so.

One day in late October, Birx and Zaidi were eating lunch at a roadside stop in Utah, beside the Bonneville Salt Flats, where the land speed records are often set. In 2016, Roger Schroer drove an electric vehicle on the flats 341 miles per hour. The salt stretched out endlessly like a frozen sea.

They had rented a blue Jeep Wrangler in Ohio, expecting they would encounter snow in Montana. "We have to go off road for just a minute," Zaidi said. Birx looked out at the great white emptiness. "As long as you don't hit anybody," she said.

20

The Hedgehog and the Fox

T HERE WAS AN erudite parlor game that Oxford undergraduates used to play in the 1930s. It derived from a fragment of Greek poetry which said, "The fox knows many things, but the hedgehog knows one big thing." Depending on their understanding of this Delphic verse, the undergraduates would divide personalities into hedgehogs or foxes. Hedgehogs are dogged and concentrated; they live their lives believing that the world is organized by universal laws, even if those laws are not entirely graspable. Foxes are scattered and contradictory, taking what they need for their journey without a real destination in mind. The game is a bit like casting a horoscope with only two astrological signs.

Isaiah Berlin took the hedgehog/fox dichotomy as a starting point for his famous lecture on Tolstoy. He later admitted he never meant it seriously. He insisted that he didn't intend the fox to be superior to the hedgehog, or vice versa, and he acknowledged that a single person could encompass both qualities. Tolstoy, for instance, confounded the distinction.

Anthony Fauci and Donald Trump, however, thoroughly embodied these opposing archetypes. They were in some glancing ways very much alike: New Yorkers, both in their seventies, immensely confident, optimistic, neither requiring more than five hours of sleep at night. In other respects, they were almost comically opposite. "We had this interesting relationship," Fauci later recalled, "a New York City camaraderie thing." That wouldn't last.

Fauci is small, trim, dapper, an "unflappable bullet of a man," as Natalie Angier once memorably described him. He has the hedgehog's intensity, working sixteen to seventeen hours a day, taking only Sundays off to be with his family. He used to run seven miles at lunchtime, no matter what the weather, but he switched to power-walking with his wife at night. He has led the National Institute of Allergy and Infectious Diseases (NIAID) through six administrations, rejecting promotions or the prosperous lure of private industry. His idea of fun is "being with my wife and children and eating fried calamari, drinking a glass of wine."

Trump has led a life marked by chaos and full of great wealth, spectacular bankruptcies, three marriages, two divorces, Playboy models and porn stars, cheated workers, showy skyscrapers, failed casinos, television stardom, tabloid fame—a life spent surfing the wave of popular culture without ever probing deeply into any defining pursuit. Even his run for the presidency was whimsical, as much for brand promotion as it was for revenge against what he perceived as Barack Obama's slights. Whimsy and grievance—what he termed his gut feelings—drove him and the nation that he dragged behind him, but it was never clear where he was taking us, nor perhaps did he know or especially care.

The relationship between Trump and Fauci was wary. They were handcuffed to each other, Fauci needing the president to allow him to do his job, Trump needing to keep the one person America trusted most in his camp. From Trump's perspective, Fauci was dangerous because he didn't have enough to lose and could not be relied upon to bend to the president's will, as had nearly everyone who remained in his administration. Unlike the CDC, HHS, and the FDA, Fauci's institution had not been bullied into submission by political appointees. Fauci and his colleagues at NIAID were outliers in the Trump-era medical research establishment, but they were also the best hope for a workable, effective, and politically timely vaccine.

To trim Fauci's vast constituency, the president pushed him off the Sunday morning news shows and onto talk radio and webinars. But Fauci's influence remained unsquashable, an ever present reminder of the peril the country was in, honestly admitting the blunders committed by the most powerful nation in the world, the one ostensibly best prepared to face such a catastrophe, but now pitied, feckless, and beaten.

Trump belittled Fauci while also envying his appeal. He retweeted that there was a conspiracy "by Fauci & the Democrats to perpetuate Covid deaths to hurt Trump." The president told Sean Hannity that Fauci was "a nice man, but he's made a lot of mistakes." He accused Fauci of misleading the country about hydroxychloroquine, which Trump continued to cling to as a miracle cure even after the FDA withdrew its emergency authorization. "He's got this high approval rating, so why don't I have a high approval rating, and the administration, with respect to the virus?" Trump wondered aloud at a press briefing. "It can only be my personality." A recent poll had showed that for information about the coronavirus, 67 percent of voters trusted Fauci, compared with 26 percent for Trump.

Fauci, a devout fan of the Washington Nationals, was invited to throw out the first pitch for the World Series champions, who were playing in an empty stadium like all teams in this spectatorless year. As Fauci was preparing to walk to the mound, wearing a Nats mask, Trump told the press that he had been invited to throw out a first pitch as well. "I think I'm doing that on August 15 at Yankee Stadium." No one had told the Yankees. Later Trump tweeted that his own busy schedule made it impossible to accommodate the August date. "We will make it later in the season!"

Covid-19 told us more about these two men than any other individuals in the country. For Fauci, science was a self-correcting compass, always pointed at the truth. For Trump, the truth was Play-doh, and he could twist it to fit the shape of his desire.

ANTHONY FAUCI CLINGS to his Brooklyn accent. "I'm New York born and raised," he boasted, as if anyone doubted. He was born on Christmas Eve 1940, and grew up in Bensonhurst, then a largely Italian American neighborhood in Brooklyn. The family later moved to Dyker Heights. His father was a pharmacist, and the family lived above the store. As a boy Tony delivered prescriptions on his bicycle. He went to a Jesuit high school in Manhattan and captained the basketball team, despite his stature (he's five feet seven inches tall). He earned a degree in classics with a concentration in premed from the College of the Holy Cross in Worcester, Massachusetts. What impressed him about the Jesuits was their intellectual rigor and seriousness of purpose. "I mean the importance of personal development, scholarly development, and the high standard of integrity and principles," he remembered in an alumni profile. "That became a part of everyday life at Holy Cross."

In the summers he worked construction in New York. Once he was part of a crew that was building a new library for the Cornell University Medical College (now the Weill Cornell Medical College). "One day during lunch break, while the rest of the construction crew was sitting along the sidewalk on York Avenue, eating their hero sandwiches and making catcalls at the nurses who were entering and leaving the hospital, I snuck into the auditorium to take a peek. I got goose bumps as I entered, looked around at the empty room and imagined what it would be like to attend this extraordinary institution," he said at the medical school's centennial celebration in 1998. "A guard came and politely told me to leave since my dirty construction boots were soiling the floor. I looked at him and said proudly that I would be attending this institution a year from now. He laughed and said, 'Right kid, and next year I am going to be Police Commissioner.'"

Fauci was first in his class when he gained his MD from Cornell in 1966.

Although immunology was not a popular field at the time, Fauci was interested in infectious diseases as "an exciting, dramatic historical specialty." He found his way to the National Institutes of Health in 1968, where he had early success in curing several fatal diseases.

He met Christine Grady when she was a clinical nurse at NIH (she became head of the NIH's Department of Bioethics). Fauci was attending a patient suffering from vasculitis who spoke only Portuguese. Grady had learned the language while working for Project Hope in Brazil. "And so they said, 'Could you come translate for Dr. Fauci?' whom I had not met, the inimitable Dr. Fauci everybody was afraid of," Grady recalled in an NIH oral history. Fauci sternly instructed the patient that, when he left, he should rest, sit with his leg up, and change his dressings every day. When Grady translated, the patient replied, "You are kidding. I am so sick of being in this hospital. I am going to go home, I am going to dance all night." Grady turned to Fauci. "He said he would do exactly as you said."

That afternoon, Fauci asked Grady for a date. They married in 1985. They have three daughters.

ON JUNE 5, 1981, the world of public health took note of an article in the *Morbidity and Mortality Weekly Report* about five men in Los Angeles suffering from an exotic infection called pneumocystis pneumonia. "Curiously, they were all gay men," Fauci recalled. "I thought it was a fluke. I thought that, well, maybe they took a toxic drug or something that suppressed their immune system." One month later, another *MMWR* reported on twenty-six men, not only from Los Angeles but also New York and San Francisco, who presented an assortment of dreadful infections. "I remember sitting there in my office, saying, 'Oh my goodness, this is a brand-new disease.'" Fauci soon became the public face of the government's underfunded, under-resourced effort to fight a highly stigmatized, invariably fatal new plague.

"I call you murderers: An open letter to an incompetent idiot, Dr. Anthony Fauci of the National Institute of Allergies and Infectious Diseases," was the headline in the magazine section of the *San Francisco Examiner* on June 26, 1988. The letter was written by Larry Kramer, the playwright and gay rights activist. Kramer was protesting an honorary dinner for Fauci, who had started the HIV/AIDS program at NIH before HIV was even diagnosed. "You are responsible for all government funded AIDS treatment research. In the name of right, you make decisions that cost the lives of others," Kramer wrote. "With 270,000 dead from AIDS and millions more infected with HIV, you should not be honored at a dinner. You should be put before a firing squad." Fauci was thunderstruck. "No one had ever done that to me or any other scientist," he recalled.

Kramer was the founder of ACT UP, which used highly confrontational tactics to gain attention for a disease that straight society largely ignored. Their main grievance was that people in the gay community had no influence over the research into the HIV/AIDS pandemic. ACT UP took their campaign to the doorstep of Fauci's building at the National Institutes of Health. "Not very many people were listening to them," Fauci said. "They were dressed funny; they had all these strange outfits; and they were screaming and cursing and yelling. And I looked at them, and I saw people who were in pain."

The police were about to arrest the protesters, but Fauci directed they be left alone. He invited several of the activist leaders to his office to talk. "What they were saying was actually making a lot of sense," he said. He set about trying to understand the gay culture. He visited the gay bathhouses in San Francisco, the epicenter of the outbreak. It was quite an education. "This is something that's going to require a lot more than just saying no," he decided. But even as he was learning about gay lifestyles, the disease refused to reveal itself. "Here I am," he thought. "I've studied infectious disease, I've studied the immune system. I have no idea what this infection is. It's probably a virus, but I've never seen anything like it before."

He was not only working in his lab, he was treating AIDS patients in the NIH clinic. "With AIDS in those days, I saved no one," he recalled. "It was the darkest time of my life." He advocated for activists to be included in the international AIDS conferences, where the latest papers were presented; he also made it possible for patients to get into clinical trials so they could be given experimental drugs. He managed to bring the scientists and the sufferers together.

And he reached out to Kramer. They developed "a dear, deep friendship," although Kramer rarely missed an opportunity to criticize him in public. "I was on a C-SPAN program a couple of months ago with Tony, and I attacked him for the entire hour," Kramer told the *New York Times* in 1994. "He called me up afterwards and said he thought the program went very well. I said, 'How can you say that? I did nothing but yell at you.' He said, 'You don't realize that you can say things I can't. It doesn't mean I don't agree with you.'"

Fauci helped Kramer get a liver transplant in 2001, which gave him nearly two decades more life. Shortly before Kramer died, in May 2020, at the age of eighty-four, Fauci called him. Kramer was fading. "The last thing he said to me when he hung up the phone was, 'I love you, Tony,' and I said, 'I love you, too, Larry.'"

———

WHEN FAUCI AND I first spoke, in July 2020, I pointed to the Johns Hopkins study in October 2019, which stated that America was the best-prepared nation in the world for a pandemic. So what happened? "It's really, in many respects, befuddling," he responded, with a despairing laugh. "How we as a nation, with all our resources, continue to fare so poorly? We never got back to baseline"—the point where the contagion had been sufficiently reduced so that contact tracing could minimize the spread. "If you look at the curves, Europe got hit badly, and yet when they finally controlled it, they got down to baseline, which was very few cases. We went up, and then we sort of plateaued around 20,000 a day. And now we're up to 30, 40, 50,000 a day. So we're not going in the right direction."

He offered several explanations. "It could be the fact that we didn't have a uniform strategy," he said. "It could be our own culture right now, of people not wanting to be told what to do. The guidelines say 'Don't go to bars. Wear a mask.' And you look at the pictures in the newspaper and on TV and you see large crowds of mostly young people, not wearing masks."

Later in the conversation, he returned to the question. "I would think if you did a real analysis, it would be multifactorial," he said. "We have a big, big country. It's very heterogeneous. What goes on in the metropolitan areas of New York City is so different from what goes on in Montana, or New Mexico, or the panhandle of Florida. We're just very, very different, and people approach the outbreak in different ways. And the sum total of it all is we have not been very successful. All you have to do is look at the numbers."

Fauci said he had never seen such distrust and anger in the country. "Political divisiveness doesn't lend itself to having a coordinated, cooperative, collaborative response against a common enemy. There is also this pushback in society against anything authoritative. And scientists are perceived as being authority, so that's the reason I believe we have an anti-science trend, which leads to an anti-vaccine trend." Even with effective vaccines, social resistance could delay the longed-for herd immunity.

The anti-science, anti-authority trend in America has led to a number of attacks on healthcare workers. Amy Acton, health director for Ohio, was the spokesperson for the state's response to the contagion. On

March 22, as Governor Mike DeWine issued stay-at-home orders, Acton spoke to Ohioans of the ordeal ahead: "This is a war on a silent enemy. I don't want you to be afraid. I am not afraid. I'm determined. But I need you to do everything. I want you to think about the fact that this is our one shot in this country." Steady and reassuring, her daily briefings became a sensation, especially for children. The "Dr. Amy Acton Fan Club" page on Facebook garnered more than 130,000 members. Her sayings were printed on T-shirts. Little girls wore white jackets and played "act like Amy." Acton went on CNN with *Sesame Street* characters to communicate the gravity of the challenge and the responsibility that even children have to stay home and keep their distance to protect their families—this, coming from a woman who was abused and homeless in Youngstown, Ohio, when she was a child.

Ohio's forceful response to the contagion was seen as a model for other states, but some Ohioans bristled at the restrictions, holding Acton responsible. In May, worried about holding the presidential primary in the onslaught of the virus, the governor tried to postpone it, but the legislature and the courts refused to go along. He turned to Acton, who was endowed with sweeping powers during a health crisis. The day before the vote, she shut down the primary. She was attacked as a "medical dictator" in the legislature. Protesters showed up at her home, some with bullhorns, some with guns, shouting sexist obscenities and anti-Semitic rhetoric (Acton is Jewish). Neighbors and members of the Amy Acton fan club interposed themselves. You could tell which side people were on by whether they wore masks.

In June, Acton resigned, one of at least twenty-seven top health officials in thirteen states who had quit, retired, or been fired since April.

I had heard that Dr. Fauci's home was under guard. I asked if he had been threatened. "Oh, my goodness," he said. "Harassing my wife and my children. It's really despicable. It's this Dark Web group of people who are ultra-ultra-ultra far-right crazies. They somehow got the phone numbers of my children, they've tracked them where they work, they've harassed them with texts, some threatening, some obscene. We have gotten multiple death threats, my wife and I." He sighed and uttered the native New Yorker's lament. "It is what it is."

Because of the threats, Fauci was assigned a security detail. One day, he was opening a letter, and a puff of white powder dusted his face. It could have been anthrax or ricin. A team of people in hazmat suits came to his office and sprayed him down. It was a hoax, but it could have been a murder.

SOON AFTER TRUMP moved into the White House, in January 2017, South Dakota's single U.S. representative at the time, Kristi Noem (who became the state's governor), was invited to the Oval Office. She related the story while taping a carpool karaoke video for the annual banquet of the Vermillion Area Chamber and Development Company. "I might have to write a book someday that says 'funny things President Trump said to me,'" Noem remarked, as the host, Mitchell Olson, who is seven feet tall and was a contestant on the second season of *Survivor*, drove them around town. "The first time, we were in the Oval Office, he said, 'Kristi, come on over here, shake my hand.' So I shook his hand and I said, 'Mr. President, you should come to South Dakota sometime. We have Mount Rushmore.'" Relating the story, Noem claps her hands and widens her eyes in imitation of the president. "And he goes, 'Do you know it's my dream to have my face on Mount Rushmore?'"

Noem and Olson crack up. "Is he aware that's not really an option?" Olson exclaims.

"Well, I started laughing. And he wasn't laughing," Noem continued. "I said, 'Come pick out a mountain.'"

A few months later, at a rally in Ohio, Mount Rushmore was still on the president's mind. "Now, here's what I do," he said to the crowd. "I'd ask whether or not you think I will one day be on Mount Rushmore." The crowd cheered. "But here's the problem," the president continued. "If I did it—joking, totally joking, having fun—the fake news media will say, 'He believes he should be on Mount Rushmore.' So I won't say it, okay? I won't say."*And yet there he was, on July 3, 2020, standing at the foot of the imposing monument, accompanied by the first lady in a stylish summer frock, the Blue Angels roaring by overhead. The president

---

* One of the president's aides did inquire about the process to get Trump's likeness on the monument. Tim Elfrink, "Trump denies that White House asked about adding him to Mount Rushmore, but adds it 'sounds like a good idea!'" *Washington Post*, August 10, 2020.

even tweeted a photo that snugly fitted his profile next to the visage of Abraham Lincoln, the first Republican president. It was Donald Trump's party now.

The U.S. Covid daily case count had reached a single-day high of 55,595 new infections. It was still climbing, concentrated now in southern and western states. Dr. Anne Schuchat, the CDC's principal deputy director, declared that the virus was no longer controllable. "We are not even beginning to be over this," she admitted. But Covid-19 wasn't on the president's mind. His topic was "violent mayhem" in the streets of American cities. "Our nation is witnessing a merciless campaign to wipe out our history, defame our heroes, erase our values, and indoctrinate our children," he said. "Make no mistake: this left-wing cultural revolution is designed to overthrow the American Revolution."

One wonders what Washington, Jefferson, Lincoln, and Teddy Roosevelt would have thought, as they gazed from their granite perch at the country they had made, and at the man who then occupied the office they once graced. Each of them had faced grave challenges. The founders, Washington and Jefferson, created a nation and then built a state to run it. Lincoln guided the country at its moment of greatest disunion. Roosevelt used the power of the presidency to break up industrial monopolies, conserve natural resources, create national parks, and prod America into taking its place on the global stage. (It didn't hurt the prospects for building the Rushmore memorial in South Dakota that Roosevelt had been a cowboy in the Dakota Territory). Each of these men knew how to use government for the good of the people.

The president always encouraged fringe groups—conspiracy theorists, such as Alex Jones and QAnon followers, and the white supremacists that he tacitly endorsed. Perhaps he believed their dogma. Perhaps he just liked to toy with irrational and polarizing ideas because they stirred up chaos. He had assumed office with little understanding or interest in governing; he demanded loyalty above all, and filled the offices of government with people whose sole mission was to please him. They became a kind of occupying army to subjugate what Trump called the Deep State. Suspicious of experts, the president relied on his "instincts," which allowed him to entertain alternative realities and convenient delusions. He gave inspiration to conspiracists of all kinds, weaving a theme with many threads spun on 8chan, InfoWars, and Fox News, and cut to fashion by eager hackers in Russia, China, Iran, and North Korea. He fanned the adulation of people who called themselves patriots but who were basically traitors, taking up arms against other Americans in order to stifle democracy. Trump's legacy was the deep anti-state.

21

Dark Shadows

BIDEN SAYS he's going to calm things down," Laura Ingraham said on Fox News, on August 31. She and President Trump were discussing the protests in Portland, which had been going on nightly since George Floyd's murder. A Trump supporter was shot and killed in downtown Portland two days before the show. Shortly before that, three people had been shot and two died in Kenosha, Wisconsin. A seventeen-year-old Trump supporter, acting as a vigilante, was charged with the killings. Trump had defended him.

"Biden won't calm things down," the president responded. "If Biden gets in, they will have won. He's a weak person. He's controlled like a puppet."

"Who do you think is pulling Biden's strings?" Ingraham asked. "Is it former Obama people?"

"People that you've never heard of. People that are in the dark shadows."

"That sounds like a conspiracy theory," Ingraham said worriedly. "Dark shadows—what is that?"

"There are people that are controlling the streets," Trump explained. "We had somebody get on a plane from a certain city this weekend, and in the plane, it was almost completely loaded with thugs wearing these dark uniforms, black uniforms, with gear and this and that."

"Where is—?"

"I'll tell you sometime, but it's under investigation right now. But they came from a certain city, and this person was coming to the Republican National Convention. And there were like seven people on the plane like this person. And then a lot of people were on the plane to do big damage."

"Planning for Washington," Ingraham surmised. "But the money is coming from somewhere. How can it be tracked?"

"Money is coming from some very stupid rich people," Trump said. "They will be thrown to the wolves like you've never seen before."

THERE WAS a singular genius at work, one that understood the American people better than we understood ourselves. Despite the pretense of morality nearly all candidates cling to, Trump knew that we are essentially a vulgar nation. In 2016, he faced sixteen competitors for the Republican nomination—at the time, the largest field of candidates in presidential history, and the most diverse—each of them with the requisite degree of rectitude and piety we thought we demanded from our public servants. He mowed them down, one by one, receiving about 14 million votes in the Republican primaries, the most in party history.

When, a month before the general election against Hillary Clinton, he was heard to say that because he is famous he is allowed to grab women "by the pussy," we thought that his chances were finished. And yet, women voted for him at about the same rate as they did for Mitt Romney in the election prior to that—actually voting against the first woman presidential nominee in favor of a sexual predator in the #MeToo era. We thought that blue-collar workers and those without college degrees would be repelled by a plutocrat who didn't pay his contractors and left lenders holding his bankrupt properties, and yet he carried non-college graduates by the widest margin in thirty-six years. We thought religious people would be outraged by his impiety and agnosticism, not to mention his divorces and habitual lying, but Trump carried Protestants, Catholics, and Mormons by significant margins, and evangelicals by 80 percent. What Trump proved to us is that we weren't the people we thought we were; the things we said we cared about weren't the things we really cared about.

Part of Trump's attraction was the sheer spectacle of his will. He was brutish, cruel, and demeaning, but he lived without apparent regrets. This was read as strength. He attacked the violence in "Democrat" cities, and yet he incited his own followers, urging them to beat up protesters at his rallies and threatening the reporters who covered them. The rallies played a similar role in the Trumpian saga as his dalliance with professional wrestling, but in that arena, no one was really hurt.

His opulent lifestyle was a cartoon of the American dream, but it dazzled, as did his appetite for attention. Another aspect of his genius was his near-magical ability to constantly turn people's heads in his direction, even if we hated ourselves for it; every day, every hour, every tweet, a new provocation arrived, and we stood there, like the knife-thrower's assistant as the blades flew, praying that the next one wouldn't be a mortal mistake. Still, how thrilling.

Subterranean currents disclose themselves during elections, perhaps more so in the 2016 election than in any other contest in recent history, given the widespread expectation that Trump was certain to lose, probably by a landslide. Russian meddling certainly had a hand in the outcome. Clinton blamed FBI director James Comey's last-minute decision to inform Congress that there were new developments in the investigation into her private email server. Either of these events may have tipped an election that was far closer than the polls had indicated. The question is why it was close, when the New York Times had forecast Clinton was on the verge of having an "unbreakable lead."

One could argue that a major factor in Clinton's loss was a public health crisis that particularly affected working-class white men, who voted two to one for Trump. That is, the opioid epidemic. Drug overdoses had become the leading cause of death for Americans under fifty; about two-thirds of those deaths were caused by opioids. The epidemic actually lowered the life expectancy of less-educated white men, and yet it remains largely unaddressed. Over 300,000 Americans died from opioid-related deaths from 1999 to 2015, a rate that reached about 115 opioid deaths a day in 2016. Two million Americans lost their jobs due to international trade during that same span of time, many of them higher-paying, union, manufacturing jobs. The highest concentration of job losses tended to be in the same counties with high levels of opioid overdoses. Those counties were far more likely to vote for Trump.

An intriguing paradox was at the heart of Trump's victory in 2016.

People in good health have traditionally been more likely to vote Republican, but the trend reversed in that presidential year. This was despite the fact that the Affordable Care Act was a centerpiece of the debate in that election. The shift was particularly notable in the traditional Democratic strongholds of Pennsylvania, Wisconsin, and Michigan—all states that went for Trump. Counties with higher mortality rates from drugs, alcohol, and suicide were more likely to vote for Trump in 2016 than they did for Romney in 2012. It was a shift born of despair. If the unacknowledged factor in 2016 was health, it would become an overriding factor four years later.

For most of Trump's presidency, a buoyant economy made its own powerful argument in his favor. But the Covid contagion broke the economy, and there were no other standards to raise. The country was drowning in acrimony and grief. Trump's inner demons had been set loose. The killers were off the leash.

"IF YOU CARRY GUNS, buy ammunition, ladies and gentlemen, because it's going to be hard to get," Michael Caputo advised in a rambling Facebook Live event on September 13, 2020. Caputo was an assistant secretary for the Department of Health and Human Services for public affairs. In that office, he controlled the flow of information from America's public health establishment—the CDC, FDA, and NIH.

The president had personally appointed Caputo to this post in April, when the disease was spreading out of hand and transparency and competence were needed to restore public trust. Instead, Trump chose a man with no expertise in science or public health. Caputo claimed that his best friend was Roger Stone, the political trickster who was convicted, among other offenses, of lying to Congress during its investigation into Russian interference in the 2016 election. (Stone's forty-month sentence was later commuted by the president.) Caputo himself had been a subject of interest in that investigation, having worked in Russia, both for the U.S. Agency for International Development, and later for Gazprom media, where his job reportedly was to brush up Vladimir Putin's image in the U.S.

The president wanted Caputo to reinforce his message that the pandemic wasn't as dangerous as scientists claimed, and that the crisis was totally under control. After Caputo meddled with CDC guidelines to get the case numbers down and stanch the flow of bad news, Trump asked him to lead a campaign to "defeat despair," which would encourage celebrities to endorse the administration's laissez-faire approach to the coronavirus. Well-known personalities were vetted to determine their political views. It was discouraging work. Justin Timberlake "publicly endorsed Obama and supports gay marriage." Scarlett Johansson "supports Elizabeth Warren," while Brad Pitt "Slammed GOP" during his speech at the Oscars. Jennifer Lopez criticized the president's immigration policies during her performance at the Super Bowl. Some highly desired figures—Lady Gaga, Beyoncé, Cardi B, Eminem—were labeled "superspreaders" apparently because of their broad appeal, not because of their capacity to spread disease; in any case, none signed on. Only ten celebrities finally passed muster, including Dennis Quaid, Dr. Oz, and Garth Brooks, but they all backed out. To fund the fruitless campaign, Caputo snatched $300 million from the CDC's budget.

Caputo's efforts met with resistance from Fauci and others, and he felt under siege. In the Facebook video, he was sitting outside his house in Buffalo, wearing a khaki T-shirt, a deep-green canopy of end-of-summer foliage behind him. He had a large round head with short-cropped white hair and a resonant baritone voice. He appeared not to have shaved in several days.

"There are scientists working for the government who do not want America to get better," he said, waving his index finger at the camera. "Nor can they allow America to hear good news. It must be all bad news from now until the election. Frankly, ladies and gentlemen, that's sedition. They are sacrificing lives in order to defeat Donald Trump." He stared into space. "I'm sorry to tell you this," he said. "But understand: this is war. Joe Biden is *not going to concede*. The Antifa attacks, the murders that have happened, the rallies that have turned into violence—this is all practice. We know it. We know it, my friends. In law enforcement, in federal law enforcement, they tell me they recognize this as drills. Remember the Trump supporter that was shot and killed? That was a drill! That was a hit squad. And the guy that shot him went down fighting. Why? Because he couldn't say what he had inside him: There are hit squads being trained all over the country. It's a fact." He concluded:

"They're going to have to kill me, and unfortunately, I think that's where this is going."

He sighed deeply. "Some of you who know me know my health is failing." (He would soon be diagnosed with cancer.) "My mental health is definitely failing. I don't like being alone in Washington. The shadows on the ceiling in my apartment, there alone, those shadows are so long."

Soon afterward, Caputo went on medical leave.

SUCH EMBATTLED THOUGHTS were shared by many who kindled to the violent fantasies of the president and his supporters. In a strip mall in Grand Rapids, Michigan, there is a shop called the Vac Shack. It sells and services vacuums. A former employee, Adam Fox, had been kicked out of his girlfriend's house and found himself and his two dogs homeless. The owner of the shop allowed Fox to sleep in the basement storage room. It was so full of boxes and filing cabinets and spare parts that there was scarcely room for the dog cages. It was there that Fox allegedly conceived the plot to kidnap Governor Gretchen Whitmer.

Fox, thirty-seven, is a powerfully built man with a trim brown beard and a square face. His ex-wife described him in a request for a protective order as "reckless when drunk." Fox was a leader of a militia called the Michigan Three Percenters—a reference to their belief that only 3 percent of American colonists took up arms against Britain in the Revolutionary War. Michigan is a hotbed of such groups. They were infuriated by Whitmer's Covid restrictions, but even before the lockdown they were prone to anger. Fox had been kicked out of another militia, the Michigan Home Guard, for having "rage issues." One of the conspirators complained, "I'm sick of being robbed and enslaved by the state," after receiving a ticket for driving without a license.

In June, at a gun rights rally at the state capitol in Lansing, Fox met with members of another militia, the Wolverine Watchmen. Much of the mythology from extremist groups springs from popular culture, especially movies and television shows that stir the dark materials of violence and paranoia. Michigan is sometimes called the Wolverine State, but the reference also comes from a movie, *Red Dawn*, about a group of teenagers who adopted the name of their high school mascot in defending their hometown against a Soviet invasion. The plan of the Wolverine Watchmen was to track down and kill police officers in their homes, then seize control of the government. They apparently called themselves "watchmen" after an HBO series of that name, which follows exactly that plot. The series is set in Tulsa, in 2019, but it begins with the 1921 massacre there. In the series, the militia group kills the police officers as a protest against reparations for victims of racial injustice. The Wolverine Watchmen were a mashup of pop culture figures and social media memes, animating the imagination of men who lived marginal lives.

Some of the militias focus primarily on grievances against the government, others on racial politics, but the boundaries are soft. Fox was an anti-government man. He was mainly motivated by the fact that, in the face of the pandemic, the state had shut down the gyms. The Watchmen were white supremacists. Their goal was to prepare for the "boogaloo"—a civil war that would lead to the collapse of society and the restoration of white dominance. The reference is to a cult movie from 1984, *Breakin' 2: Electric Boogaloo*. In the racist shadow world, the title was transmuted into *Civil War 2: Electric Boogaloo*. Somewhere along the line, "boogaloo" got coded into "big luau," which is why many of the members wear Hawaiian shirts.

Fox allegedly told the Watchmen he was recruiting for an operation targeting the state capitol. He needed two hundred men to storm the building and abduct politicians, including the "tyrant bitch," Whitmer. They would try her for treason. All this had to be completed before the presidential election, less than five months away.

One can speculate on the farce of a man living in the basement of a vacuum shop nominating himself to overturn the social order of the state, but the prospect of a total reversal of fortunes animated his dream. Adam Fox was unwanted—by his ex-wife, by his girlfriend, by the society that wouldn't give him a prestigious job—and the distance between who he was and who he wanted to be was so great it could only be closed by force. Governor Whitmer was a woman, attractive, powerful, popular. There was talk she might be picked as Joe Biden's running mate. Fox would strip her of her authority. He would take charge, subjugate her. It was a kind of rape fantasy, one that Whitmer would recognize: she had been raped when she was young.

Although the plotters were mostly unemployed or in low-paying jobs, they invested thousands of dollars in a Taser and night-vision goggles and were planning to spend thousands more on explosives. They were already heavily supplied with arms. Their weapons were a signal of the group's seriousness but also compensated for their despair and perceived powerlessness. They were plainly inspired by Trump's tweets disparaging Whitmer for shutting down her state during the pandemic and his call to "LIBERATE MICHIGAN!" They also considered kidnapping Virginia governor Ralph Northam, who had been similarly targeted by Trump, who also had tweeted "LIBERATE VIRGINIA!" Adam Fox and most of his followers were answering the president's summons. On the other hand, one of the gang was an anarchist who called the president a tyrant, and another attended a Black Lives Matter protest because he was upset about police killings. What united them was a combination of weakness and grand delusions.

The plotters squeezed into Fox's basement to sort out their plan. Fox made them surrender their cell phones to prevent any monitoring, but two FBI undercover operatives had already penetrated the group, and there were a couple of informers as well, so their schemes were secretly recorded. Over the next weeks, the plan of assaulting the capitol fell aside, given their limited numbers. Instead, Fox proposed that they capture Whitmer at her vacation home. "Snatch and grab, man," he said. "Grab the fuckin' governor. Just grab the bitch. . . . We do that, dude—it's over." Another plan was to mail a bomb to Whitmer's office. "I just wanna make the world glow, dude," Fox said. "I don't fuckin' care anymore. I'm just so sick of it. That's what it's gonna take for us to take it back, we're just gonna have to—everything's gonna have to be annihilated, man. We're gonna topple it all, dude. . . . We're just gonna conquer every fuckin' thing, man." They entertained the idea of abandoning the governor in a boat in the middle of Lake Michigan. What they would do with the state once they took over was not a matter of interest.

While this plan was brewing, the FBI and the Michigan State Police kept the governor and her family on the move between undisclosed locations. When the plotters were arrested, in October, Whitmer singled out the president, who only days before, in a debate with Joe Biden, had refused to explicitly condemn right-wing, white supremacist violence. "Words matter," Whitmer said. "When our leaders meet with, encourage, or fraternize with domestic terrorists they legitimize their actions—they are complicit. When they stoke and contribute to hate speech—they are complicit."

Mike Shirkey, the Republican leader of the state senate who had failed to return Whitmer's call when her home was besieged, now tweeted, "a threat against our governor is a threat against us all. We condemn those who plotted against her and our government. They are not patriots, there is no honor in their actions. They are criminals and traitors and they should be prosecuted to the fullest extent of the law."

The president tweeted: "My Justice Department and Federal Law Enforcement" had foiled the plot against the governor. "Rather than say thank you, she calls me a White Supremacist." He commanded, "Governor Whitmer—open up your state, open up your schools, and open up your churches!"

This aborted plot was a prelude for the insurrection that was brewing all across the country, and would soon converge in Washington, at the Capitol.

22

The Rose Garden Cluster

O N HER DEATHBED, Supreme Court Justice Ruth Bader Ginsburg dictated her final thoughts to the public through her granddaughter Clara Spera: "My most fervent wish is that I will not be replaced until a new president is installed." But on September 26, eight days after Ginsburg's passing, the president presented his third nominee for the high bench, Amy Coney Barrett, in a ceremony in the White House Rose Garden. The Reverend John Jenkins, the president of the University of Notre Dame, where Barrett had taught law, recalled, "We were required to wear a mask at entry and, after going through security, were immediately taken to a room and administered a nasal swab for a Covid test." Once a negative result came back, guests could remove their masks. "I assumed that we could trust the White House health protocols," Jenkins said. He regretted his decision: "I unwittingly allowed myself to be swept up very publicly into the image of a White House that sometimes seemed to disregard scientific evidence and minimize the threat of the pandemic."

That day, 769 American deaths from Covid were recorded—down from the spring peak, on April 15, of 2,752. Despite the absence of miracle drugs, the death rate for hospitalized patients had fallen significantly. In part, this was because the average age of patients was lower, but the improved chances of survival were also the result of flattening the curve, which gave doctors and scientists the time to devise more effective treatments. The infection rate, however, was harder to slow. The number of cases per day, which had topped 75,000 in mid-July, had faded a bit in the late summer, but it was again rounding upward. After months of being more careful, Americans had apparently let down their guard.

It was a pleasant autumn day; somewhat overcast, the leaves were beginning to turn but had yet to fall. Guests were ushered to the Rose Garden, where there were two hundred assigned seats. "The flag of the United States is still flying at half-staff in memory of Justice Ruth Bader Ginsburg, to mark the end of a great American life," Judge Barrett said in her brief, gracious remarks. She referenced the friendship between Ginsburg and Barrett's own mentor, Justice Antonin Scalia. "These two great Americans demonstrated that arguments, even about matters of great consequence, need not destroy affection." She was gesturing toward a bygone and perhaps mythic America, one often invoked but increasingly distant from reality.

"Movement conservatives were very happy," Mike Lee, the Republican senator from Utah, recalled. Friends who hadn't seen one another for months reunited, he said, which "added to the jovial atmosphere." As Barrett spoke, the virus was circulating among the crowd, who were sitting closely pressed together, few wearing masks. When the speech was done, the hobnobbing began, with Senator Lee and Chris Christie, among others, embracing old friends. Health and Human Services Secretary Alex Azar was among the unmasked glad-handers.

Perhaps the president was already infected. The White House refused to give the last date when the president was tested before the Rose Garden event. "I don't want to move backwards," the president's doctor, Sean Conley, explained. Trump had just made multiple campaign stops the previous day, in Florida, Georgia, and Virginia. Some Covid carriers can go as long as two weeks before they start to show symptoms, and without knowing when the president last tested negative, it's impossible to know when he contracted the disease and how many other people he might have infected.

More than a dozen guests—including Senator Lee, former governor Chris Christie, former White House adviser Kellyanne Conway, and Father Jenkins—would soon test positive. All had been negative when they arrived, and none wore a mask. The only people in the Rose Garden who might not have been tested were the president and the first lady.

The audience returned to their lives, some carrying the virus with them. The White House ignored the CDC's request to do contact tracing, saying that it would be done internally, but statements by attendees said they had not been contacted. The full extent of the contagion from the Rose Garden cluster will never be known. Dr. Fauci labeled it a superspreader event.

Still untested, Trump flew to Pennsylvania that evening for two campaign events. Kayleigh McEnany, his chief spokesperson, and Michael Shear, a White House correspondent for the *New York Times*, were on Air Force One. They would both be infected. The president chatted with reporters on the flight for about ten minutes. "He was not wearing a mask," said Shear. He added that, after testing positive, "Nobody from the White House has said 'boo' or asked anything about where I was or who I talked to or who else I might have infected."

Thousands of supporters, many unmasked, greeted the president at an airport hangar in Middletown. Tom Wolf, the governor of Pennsylvania, complained that the Trump campaign had violated state guidelines by "disregarding gathering limits, mask orders, and social distancing guidelines."

The next morning, the president went to the Trump National Golf Club in Potomac Falls, Virginia. It was the 291st time he had visited one of his seventeen golf clubs while in office. Back in the White House, he prepared for his debate with Joe Biden. There were five or six people in the room with the president: Chris Christie, who may already have been infected, as well as the president's close advisers Rudolph Giuliani, Hope Hicks, and Stephen Miller. Miller and Hicks would test positive. Later that day, the president held a news conference, where Al Drago, a *Times* photographer, may have been infected, and a reception for Gold Star families, attended by Admiral Charles W. Ray, vice commandant of the Coast Guard; his infection would cause most of the Joint Chiefs of Staff to quarantine themselves and much of the Pentagon to clear out.

The presidential debate was Tuesday, September 29, in Cleveland. Trump's family and entourage who were in the audience rejected the masks they were offered and which the Cleveland Clinic required. The Trump party reportedly had not arrived in time to take the mandatory tests, which might have shown that the president and members of his party were already infected. Later, when pressed on the subject of whether he had tested negative for the coronavirus that day, Trump responded, "Possibly I did, possibly I didn't."

The next day the president traveled to Minnesota, where he attended a private fundraiser and a massive rally at the airport in Duluth. "I really enjoyed last night's debate with Sleepy Joe," he said, clouds of his breath lingering in the chilly air. He claimed that the debate, widely considered a disastrous performance on his part, had the "highest ratings of any show in the history of cable television and it had the second-highest ratings of overall television in the history of television." (About 73 million people watched the debate, about 13 percent fewer than watched the first presidential debate four years before.) He also claimed that Mexico was paying for the border wall. He spoke for about forty-five minutes, about half the time of his usual campaign speeches. Bill Stepien, Trump's campaign manager, may have become infected on this trip, if he hadn't already been infected in Cleveland.

While Trump slept on the flight back to Washington, Hope Hicks isolated herself. She tested positive the next morning. Despite the fact that the president now knew for certain he had been in contact with the virus, he did not immediately get tested; instead, he attended a fundraiser at his club in Bedminster, New Jersey, which included meeting supporters in close quarters, where he did not wear a mask. No one told the four hundred staffers in the White House that Hope Hicks had tested positive; that news was broken by a Bloomberg reporter. The president and the first lady each took a rapid test, and both were positive. He then took a PCR test to confirm the diagnosis. He was tired and congested. He was coughing. At 1:00 a.m., he tweeted, "Tonight, @FLOTUS and I tested positive for COVID-19. We will begin our quarantine and recovery process immediately. We will get through this TOGETHER!"

FOR AN OBESE MAN, age seventy-four, with mild heart disease and high cholesterol, Trump's chances of dying were 1 in 25; but he was not a statistic, he was the president of the United States.

Dr. Conley said the president had a high fever and that his oxygen levels had dropped into the 80s, at the point the disease is considered severe. He was given supplemental oxygen and an experimental monoclonal antibody cocktail made by the biotechnology company Regen-

eron, along with zinc, Vitamin D, aspirin, melatonin, a heartburn drug
called famotidine, and remdesivir, an antiviral drug that has been shown
to moderate symptoms of Covid-19 but has not had an effect on mortality. He was not given hydroxychloroquine. His lungs were inflamed
and filled with substances that could indicate an acute case of the disease. At first, he declined to leave the White House for treatment, but he
was asked to imagine the alternative of the Secret Service carrying him
out if the disease progressed. That evening he was helicoptered to Walter Reed hospital, where the presidential suite awaited him. There his
oxygen levels dropped again, and he received a steroid, dexamethasone,
which was being used experimentally to diminish the inflammation
caused by the body's reaction to the disease. He reportedly had heart
palpitations. "The president's vitals over the last twenty-four hours were
very concerning, and the next forty-eight hours will be critical in terms
of his care," Trump's chief of staff, Mark Meadows, told reporters the
next morning. "We are still not on a clear path to a full recovery."

In the alternative reality that Trump embodies, a too-familiar voice
spoke. "President Trump is in great danger," Alex Jones said on his
InfoWars show. "Evidence is mounting that he's being deliberately killed
at Walter Reed Military Hospital." As soon as the deed was done, Jones
warned, the "corrupt establishment could claim total victory, lock down
the entire country, start going after the patriots, and destroy whatever's
left of our birth right."

Meantime, the first lady chose "a more natural route," in terms of
treatment, by which she meant "vitamins and healthy food." She experienced "a roller coaster of symptoms," including body aches, cough,
headaches, and extreme fatigue. Their fourteen-year-old son, Barron,
was infected but did not show symptoms.

"Recovering from an illness gives you a lot of time to reflect," Melania Trump wrote in a blog post. She thought about "the hundreds of
thousands of people across our country who have been impacted by
this illness that infects people with no discrimination. We are in unprecedented times—and with the election fast approaching, it has been easy
to get caught up in so much negative energy." She added: "I want people to know that I understand just how fortunate my family is to have
received the kind of care that we did."

Despite his germophobia, the president is proud of his immune system, boasting on multiple occasions that he's never even had the flu. But Covid struck him hard—hard enough for him to admit "I could be one of the diers." He had lost a friend to the disease, Stanley Chera, whom Trump knew in the real estate world. "He went to the hospital, he calls me up," Trump recounted after Chera's death. "He goes, 'I tested positive.' I said, 'Well, what are you going to do?' He said, 'I'm going to the hospital. I'll call you tomorrow.' He didn't call." Now, the president himself was in the hospital with heart palpitations. He asked his aides, "Am I going out like Stan Chera?"

One wonders if he had ever seriously considered his own mortality until then, or if, in fact, he thinks about it all the time. His fear of germs was accompanied by a dread of seeing blood. "I'm not good for medical," he once admitted on the *Howard Stern Show*. "If you cut your finger and there's blood pouring out, I'm gone." He told an anecdote about a charity event at Mar-a-Lago. "The Marines were there, and it was terrible because all these rich people, they're there to support the Marines, but they're really there to get their picture in the *Palm Beach Post* . . . so you have all these really rich people, and a man, about eighty years old—very wealthy man, a lot of people didn't like him—he fell off the stage. . . . So, what happens is, this guy falls off right on his face, hits his head, and I thought he died. And you know what I did? I said, 'Oh my God, that's disgusting,' and I turned away. . . . He's bleeding all over the place, I felt terrible. You know, beautiful marble floor, didn't look like it. It changed color. Became very red. And you have this poor guy, eighty years old, laying on the floor unconscious, and all the rich people are turning away." The Marines sprang into action—"they grab him, they put the blood all over the place, it's all over their uniforms"— and rushed the injured man out of the ballroom. "I was saying, 'Get that blood cleaned up! It's disgusting!'" Blood, he concluded, "it's just not my thing."

One can see in this ingenuous story Trump's disdain for the class of people he entertains, but also, once again, his horror of contamination. Death stalked him, as it does us all; his wealth was no defense, nor was celebrity. With age, thoughts of death intrude more forcefully; one tries to put them aside, but then, with a sudden gush of blood or the onset of illness, mortality barges in.

So often, hospitals are portals to the graveyard, and that was doubly true during the pandemic. But President Trump was ready to return to the White House after three days. As he was preparing to leave the hospital, he imagined hobbling out as if he were really frail, rather than hopped up on steroids, then yanking open his shirt to reveal a Superman jersey. In the event, he saved his drama for the moment he stood again on the Truman Balcony and defiantly ripped off his surgical mask.

"Don't be afraid of Covid," he tweeted. "Don't let it dominate your life." Like Superman, he was feeling invulnerable. Unlike Superman, he wasn't.

23

The Search for Patient Zero

THE INITIAL THEORY of the origin of the new coronavirus—an
infected animal, possibly a pangolin, at Huanan Seafood Wholesale Market in Wuhan, passed the disease to a human—soon fell
apart, and was disavowed by leading Chinese scientists. The first person nominated to be Patient Zero for Covid-19 was a seventy-year-old
man with Alzheimer's, who showed symptoms on December 1, 2019.
It turned out he had had no contact with the market. No one knows
where or how he contracted it. In any case, prior infections may have
taken place in November and possibly as far back as September, without
evident contact with the wet market. George Gao, director of the China
CDC, admitted, "It now turns out that the market is one of the victims."

So how did the pathogen arise? The question was fraught with blame
and political opportunism, and yet China's behavior invited suspicion.
Two labs, the Wuhan Center for Disease Control and Prevention and the
Wuhan Institute of Virology, are world leaders in the study of bat diseases, including coronaviruses. Could the new disease have accidentally
escaped from one of those laboratories? The novel virus spread with
shocking efficiency, seeming to be perfectly adapted to the human host
from the beginning, with little evidence of adaptation. Was a bat virus
purposely engineered to be a super-contagious human disease? Was
it designed to be a weapon? Such questions would be posed by China
hawks in the Trump White House. The Chinese government protested

the motivations of those who made such charges, while stalling an international investigation into the origin of the virus.

"China created this pandemic," White House economic adviser Peter Navarro said on CNN. "They hid the virus, they created that virus, and they sent over hundreds of thousands of Chinese citizens here to spread that around, and around the world. Whether they did that on purpose, that's an open question."

"Did you say China created this virus?" the host, Jake Tapper, asked.

"That virus was a product of the Chinese Communist Party, and until we get some information about what happened in those labs, what happened in that wet market, we know that the virus was spawned in China. That's what I mean. Spawned in China." Navarro was one of the first voices to allege that the new virus was created in one of the two government laboratories in Wuhan. His theory was backed by Secretary of State Pompeo, who said that there was "enormous evidence" that the virus leaked from the Wuhan Institute of Virology.

Navarro had been one of the most durable members of the Trump team. The president called him "my Peter," because Navarro reinforced Trump's combativeness on trade issues. Navarro has a PhD from Harvard and served for nearly three decades as a professor of economics and public policy at the University of California, Irvine. Although he had no previous experience in government (one thing he had in common with many White House colleagues), he had run for office four times in the 1990s, losing races for mayor of San Diego and the San Diego city council, among others. His political affiliation moved from nonpartisan, to Republican, to Independent, to Republican again. He presented himself as a pro-choice, environmentalist Democrat when he ran for Congress in 1996, and was endorsed by Hillary Clinton. "I lost the race because I had run too many times and offended too many people in the process," he wrote in a rueful account called *San Diego Confidential* about how his political ambitions had ruined his life. "On that bright, sunny day in 1992 when I declared my candidacy for mayor, I had a fine reputation, a solid marriage, a spacious home, a new car, and a net worth of almost a million dollars. Today, after losing four political races, at least half the people in San Diego think I'm a jerk, a carpetbagger, a criminal, or worse. I'm divorced and living in a place the size of a postage stamp." During the 2016 presidential campaign he labeled himself a "Trump Democrat."

He was still looking for a platform and a cause when Jared Kushner called.

Kushner had been scrolling through Amazon, looking at books on China that might fortify Donald Trump's foreign policy. One title struck him: *Death by China*, which Navarro co-wrote (with Greg Autry). Kushner phoned Navarro out of the blue and offered him a position as a White House economic adviser. In July 2018 at Navarro's urging, the president imposed an initial 25 percent tax on $34 billion worth of Chinese goods, and the world's two biggest economies went to war. China suffered slower growth and a decline in manufacturing, but retaliatory actions also hurt American farmers, contributing to a spike in bankruptcies in 2019. Moreover, American consumers wound up paying the cost of the tariffs. The struggle left both countries bitter and suspicious and full of recriminations.

Hanging over the discussion within the Trump White House was the belief that the Chinese were engaged in what is termed "dual use"— that is, taking advantage of legitimate scientific research to create bioweapons. "The Wuhan Institute of Virology has engaged in classified research, including laboratory animal research, on behalf of the Chinese military since at least 2017," a spokesman for the NSC told me. "There is much that we still don't know—and which Beijing will not let the world know—about the activities, both military and civilian, that have taken place in that lab."

It is against that backdrop that the theory of the virus's origins in a Wuhan lab arose.

THE LIMESTONE HILLS of Yunnan Province, in southern China, are pocked with caverns hosting millions of bats of many different species. The SARS virus that caused the 2002–2003 epidemic was traced to horseshoe bats in Yunnan. Among the caverns is an abandoned copper mine. In the spring of 2012, six men who had worked in the mine reported to the hospital suffering from high fevers, coughs, and severe pneumonia. The job of these six men was to sweep up bat droppings from the mine. The first victim, named Zhou, was sixty-three, the oldest of the six. He was dead in twelve days. "The disease was acute and fierce," a student doctor recorded in a master's thesis about the incident. The next to die was Lu, age forty-two. Confounded, the doctors tested the survivors for influenza, encephalitis, and dengue, as well as SARS, but found no match. They turned to Professor Zhong Nanshan, who is sometimes described as China's Dr. Fauci. He suggested that the survivors also be tested for SARS antibodies, even though they had shown no reaction to the diagnostic test. They proved to be positive for a different, unknown coronavirus. A third victim in Yunnan succumbed in August of that year.

A team of scientists led by Shi Zhengli at the Wuhan Institute of Virology went to investigate the mine. Shi, known as China's Bat Woman, is one of the most famous scientists in the country and is largely responsible for enlarging the study of bat coronaviruses. At dusk, Shi's team placed nets in front of the mine opening and captured the bats as they emerged to feed, extracting blood and saliva samples, along with fecal swabs, from nearly three hundred bats from six different species. In the morning, the scientists picked up droppings and urine samples. Back in the lab in Wuhan, the scientists discovered hundreds of varieties of coronavirus in the samples. Some bats were infected with multiple coronaviruses simultaneously. Viruses have the ability to shuffle their genetic decks inside a host and create entirely new strains. The mine was a virus factory.

Most of the viruses were harmless to humans, but one resembled a SARS-type coronavirus. It was labeled RaTG13. The question of what exactly happened with that sample is unresolved, but the answer is key to understanding how the pandemic arose and what must be done to keep it from happening again.

Let's start with the question of the need for an intermediary animal. MERS is a coronavirus thought to have originated with Egyptian tomb bats, which infected camels sometime in the distant past; in 2012, it jumped to humans but struggled to adapt and never exploded into a pandemic. SARS has been found in palm civets, a small, gray, cat-like creature with a tail like a monkey and a mask like a raccoon. They were sold in the exotic-game markets in China and served in restaurants. Civets were thought to have been a viral stepping-stone into humans, and because of that, about 10,000 of these animals were slaughtered, many of them drowned or electrocuted. Later research failed to discover SARS in civets outside of the markets, so it is likely that the civets were incidental victims that had been infected by other animals or by humans.

In the laboratory, RaTG13 doesn't bind effectively to ACE2 receptors and seems a poor candidate for infecting humans. Many scientists, including Dr. Fauci, believe that the most likely origin story is that a bat infected another mammal, which then infected a human, and the virus circulated in people without being detected as it adapted to the new host. If earlier strains of the disease are found in banked human samples, that would be strong evidence of a process of natural selection.

With SARS-CoV-2, the intermediary animal was thought to be a pangolin. Also known as scaly anteaters, pangolins are nocturnal mammals living across much of tropical Asia and sub-Saharan Africa; their meat is favored in China as a delicacy and their scales for use in traditional medicine. This has edged them close to extinction. In 2019, Hong Kong authorities seized a shipment from Nigeria containing eight tons of pangolin scales. That same year, Chinese customs intercepted twenty-nine smuggled pangolins. "These animals were sent to the wildlife rescue center, and were mostly inactive and sobbing, and eventually died in custody despite exhaustive rescue efforts," scientists reported. They took tissue samples from the dead pangolins and discovered many were infected with a SARS-type coronavirus.

It is possible that infected, smuggled pangolins were sold at the wet market in Wuhan, but it turns out there were no pangolins in the market. In fact, no SARS-CoV-2 isolates were detected in any of the animals or fish in the market, although it was found in the sewage.

Perhaps the virus didn't need an intermediary; perhaps it was already close enough to become transmissible between people. Ebola is thought to have made just such a species jump, from bats to people. After fourteen years of dogged research into bat viruses, Shi Zhengli and her colleagues collected gene samples that precisely matched SARS. In southern China, as in some other regions of the world, bats are hunted and eaten. The feces are dried and used in Chinese traditional medicine to treat eye problems. Bats make up 20 percent of all known mammal species on earth, and they carry an extensive inventory of coronaviruses. So far, no naturally occurring bat virus sufficiently similar to SARS-CoV-2 as to be a human disease has been discovered. But such viruses have been created in laboratories.

———

THE RATG13 BAT VIRUS that Shi collected from the copper mine is highly similar to SARS-CoV-2, with 96 percent of its genome being identical. (The first SARS and SARS-CoV-2 are only 82 percent alike.) Scientists determined that they came from a common ancestor. A few modifications could easily transform this strain into a human disease.

After the original SARS outbreak, Shi collected SARS-like corona-viruses from Yunnan caves, the first evidence that demonstrated a likely bat origin. She was accompanied by a British zoologist, Dr. Peter Daszak, who is president of EcoHealth Alliance, which studies emerging diseases, particularly those that jump from one species to another. The NIH, along with the Pentagon's U.S. Defense Threat Reduction Agency, funded Eco-Health's research grant. Shi and Daszak collected about 15,000 samples from bats that contained 400 previously unknown coronaviruses, work that was innovative and absolutely vital. Daszak warned the WHO in 2015 that SARS was "alive and well in bats in Yunnan Province!" They also found coronavirus antibodies in villagers nearby, which they specu-lated came directly from bats. Daszak estimated that as many as seven million people a year in rural China and Southeast Asia are exposed to such viruses. It is probable that's what happened with the miners.

When an animal infects a person, it usually goes no further; but occasionally the virus adapts itself to the new host, a process called a cross-species jump. This period is usually marked by mutations as the virus struggles against destruction by the human immune system. Even if it succeeds in colonizing one person, it still needs a strategy to leap to another. The sole mission of the virus is to replicate itself, which it cannot do alone. As the virus replicates, using energy from the host cell, it adapts, just as HIV did in its evolution from a non-human primate pathogen into one that primarily infects people. An ember becomes a flame that becomes a forest fire. This is how novel diseases turn into pandemics.

The surprising thing about Covid-19 is that it seems to have been an uncannily successful human disease from the start—binding a thousand-fold more tightly to the ACE2 receptors than did SARS. With the first SARS, there was considerable genetic diversity in its early stages. Cana-dian and American researchers observed that the SARS-CoV-2 pandemic "appears to be missing an early phase during which the virus would be expected to accumulate adaptive mutations for human transmission." It looked like a mature human virus from the moment it appeared, which is why Dr. Redfield believes it came from a lab.

Perhaps one of the infected miners was Patient Zero. This theory has been promoted by Jonathan Latham, a virologist who runs the Bioscience Resource Project, an advocacy organization for agricultural research. He suggests that at least one of the miners was infected, not only with the RaTG13 virus but with another coronavirus simultaneously, and that they recombined inside his lungs, thereby creating a disease exquisitely suited for its new human host.

The miners' serum and other samples were frozen and stored in Shi's lab at the Wuhan Institute of Virology. It is possible that one of them—possibly Patient Zero's—was finally pulled out of the freezer and used for research, and this already human-adapted disease infected someone in the lab. That person may not have shown symptoms. But in this scenario, the disease that killed half of the miners who contracted it in 2012 was inadvertently let loose in Wuhan and from there upon the world.

Although Chinese officials indignantly deny that the virus came from the Wuhan Institute of Virology, pathogens do escape from labs, even highly secure ones, such as the CDC and the U.S. Army Medical Research Institute of Infectious Diseases in Fort Detrick, Maryland. Among the escapees were Ebola and Marburg. Smallpox has escaped from labs in the U.K. on at least three occasions, and SARS broke loose from the National Institute of Virology in Beijing four times. Many of these labs, containing the most dangerous diseases ever known, are located in densely populated urban centers. In 2014, the *Bulletin of the Atomic Scientists* examined the public health danger of escaped viruses. "It takes only one superspreading graduate student or maintenance worker to start a pandemic," the author concluded.

Another lab, the Wuhan Center for Disease Control, also studies coronaviruses from bats and operates at a lower level of safety. It had moved just six hundred yards from the wet market that was originally implicated in the outbreak the same month the first cases were discovered.

To their credit, Shi and Daszak have been warning for years that new pandemics could emerge from the bat caves of southern China. However, Shi has downplayed the likelihood that the miners who died in 2012 were infected by a coronavirus, claiming that they were sickened by a fungus that caused pneumonia. And yet her own lab had discovered the coronavirus antibodies in the miners. The doctor who treated them listed the probable cause of death as a SARS-like coronavirus from a horseshoe bat.

THERE IS ANOTHER scenario that might account for the precocious adaptability of the coronavirus in humans. There is an experiment called "gain of function." Suppose you have an animal virus that is potentially deadly but not yet contagious in humans. What would cause it to evolve that capability? In 2011, two virologists, Ron Fouchier at the Erasmus Medical Centre in the Netherlands and Yoshihiro Kawaoka at the University of Wisconsin, undertook such an experiment with an avian influenza, H5N1, that has killed 60 percent of the people who contracted it from birds. Working separately, they cultured the disease through repeated infections of ferrets, who are often used as human stand-ins. The scientists created an airborne respiratory disease after only a few mutations. They might as well have created a hydrogen bomb. A fiery debate about whether such experiments should ever be done led to a "pause" in 2014 of gain-of-function trials by virologists in the U.S., but three years later the pause was lifted. Gaining such knowledge might give science a head start on creating vaccines for diseases that could evolve in nature, but it's also possible that a slip in the lab would cause the very pandemics the research is meant to deter. Shi described doing "virus infectivity experiments" to determine if bat coronaviruses could be made more contagious in humans. NIAID, Dr. Fauci's shop, funded some of the research.

On several occasions in late 2017 and early 2018, the U.S. Embassy in Beijing dispatched American scientists to the Wuhan Institute of Virology. They were alarmed by what they saw, noting "a serious shortage of appropriately trained technicians and investigators needed to safely operate this high-containment laboratory." One of their cables to the State Department added that "the researchers also showed that various SARS-like coronaviruses can interact with ACE2, the human receptor identified for SARS-coronavirus. This finding strongly suggests that SARS-like coronaviruses from bats can be transmitted to humans."

When Shi heard that a novel virus had surfaced in Wuhan in December 2019, she frantically went through the lab's records to see if there had been any mishandling of materials and comparing the sequences of the new virus with the ones she had collected. She said that none of them matched. "That really took a load off my mind," she said. "I had not slept a wink for days." Chinese social media continued to cast a suspicious eye on her lab as a probable source of the new virus, however, even singling out one of her former graduate students as Patient Zero.

After a lengthy period of silence, leading to speculation that Shi had disappeared or defected, she responded to questions from *Science* magazine. She said that her lab has experimented with three SARS-related coronaviruses that are similar to SARS-CoV-2, but RaTG13 wasn't one of them. She denied that anyone in her lab has been infected. Her theory of the emergence of SARS-CoV-2 was that it came through an intermediary animal, possibly a pangolin.

Researchers in another lab, in Beijing, including some affiliated with the Chinese military, have created humanized mice with lung cells containing ACE2 receptors. Some American officials speculate that such mice were used in gain of function experiments with coronaviruses. President Trump declared that he has a "high degree of confidence" that the virus came from the Wuhan Institute of Virology, but said he can't provide specifics. Shi responded: "President Trump's claim that SARS-CoV-2 was leaked from our institute totally contradicts the facts. It jeopardizes and affects our academic work and personal life. He owes us an apology." She denounced as "absolutely absurd" Trump's termination in April of funding by the NIH for the collaboration with EcoHealth Alliance, Dr. Daszak's organization, pointing out that future diseases from bats are inevitably going to spill into the human population.

The U.S. intelligence community said that it does not believe that SARS-CoV-2 is a manmade virus. Francis Collins, the director of the NIH, agreed, saying, "Nature created this virus, and has proven once again to be the most effective bioterrorist." But Collins added that there was no way of knowing whether it might have escaped from a lab in Wuhan. In May 2020, seventy-seven Nobel laureates and thirty-one scientific societies sent letters to Collins protesting the decision to terminate the grant to EcoHealth for its project with WIV. In July, the NIH offered to restore funding for EcoHealth and the Wuhan Institute of Virology on the condition that the lab provide a sample used to sequence the SARS-CoV-2 virus and permit an independent investigation to determine if the lab possessed the virus before December 2019. The NIH also demanded to know the whereabouts of the scientist who was pegged as Patient Zero in Chinese social media. In the meantime, Dr. Fauci's institute, NIAID, awarded a larger grant to EcoHealth Alliance for research outside of China. It is part of an ambitious global initiative called the Centers for Research in Emerging Infectious Diseases. "The CREID network will enable early warnings of emerging diseases whenever they occur," Fauci said. "The knowledge gained through this research will increase our preparedness for future outbreaks."

In the summer of 2020, the WHO sent a team to discuss a prospective investigation into the origins of the virus. "Science must stay open to all possibilities," Mike Ryan, the executive director of WHO's Health Emergencies Program, said. "We need to lay out a series of investigations that will get the answers that I'm sure the Chinese government, governments around the world, and ourselves really need in order to manage the risk going forward." But China forbade WHO officials to actually conduct an independent investigation, agreeing only to allow the team to review studies produced by Chinese scientists and examine possible animal hosts. There was no mention of examining lab books at the Wuhan Institute of Virology or the Wuhan CDC. Not until January 2021, a year after the outbreak, did China permit a WHO team into the country to begin investigating the origins of the virus. This came as China itself was experiencing a resurgence of the contagion and parts of the country were once again locked down. China had the opportunity to completely open itself to the scrutiny of impartial scientists, but during what was described as heated exchanges it refused to share raw data, such as detailed patient records; instead, Chinese officials once again offered their own analyses. "Sometimes emotions have run really high," said Thea Kølsen Fischer, a Danish epidemiologist on the team. "I am a scientist and I trust data, I don't just trust what anyone tells me."

The WHO team pressed China to examine blood samples to determine if there was evidence of disease earlier than December 2019, which the Chinese have resisted. If the disease had been discovered to be circulating earlier, there would have been greater opportunity to halt its spread. Based on the evidence the WHO team was able to see, the outbreak began spreading in Wuhan in November, and perhaps as early as September, before catching fire in December.

The Chinese floated a theory that the virus entered China from else-where, possibly in frozen food, especially wildlife. There is some evidence that SARS-CoV-2 can remain infectious on frozen or refrigerated meat for as long as three weeks. In September 2020, Chinese scientists found the virus on the packaging of frozen cod coming into the port of Qingdao. The WHO team thought the transmission through frozen food was a "reasonable hypothesis," but not a likely source of the pandemic.

"It was my take on the entire mission that it was highly geopolitical," Dr. Fischer said. "Everybody knows how much pressure there is on China to be open to an investigation and also how much blame there might be associated with this." In the end, the team leader of the investigation, Peter Ben Embarek, said that although the lab origin theory was unlikely, it was "definitely not off the table." The WHO director-general, Tedros Adhanom Chebreyesus, later admitted that China had withheld data from the team.

Scientists have examined a multitude of newly discovered coronaviruses in bats across Asia similar to SARS-CoV-2, making a strong case that the pandemic strain evolved naturally. Several bats taken from a cave in Thailand showed antibodies to SARS-CoV-2, suggesting that they must have been infected at some point by a similar virus. That was also true of confiscated pangolins who were being held in quarantine centers. The WHO investigators learned that Chinese authorities had shut down a number of wildlife farms in southern China that were raising bamboo rats, civets, pangolins, and other exotic animals for consumption. Those same farms had been supplying wet markets, suggesting that officials believed such farms might have been a pipeline for human infection.

Patient Zero, if that person is ever found, will tell us how the current pandemic arose, but the search will also uncover the many ways dangerous diseases emerge. If the evolution of SARS-CoV-2 is natural, then we can expect recurrences, as the processes that led to its interaction with humans—climate change, intensive animal farming, the encroachment of civilization into natural preserves, smuggling and consumption of exotic species—have only increased. If the virus was created in a laboratory, for whatever purpose, then it is a reminder that science is engaged in experiments that invite catastrophe with the smallest slip. In either case, Covid-19 is a harbinger.

24

Survivors

I N WUHAN, on June 12, 2020, Fu Xuejie gave birth to a son. She is the widow of Dr. Li Wenliang, the Chinese doctor who died of Covid-19 after being censured by the police for warning his colleagues about the new coronavirus. "My husband, can you see us from heaven?" she wrote on WeChat. "You have given me your final gift today. I will definitely take care of him well."

In death, Dr. Li was transformed into something more than a martyr for free speech. His social media page on Weibo, the Chinese equivalent of Twitter, became a repository for millions of postings from Chinese citizens. Initially, there was an outpouring of anger at the government, which was shamed into apologizing for his mistreatment. But as the months passed, people continued to write to him. His page has been compared to the Wailing Wall or a tree hollow where people deposit their deepest fears or fondest hopes. Some of the messages are mundane notes that one might write to a family member:

"Good morning Dr. Li, I've got an English exam tomorrow. I hope I get full marks," said one.

"Hey Li, the weather's nice today in Wuhan. Spring is here."

"Dr. Li, my boyfriend just broke up with me. Now my future is so uncertain."

Other messages reflect a profound sense of despair:

"Morning, Dr. Li. I was taking a taxi home yesterday. The driver talked about you with me, with his voice trembling. You're very missed here."

"There was a downpour in Wuhan yesterday, as if the city was crying for the deceased. Wenliang, your ash is collected by Wuhan people, by people from all over the nation."

"He was an ophthalmologist and a young father who committed a small act of bravery and then a big act of bravery," Matt Pottinger said, in a speech he delivered in Mandarin in May 2020. Li's small act was warning his colleagues via social media about the dangerous new virus that was turning up in Wuhan hospitals. That warning circulated more widely than Li intended. After being forced to sign a confession and threatened with prosecution if he spoke out again, said Pottinger, "Dr. Li did a big brave thing. He went public with his experience of being silenced by the police. The whole world paid close attention. By this time, Dr. Li had contracted the disease he'd warned about. His death on February 7 felt like the loss of a relative for people around the world."

With the news of the birth of his son, a surge of well-wishers responded, many expressing hope that the child would carry on his legacy. "Congratulations, Dr. Li! I hope the baby will grow up to be a good man just like his dad," said one. Another correspondent posed the question, "Why is our sadness toward Li Wenliang's death so sharp? Because we witnessed someone just as ordinary as you and me, a gentle and professional doctor, a friend, a son, a husband, and a father suffering for us." One cannot escape the sense that the messages to Dr. Li are a form of prayer.

WHEN AMY KLOBUCHAR dropped out of the race for the Democratic presidential nomination, she moved onto Biden's shortlist for his running mate. George Floyd's death put an end to that. Klobuchar had begun her career twenty years earlier as the district attorney in Hennepin County, developing a reputation for being tough on crime but light on police misconduct. In the mid-1990s, homicides were more than triple the national rate, earning the city the sobriquet "Murderapolis." As the county's chief prosecutor, Klobuchar drove up the number of prison inmates by 20 percent during her eight years in office, when Blacks were incarcerated at a rate eighteen times higher than that of whites.

Klobuchar could read the times. On June 18, she asked Biden to take her name off his list and select a woman of color as his running mate.

That day she learned that her ninety-two-year-old father, Jim Klobuchar, had Covid. He was a big figure in Minneapolis, a retired newspaper columnist, a Jimmy Breslin character known to everyone, especially cops and bartenders, full of adventure and often too full of alcohol, trailing a record of DWIs. On Thanksgiving Day, when Amy was fifteen, her father asked her mother for a divorce. When she heard the news, Amy ran away from home. And yet, she kept up a relationship with her father, mainly through long-distance bike rides, often well over a hundred miles a day. When Amy was a young lawyer, her father was arrested again for drunk driving. In a closed hearing, she encouraged him to take responsibility and plead guilty. He did so, and finally got sober. Now this vigorous old man, so troubled and so beloved, had Covid—and Alzheimer's. When Klobuchar visited him, at an assisted living facility, they were separated by a window. He recognized her but he couldn't figure out why they had to be apart. He sang to her, "Happy Days Are Here Again." Amy believed that it would be the last time she would ever see him, but Jim Klobuchar beat the odds once again.

ABOUT THREE THOUSAND healthcare workers in the U.S. who took care of Covid patients in 2020 have died of the disease. Nurses are the most likely to perish, as they spend more time with the patients. The first one to die at Bellevue was on April 13, near the peak of the spring surge, but the traumas continued even after the contagion receded. "One of the things we really worried about was the well-being of nurses and physicians, not during the event, but actually after, when things calm down," Dr. Doug Bails said. In June, the hospital had a conference to review how the staff were handling the psychological stress they endured. "Some of the residents had trouble listening," Bails said. "After it all happens is when you lose it emotionally." When new Covid patients appeared, healthcare workers were often triggered by memories of their lost comrades. On June 29, Bellevue staff members gathered in the garden facing First Avenue to plant cherry blossom trees in their honor. There are seven trees.

As the coronavirus withdrew from Bellevue, it left perplexity behind. Why had death rates declined? Bails wondered if the virus had mutated to a less virulent state. Dr. Nate Link thought that therapeutic treatments were working, but that might be because the patients were now younger. A WHO study of remdesivir and three other potential treatments found "little or no effect" on hospitalized patients. According to Bails: "We have no real new or effective treatment or lessons about treatment that I believe to be very impactful." Dr. Amit Uppal pointed out that the hospital was much better at managing the disease. The challenge had become how to prepare for the vaccine and determine who received the very limited emergency supply.

When a patient was discharged, it offered a rare moment for the staff to celebrate. On August 4, a beaming Chris Rogan was wheeled by his wife, Crystal, past cheering healthcare workers, in scrubs and masks. There were balloons and bouquets. After so much death, a miracle occurred.

Chris was an account manager for a health insurance firm in midtown, and Crystal was a teaching assistant. In late March, he developed a low-grade fever and stomach discomfort, but he wasn't coughing. His doctor thought he had the flu. Rogan grew increasingly lethargic. He developed pneumonia. An ambulance took him to Metropolitan Hospital, on the Upper East Side. He still felt okay, even when his oxygen level fell to 64 percent, but within an hour after he checked in, he couldn't breathe. He was placed in a medically induced coma and intubated for nine days. During that time, the ventilator clogged and Rogan's heart stopped for three minutes. When he was brought back to consciousness, a doctor asked, "Did you see anything while you were dead?"

"No," said Rogan. "I don't even remember being resuscitated."

He began experiencing what hospital staffers told him was ICU psychosis. He told Crystal that he'd been stabbed as a child. He began conversing with God. Just before he was intubated again, on April 15, he felt certain that he would die in the hospital. He didn't wake up for sixty-one days.

During that time, he was transferred to Bellevue, which was better equipped to handle him. His chart described him as "a 29 y.o. transgender male" with a history of asthma, hypertension, and hypothyroidism. Before being transferred to Bellevue, the notes say, "He had one episode of cardiac arrest" as well as hypoxia. He continued to be ventilated.

It's a mistake to think that a patient in a coma is totally unaware. Rogan swam in and out of near-consciousness. When his doctor came in, he imagined being able to talk to him: "Why am I awake? Why can't I move?" He couldn't sleep, because his eyes were partly open. "It's like being buried alive," he said.

His tenth wedding anniversary passed. Sometimes he heard Crystal's voice on video chat. "I hear you," he'd say. "I feel the tube down my throat, tell them to take me off the vent." But she couldn't hear him. A machine kept pumping oxygen into his lungs: *psht! psht! psht!* The sound pounded in his head. He would dream that he had left the hospital, then wake to find himself still there, the ventilator pumping away, ceaselessly. "It was fucking torture," he said.

He developed internal bleeding. Clots formed in his legs. He told God he didn't want to die—that he had too much left to do. In a perfectly human voice, God assured him that he was going to make it.

Crystal was charged with making choices for Chris's care. The hardest one was the decision to amputate his right leg. It took three days to get him stable enough to perform the operation, which had to be done at his bedside because he was too fragile to move. The doctors performed a rare "guillotine" amputation, just below the knee. Eight days later, they had to take off the knee.

Rogan didn't remember any of that.

When he emerged from the coma, he couldn't move his arms, but eventually his right hand became functional. After several weeks of rehab, he could walk a bit with a prosthetic leg. These days, he is sometimes elated to be alive; other times, he asks himself, "What kind of quality of life is this?" Whether or not it was ICU psychosis, he's clung to the experience of talking with God.

When he fell ill, there were 150,000 cases in the U.S. When he left the hospital there were more than four million. Chris Rogan's story was one of them.

OPERATION WARP SPEED, the government initiative to accelerate vaccine development, may prove to be the Trump administration's most notable success in the pandemic. Deborah Birx gives much of the credit to Jared Kushner for pushing it through the administration. On December 11, the FDA granted its first Emergency Use Authorization for a Covid vaccine. Created by Pfizer, in partnership with the German firm BioNTech, it used the modified protein that Barney Graham and Jason McLellan designed. In its third and final human trial, it was deemed 95 percent effective. The first employee at U.Va.'s hospital to get the Pfizer inoculation was Ebony Hilton.

Moderna's vaccine secured approval next. Its formulation proved to be 94.1 percent effective in blocking Covid-19 and 100 percent effective in preventing serious disease. Graham is happy that he chose to work with Moderna. In 2016, his lab developed a vaccine for Zika, a new virus that caused birth defects. His department did everything itself: "We developed the construct, we made the DNA, we did Phase 1 clinical trials, and then we developed the regulatory apparatus to take it into Central and South America and the Caribbean, to test it for efficacy." The effort nearly broke the staff. Moderna was an ideal partner to shoulder the load for the Covid project, and its messenger-RNA vector was far more potent than the DNA vaccine that Graham's lab had been using.

Eli Lilly received emergency authorization for a monoclonal antibody that is also based on the spike protein that Graham and McLellan designed. It is similar to the treatment that President Trump received when he contracted Covid.

Graham was in his home office, in Rockville, Maryland, when he got a call telling him that the Pfizer version of his vaccine was breathtakingly effective—far better than could have been hoped for. "It was just hard to imagine," he recalled. He walked into the kitchen to share the news with his wife. Their son and grandchildren were visiting. "I told Cynthia, 'It's working.' I could barely get the words out. Then I just had to go back into my study, because I had this major relief. All that had been built up over those ten months just came out." He sat at his desk and wept. His family gathered around him. He hadn't cried that hard since his father died.

"Almost every aspect of my life has come together in this outbreak," he told me. "The work on enhanced disease, the work on RSV [respiratory syncytial virus] structure, the work on coronavirus and pandemic preparedness, along with all the things I learned and experienced about racial issues in this country. It just feels like some kind of destiny."

THE DEATH TOLL kept mounting. Some of them were well known. Terrence McNally, the playwright, was one of the first. Ellis Marsalis was a jazz pianist and an endearingly grumpy teacher who fathered not only a musical family but a generation of New Orleans musicians. I interviewed him years ago, and he left his mark on me as well. I had also interviewed Tom Seaver, one of the greatest pitchers in baseball history, a fiery competitor, but what struck me was his graciousness. Charley Pride was the first Black singer in the Country Music Hall of Fame. Phil Spector was a legendary music producer, who died in prison after being convicted of murder. Most of the victims were elderly, or minorities, or confined, so their losses were not so visible. One has to wonder how the nation might have responded had the victims been younger, whiter, richer, or better known.

It feels odd to find myself sorted into the vulnerable population, among the elderly. I'm a year younger than Donald Trump, so his adventure with Covid-19 was of considerable interest to me. If I got ill, I wouldn't be likely to receive the kind of treatment the president did, but I'm in better physical condition, despite a bout of cancer. My wife, though, has compromised lungs. Even before the coronavirus put a target on our age group, mortality was much on my mind. Sometimes I'm dumbstruck by how long I've lived; for instance, when I'm filling out a form on the internet, and I come to the drop-down menu for year of birth, the years fly by, past the loss of parents and friends, past wars and assassinations, past presidential administrations—more than a third of American history since the Declaration of Independence has unspooled in my lifetime.

On September 9, at two in the morning, our grandchild Gioia was born. She's the dearest creature. We stare into each other's eyes in wonder. Even in this intimate moment, the menace of contagion is present. We are more likely to infect the people we love than anyone else.

Deborah Birx has recalled that, in 1918, her grandmother, age eleven, brought the flu home from school to her mother, who died of it. "My grandmother lived with that for 88 years," she said.

Uncounted in the tally of death is the grief of the survivors who spread the contagion, possibly not even knowing they were ill, leaving illness and death behind, and carrying memories they will never be able to bury.

DEBORAH BIRX HADN'T SEEN the president since the summer, when Scott Atlas seized the role of Trump's closest health adviser. But she continued to write her daily brief, and her tone was increasingly alarmed. She concluded her report on October 17 with a desperate plea: "There is an absolute necessity of the Administration to use this moment to ask the American people to wear masks, physical distance and avoid gatherings in both public and private spaces." That same day, the president held large rallies in Michigan and Wisconsin. "We are entering the most concerning and most deadly phase of this pandemic . . . leading to increasing mortality," Birx warned again on November 2. "Cases are rapidly rising in nearly 30 percent of all USA counties, the highest number of county hotspots we have seen," she wrote. "Half of the United States is in the red or orange zone for cases despite flat or declining testing." She was preaching to the wind.

Thanksgiving was Birx's first day off in months. She and her husband have a house in Washington, D.C., and her daughter's family lives in nearby Potomac, Maryland. They were a pod so they could see each other safely. Birx had purchased another house, in Delaware, and after Thanksgiving, she, her husband, and her daughter's family spent the weekend there, to fix up the new house. A few days later, a news report revealed that she had traveled over the Thanksgiving weekend, counter to the CDC's recommendation. In the press and on the internet, she was plunged into a cold bath of schadenfreude. Old photographs resurfaced online, making it look as if she were currently attending Christmas parties.

She realized it would soon be time to leave government service.

———

THE COVID RECESSION of 2020 marked the worst year of economic growth since the middle of the twentieth century, which is when modern economic statistics began. The economy shrank by 3.5 percent, compared to 2.5 percent during the lowest point of the 2008 Great Recession.

Perhaps a third of New York City's small businesses are gone for good. More than half of the nation's Black-owned businesses may not survive. "We are crushing the economy," Texas lieutenant governor Dan Patrick said on Fox News, suggesting that old people, such as himself, should be willing to sacrifice themselves for the sake of their children and grandchildren. "We've got to take some risks and get back in the game and get this country back up and running." But old people didn't cause the economy to slow down; it was the reluctance of consumers to shop, of working people to go back to the office, of families to send their children to school, of travelers to fly, and of diners to eat in crowded restaurants. Until the spread of the virus was halted or the disease cured, the economy would continue to sputter. "We don't have an economic problem, we have a disease problem," Senator Lamar Alexander told me. Reopening prematurely and trying to push people back into the public arena only led to more infections and new shutdowns. People were waiting for the coast to clear.

"We are nearing the end of the beginning," Steve Strongin at Goldman Sachs said at the end of the year. "The shared experience is declining, but the pain is not done yet. This will make the public policy debate harder and the markets less correlated.

"The good news is that there is a lot of good news coming—new medicines, new jobs, new businesses. The bad news is that it will take a long time for the good news to compensate for the very real damage that has already been done, though in many cases not yet recognized, as many damaged businesses have not yet closed and many jobs that no longer make economic sense have not yet been eliminated."

The coronavirus will change investing forever, he believed. "Covid-19 is the type of event that resets the entire economy," he wrote in a recent Goldman white paper. "For investors and companies this is an existential event where capital needs to find new homes and where yesterday's strategies will only work by accident."

THE ST. JAMES THEATRE still sat empty on West 44th Street, the doors shuttered, the marquee dark. Jordan Roth hadn't been back. "I'm not sure how it will feel," he said. He always loved being in an empty theater before a show, when it felt like the theater was "resting," saving its energy for the performance. "I always believed these buildings are living organisms. You can feel the life force in them." He confessed that he was reluctant to return while the theater remained in an altered state, a kind of limbo or stasis. "Part of me is afraid of what would be missing when we return. But I know it's still there. It's still there. It's just waiting for us." Meantime, in the St. James, as in every theater, a single bulb on a metal stand, called a ghost light, stands in the center of the stage, keeping the bygone spirits of actors and the characters they played from running riot.

Austin's economy also depends on tourism and entertainment. The city bills itself as "The Live Music Capital of the World," but the bars and dance halls that made that boast real were all closed. Threadgill's, a roadhouse on North Lamar Boulevard where Janis Joplin got her start, was being torn down. Clubs on Sixth Street, Austin's answer to Bourbon Street, were boarded up. For the past several years a band I play in has had a regular Sunday gig at the Skylark Lounge. It's a shack on the east side of town, tucked behind an auto body shop in a former lumberyard. Johnny LaTouf runs the place with his ex-wife, Mary. It's been closed since March 15, when the governor shuttered the bars.

"All small businesses have been affected, but music venues around the country were already in a struggle," Johnny told me. "Covid killed off more than people with pre-existing conditions. Lots of businesses have pre-existing conditions as well. Covid accelerated those deaths." He's had to let go his ten employees, including three family members, but that's only part of the damage. "When the musicians get laid off and the bands disperse and go their separate ways, then you've actually broken up *their* business."

Skylark brings in a mixed crowd. We usually opened for Soul Man Sam, who drew a predominantly African American audience; ours was younger and whiter. Miss Lavelle White, born in 1929, was still singing the blues at Skylark until the doors closed. "Some of our greater musicians are older, because it takes a lifetime to master the craft," Johnny said. The Skylark was like a mixing bowl, where younger musicians learned from their elders. "Now that pathway is broken." Several of those older musicians who played at Skylark have passed away, others are struggling financially. Johnny helps out with groceries, but he doesn't know how many of that crowd will return.

When the CARES Act was passed, containing money to support small businesses, Johnny wasn't able to benefit. Bars were low on the list of priorities, and by the time Johnny got to his branch of Wells Fargo he was told "There's no money."

EVEN BEFORE THE ELECTION, Matt and Yen Pottinger decided they had had enough of Washington. He was burned out on the task force, which had drifted into irrelevance as the administration embraced magical thinking. They drove west, looking for a new place to live, and settled on a little ski town in Utah. They bought a house on the spot and moved all their belongings, except an inflatable mattress, some of Matt's suits, and the food Yen left for him in the pantry. He planned to stay in Washington, living with their pet rabbit, Cinnamon Bun, and working with the transition to the Biden administration.

After he withdrew from the task force, he quietly started a series of parallel efforts in the National Security Council, including diversifying the supply chain so the nation wouldn't be so dependent on China. Pottinger required the Departments of Defense and Veterans Affairs to meet with him twice a week to pool the data about sick veterans. He also met with the Department of Energy, which runs the Oak Ridge National Laboratory in Tennessee; it contains what was at the time the fastest supercomputer in the world. "Let's just jam all that data through the supercomputer and see what we learn about this thing," he said. Something interesting did arise: a peptide called bradykinin that regulates blood pressure was wildly out of balance in Covid-19 patients, causing leaky blood vessels. The "bradykinin hypothesis" could account for many of the weird manifestations of the disease, such as the dark, swollen toes, the loss of the senses of taste and smell, and the formation of a kind of gel that clogs the lungs and causes patients to suffocate even when they are ventilated. Fortunately, there are already drugs used to treat bradykinin irregularities, and they are now in clinical trials for Covid patients.

Pottinger's experience has made him acutely aware of what he calls "the fading art of leadership." It's not a failure of one party or another; it's more of a generational decline of good judgment. "The elites think it's all about expertise," he said. It's important to have experts, but they aren't always right. They can be "hampered by their own orthodoxies, their own egos, their own narrow approach to the world." He concluded: "You need broad-minded leaders who know how to hold people accountable, who know how to delegate, who know a good chain of command, and know how to make hard judgments."

At the end of October, before heading back to D.C., Pottinger went on a trail ride in the Wasatch Range. As it happened, Deborah Birx had arrived in Salt Lake City. Utah had just hit a record high number of new cases. On the ride, an alarm sounded on Pottinger's cell phone in the saddlebag. It was an alert: "Almost every single county is a high transmission area. Hospitals are nearly overwhelmed. By public health order masks are required in high transmission areas."

Pottinger thought, "Debi must have met with the governor."

25

Surrender

A MERICA WAS BOUND to suffer from Covid-19; every nation has. Opportunities were missed, first in China, which acted to suppress critical information about the new virus and the fact that asymptomatic carriers were contagious. Had the Chinese been transparent, other nations might have gotten a head start on their preparation. A week or two or three would have allowed governments to stockpile equipment and consider travel bans. Those countries that did act quickly, such as Taiwan and South Korea, did so in part because of their previous experience with Chinese obfuscation.

Nearly a month had passed between the discovery of the virus and the admission by Chinese authorities, on January 20, that it was transmissible between people. By that time, the CDC had already designed a test at breakneck speed. The FDA took another two weeks to approve what turned out to be a flawed test kit. That cost an additional three critical weeks, when the nation was blinded to the explosive spread of the new disease. There was still time to reduce the toll of death and suffering. No other country could match the scientific and medical expertise that America had to offer. Tens of thousands of people were bound to perish. But perhaps not hundreds of thousands.

Two qualities determined success or failure in dealing with the Covid contagion. One was experience. Some places that had been seared by past diseases applied those lessons to the current pandemic. Vietnam,

Taiwan, and Hong Kong had been stricken by SARS. In Taiwan, some eight hundred people had contracted Covid-19 by the end of 2020 and only seven died. Saudi Arabia did better than many countries, perhaps because of its history with MERS (and the fact that many women routinely wear facial coverings). Africa had a surprisingly low infection rate, in part because the experience with HIV/AIDS and Ebola has schooled the continent in the mortal danger of ignoring medical advice.

The other quality was leadership. Nations and states that did well have been led by strong, compassionate, decisive leaders who speak candidly with their constituents. Early on, West Virginia, which was ranked as the state with the greatest share of adults at risk of serious illness if infected with Covid, managed to test all of its 28,000 nursing home residents in two weeks and would become a leader in the vaccine rollout. In Vermont, Phil Scott, the Republican governor, closed the state early and reopened cautiously, keeping the case load and death toll low. "This should be the model for the country," Fauci told state leaders in September. If the national case fatality rate were the same as Vermont's, some 250,000 Americans would still be alive at the end of 2020. Granted, Vermont has fewer than a million people, but so does South Dakota, which was topping a thousand cases a day in November. Scott ordered Vermont to shut down in March, causing an immediate economic contraction. Governor Noem opposed mandates of any sort, betting that South Dakotans would act in their best interests while keeping the economy afloat. Vermont's economy recovered, with an unemployment rate of 3.2 percent—about the same as South Dakota's. But South Dakota has seen twelve times as many deaths.

In Michigan, the state's chief medical officer, Joneigh Khaldun, is a Black emergency room doctor. "She was one of the first to look at the demographics of Covid and highlight that we have a real racial disparity here," Governor Whitmer told me. "Fourteen percent of our population is Black and forty percent of the early deaths." That led to aggressive outreach to Black communities in the state. By August, the rates of both cases and fatalities for Blacks were the same as—or lower than—those for whites. The vast differences in outcomes among the states underscore the absence of a national plan.

Seattle, the first city struck by the coronavirus, wound up with the lowest death rate among large metropolitan areas. Despite its rigorous restrictions on public gatherings and business openings, Washington state's economy suffered but wound up outperforming places, such as Texas and Arizona, that rushed to reopen. Seattle's success has many probable reasons, among them a healthy workforce that could largely work remotely. Unified messaging from political officials and public health authorities was essential. Paul Pottinger points to the "unusual nature of our public health and university system," which worked together to patrol the outbreak. "But frankly I am very humble about Seattle's success, because so much of it has come down to the decisions and actions of ordinary citizens," he wrote me. "I recall coming to work on March 5, 2020, the first day when the governor's 'stay home' order was in place. The streets were EMPTY. It was very striking and eerie. And so uplifting, because people understood what was at stake." This was at a time when New York's mayor was still urging citizens to go out on the town. Seattle's death rate from Covid-19 was 64 people per 100,000, compared with 294 for New York and 201 for Los Angeles. Detroit, the city closest in size to Seattle, suffered 202 deaths per 100,000.

By the end of 2020, the death rate per 100,000 for the United States as a whole was 134.89; in other words, more than one American died for every thousand people in the country. That was nearly two and a half times the rate in Canada, at 53.98. Only Italy and the U.K. had higher rates than the U.S. among countries most affected by Covid. In the first half of 2020, life expectancy in the U.S. fell by a full year, from 78.8 years to 77.8, the largest drop since the Second World War. By the end of the year, the United States had more cases and more deaths than any other country. The actual tally will never be known, but a retrospective serological study estimated that 35 percent of Covid deaths went unreported. Total deaths increased by 15 percent, making 2020 the deadliest year in recorded U.S. history. The figure that will haunt America is that the U.S. accounts for about 20 percent of all the Covid fatalities in the world, despite having only 4 percent of the population.

At the beginning of the pandemic, China's unprecedented lockdown, compared to the initial halting reaction in Italy, suggested that autocratic systems had an unbeatable advantage in dealing with a contagion like that of SARS-CoV-2. Over time, however, democratic regimes found their footing and did marginally better than authoritarian ones. Advanced countries performed better than developing ones, but not by as much as might have been expected. Due to the high volume of air travel, richer countries were quickly overwhelmed, while poorer countries had more time to prepare for the onslaught. High-tech medical advantages proved of little use when the main tools for countering the spread of the disease were social distancing, hand washing, and masks. This can be seen in the rankings by the Lowy Institute of the performance of countries managing the pandemic. The top ten countries are:

New Zealand
Vietnam
Taiwan
Thailand
Cyprus
Rwanda
Iceland
Australia
Latvia
Sri Lanka

The United States ranked number 94 out of 98, between Bolivia and Iran. China was not included in the rankings because of the lack of transparency in its testing.

The Pew Research Center surveyed fourteen advanced countries to see how they viewed the world during the pandemic. In Denmark, 95 percent of the respondents agreed that their country had handled the crisis capably. In Australia, the figure was 94 percent; Germany was 88 percent. The United Kingdom and the U.S. were the only countries where a majority disagreed. In Denmark, 72 percent said that the country had become more unified since the contagion emerged. Only 18 percent of Americans agreed with the statement. In every country surveyed, people ranked the U.S. response lowest. And respondents in most countries said that China was now the leading economic power, not the U.S.

Each of these categories is a measure of leadership.

IN THE EARLY MONTHS of the contagion in America, President Trump did show leadership. He shut down travel from China and then from

Europe at a time when such bans were rare and unpopular. Matt Pottinger believed that if Trump hadn't ended travel from Europe, there would be up to a million dead Americans. On March 16, the president followed the guidance of his public health advisers and issued nationwide recommendations for school closures, shutting down bars and restaurants, and limiting unnecessary travel and social gatherings. But that same day marked a turning point. In his conversation with governors that morning, he abandoned any effort to coalesce a national plan, and his administration began undercutting governors' attempts to acquire the personal protective equipment that their frontline workers needed. Then, on April 3, at a press briefing, the president introduced the new CDC guidance for masks. "It's going to be, really, a voluntary thing," he said. "You can do it. You don't have to do it. I'm choosing not to do it, but some people may want to do it, and that's okay. It may be good. Probably will. They're making a recommendation. It's only a recommendation. It's voluntary."

By his words and his example, the president became not a leader but a saboteur. He ridiculed mask-wearing. He campaigned against taking the pandemic seriously. He subverted his health agencies by installing political operatives who meddled with the science and suppressed the truth. His unmasked political rallies were reckless acts of effrontery. In his Tulsa speech, he frankly admitted that he had told his health officials to "slow the testing down please," so the numbers, the growing constituency of the infected, would be hidden from view. When he finally, inevitably, contracted the disease, he almost certainly spread it. Every guest at the Barrett reception tested negative for the virus before entering. Most likely, Trump was the superspreader in the Rose Garden. He failed to isolate himself after his close adviser, Hope Hicks, tested positive. Instead, he went to his golf club in Bedminster, New Jersey, for a fundraiser, unmasked. That night, he and the first lady tested positive and the next day Trump was flown to Walter Reed. If he were not president, he might have died. The disease killed many like him, an overweight older man; instead, he was treated aggressively with experimental drugs that few Americans had access to. His recovery was a victory for medical science and a sharp reminder of the disparity in treatment Americans can expect, depending on their race and influence.

There was another path he might have taken. He could have chosen to bring the country together to fight this deadly disease. In the same press conference where he announced he would not be wearing a mask, he praised the efforts of Democratic governors in New York and New Jersey; he expressed sympathy for the people of Michigan, who are "getting hit very, very hard." He announced federal efforts to aid New York City. "America is engaged in a historic battle to safeguard the lives of our citizens, our future society," he said. "Our greatest weapon is the discipline and determination of every citizen to stay home and stay healthy. . . . We will heal our citizens and we will care for our neighbors, and we will unleash the full might of the United States of America to vanquish the virus." The man who said those words might have been the president the country needed. But he was not that president.

Instead, with voters already mailing in their ballots or standing in long lines at the polls, he campaigned against the disease. "When the year started, he appeared unbeatable," Senator Lee told me. "My Democratic colleagues were discouraged about their chances. By the end of the impeachment trial, when we began hearing about the virus, we were not sure it would be a big deal. But it put an end to one of the things the president is best at—those big rallies." When Trump finally resumed them, defying medical advice and leaving a trail of infections behind him, his fury was volcanic. "People are tired of hearing Fauci and all these idiots," he grumbled on October 19, when the number of new cases topped 65,000. "Covid, Covid, Covid, Covid, Covid, Covid! A plane goes down, five hundred people dead, they don't talk about it," he complained at a rally in North Carolina, five days later. He added: "We're rounding the turn, we're doing great. Our numbers are incredible." That day nearly 80,000 new cases were reported, overshadowing the highest levels of the summer. "You notice the fake news, now, right? All they talk about is Covid, Covid, Covid, Covid, Covid," he said at a rally in Omaha on October 27. "I'm here, right? . . . I had it." Hospitalizations were up 46 percent that month.

"Hey, excuse me, I'm sure you didn't hear," Trump said on October 29, in Tampa. "Nobody heard this, right? I had it. Did you know that? I had to get back on the trail. I said, 'This is not good timing.' And I got better very quickly." He indicated his wife, Melania, who was present at the speech. "She had it and she got better very quickly." Their fourteen-year-old son, Barron, also tested positive, but he got over it, "like twelve minutes later." The president attacked Democratic governors, ignoring the fever sweeping through the Mountain West and the Great Plains— Trump country. He boasted, "If I can get better, anybody can get better." More than a thousand Americans died that day.

In counties where the president held a rally, an increase in Covid cases often followed. The surging number of infections and deaths mocked his assertion that "we're rounding the turn." Instead, the disease stalked him; it encircled him. Trump's own chief of staff, Mark Meadows, conceded, "We are not going to control the pandemic." The administration had yielded to a force far better adapted to its purpose.

Covid didn't kill Donald Trump, but it would defeat him.

Five days before the election, Joe Biden spoke at a drive-in rally in Tampa. "So much pain, so much suffering, so much loss in America," he said. "More than 225,000 people dead, 225,000. The estimates are, if we'd have acted responsibly, there'd be 160,000 fewer dead than there are today. . . . Donald Trump has waved the white flag, abandoned our families, and surrendered to the virus." Honking cars punctuated his remarks. That day new confirmed cases topped 90,000.

The next day, Fauci warned, "We're in for a whole lot of hurt. It's not a good situation." New cases surpassed 98,000. "All the stars are aligned in the wrong place as you go into the fall and winter season, with people congregating at home indoors. You could not possibly be positioned more poorly."

Halloween was a beautiful night, graced with a blue moon. We set out a bowl of chocolate bars and Dum-Dums, but there were scarcely any trick-or-treaters. As dusk settled over the city, when our neighborhood would normally be filled with fairies and vampires, a deer galloped down the street.

AMERICA IS FULL of strivers whose dreams seem just out of reach. Iris Meda was one of them. She had a big smile but sad eyes. She grew up in Harlem, the oldest of six children. Her mother was a domestic who was home only one day a week; her stepfather was a longshoreman. Iris's first bed was an ironing board.

For most of her childhood, she was the family caretaker, walking her siblings to school before she went herself. Like many of her high school friends, she dropped out, after a bout of depression. She married and had two daughters. Iris eventually got a GED and surprised herself by graduating at the top of her class from Bronx Community College. In 1984, she earned a nursing degree from City College. Medicine fascinated her. She would go home and talk about watching a surgeon crack open a patient's chest and massage his heart. She worked for a while in a children's burn unit. She was drawn to those who were wounded or hurting—people who felt that the world wasn't big enough for them. For years, she was a nurse at the Rikers Island jail. She cared about the prisoners, and they knew it. When her husband was transferred to Dallas, she gave notice, and on her last day the inmates clapped her out. "She was always looking for an underdog to pull up, because she was an underdog," her daughter, Selene Meda-Schlamel, said.

Iris Meda retired in January 2020, after two years in the North Texas Job Corps. She had been in charge of on-site care, meaning that she was on call nights and weekends, and when she turned seventy she decided that she'd had enough. She and Selene had big plans. Iris wanted to travel; she hoped to ride in a convertible for the first time; she talked about writing a book. "In March, it all came to a screeching halt," Selene said, referring to the lockdown. Her mother was still a proud New Yorker, so she spent a lot of time during the shutdown in front of the TV watching Dr. Fauci and Governor Cuomo. "Her knowledge of science kept her ahead of the news reports," Selene said. Iris, having worked in nursing homes, hospitals, and jails, knew that Covid would be devastating for people who were confined and for those who took care of them.

Idled by the crisis, Iris longed to teach. "She wanted to encourage younger nurses to continue their education," Selene said. "She wanted them to reach their full potential in a way she almost didn't." Iris successfully applied for a job at Collin College, in Allen, Texas, a suburb of Dallas. At the time, courses were being offered virtually, and Iris imagined that she would be teaching online in the fall, but when the semester began, she learned that her class was in person. The college's president, H. Neil Matkin, had made his views of the virus known in an email to trustees: "The effects of this pandemic have been blown utterly out of proportion across our nation."

Iris hoped to be in a large classroom where students could be widely spaced, but she was assigned to teach a lab for a nurse's aide course. There would be no social distancing. On October 2, a student was coughing and sneezing, complaining of allergies. That was the day Trump announced that he had Covid. Iris was repulsed when the president insisted on taking a car ride to wave at his supporters outside the hospital, with Secret Service agents in the car with him. Iris texted Selene: "He's putting all those people at risk just for a photo."

On October 7, Iris learned that the student had tested positive. The college chose to continue in-person classes even after one student died. By this time, Trump was out of the hospital, saying he felt "better than twenty years ago."

Iris became feverish on October 12. Two days later, she tested positive and went to the ER, but her oxygen level was not low enough for her to be admitted. On October 17, Selene took her mom back to the hospital. By now, she was seriously ill, but the staff, worried about Covid, kept her waiting outside, slumped over on a bench in the ER drive-through. When the triage nurse finally waved Iris in, Selene wasn't permitted to join her, because she had been exposed. Iris's oxygen level was now so low she couldn't speak. Selene didn't see her again for thirty days.

During that period, Iris was able to talk only once on the phone. Most days, she texted with Selene. Once she asked Selene to call a nurse who she thought was doing an excellent job. "She's having a hard day," Iris texted. She worried about her students and wondered if anyone else had caught the virus. (None showed symptoms.)

The disease progressed inexorably. Selene could tell that doctors were doing everything they could, but her mother's lungs wouldn't rebound. Selene wondered if things would be turning out differently had her mother received treatment earlier.

On November 14, Selene got a call advising that her mother's blood pressure was plummeting. "Based on how she's declining, how long do we have?" Selene asked, thinking that she would pick up her father so that he could say goodbye. "A couple hours," the doctor said. Ten minutes later, a nurse called and said, "Get here now."

"They put me in a helmet," Selene recalled. "There was a plastic flap that closed around my neck. Inside the helmet there was a fan at the top that blew air down, so that any air that got in would be flushed away.

And they put a gown on me, and double gloves, and they let me go in and say goodbye to her. That was the biggest shock, to see her, and to see how she looked. She was twice her size, because she was swollen from steroids. Her tongue was hanging out the side of her mouth because she was on the ventilator—she'd been intubated. They had to brace her head to keep it straight on the pillow, and they had tape around her mouth to keep the tube in. I'll never forget it. But I think the thing that will haunt me is the smell. It's like the smell of decay, like she had already started to die.

"The thing that made it so hard to see that was to juxtapose it against President Trump out there, saying he felt like he was twenty-eight years old again and he never felt better. So how could the same thing that did this to her, how could someone ever take it for granted that this was nothing, you have nothing to be afraid of?"

Selene gathered her mother in her arms as the machines went silent.

COVID-19 HAS BEEN hard on Little Africa. "Some of our church members have passed and quite a few of our friends," Mary Hilton, Ebony's mother, told me. One of her cousins was in the hospital as we talked. "We just buried one yesterday. They're dropping everywhere. It's so scary."

"One out of eight hundred Black Americans who were alive in January is now dead," Ebony told me, as the year came to a close. "There would be another twenty thousand alive if they died at the same rate as Caucasians." She and two colleagues have written a letter to the Congressional Black Caucus proposing the creation of a federal Department of Equity, to address the practices that have led to such disparate health outcomes.

Doctors everywhere have learned better ways of treating the disease, but deaths still batter morale. When we spoke, Hilton had recently attended the hospital's first lung transplant, a fit man in his forties, who contracted Covid. He survived. But more young people, including children, were populating the Covid wards. Hospitals and clinics all over the country were struggling financially, and many healthcare workers, including Hilton, took pay cuts.

Thanksgiving in Little Africa is usually a giant family reunion. Everyone comes home. There's one street where practically every house belongs to someone in Hilton's family; people eat turkey in one house and dessert in another. Hilton hadn't seen her family since March. She spent Thanksgiving alone in Charlottesville, with her dogs.

ON THE EVE of the election, Tucker Carlson posed a question on his Fox News show, asking why Donald Trump's voters love him so much. He showed a picture of a mass rally for the president in Butler, Pennsylvania, one of the many former industrial towns that have been gutted by the unwinding of American industry. "They made Pullman rail cars there for many years," Carlson observed. It had been losing population for decades. "The men of Butler may have built this country, and they did, but they mean nothing to our leaders now. You can be certain of that because when large numbers of people in Butler started killing themselves with narcotics, no one in Washington or New York or Los Angeles said a word about it." In 2017, there were so many opioid deaths in the little town of Butler—eighty-seven—that a makeshift monument was erected in the center of town in their memory. The number of drug overdoses in America continued to rise during the Trump era, reaching their highest levels ever in 2020. It was an epidemic within a pandemic.

"So, given all of that, it was interesting to see how people around Butler feel about Donald Trump," Carlson continued. "Pictures of the rally site showed a sea of people obscuring the horizon, the kind of image you would see in a visit of the pope." There were people wearing red MAGA hats waving PROMISES MADE, PROMISES KEPT signs. "They must have known that Donald Trump is the most evil man who has ever lived," Carlson said. "They've heard that every day for five years. They know that people who support Donald Trump are also evil, they're bigots, they're morons, they're racist cult members. . . . Only losers and freaks support Donald Trump.

"People in Butler knew all that. But on Saturday, they went to the Donald Trump rally anyway. Why exactly did they do that?" The answer, Carlson said, is they love him. "They're not deluded. They know exactly who Trump is. They love him anyway. They love Donald Trump because no one else loves them."

ELECTIONS REVEAL WHO we really are. They dispel illusions. They also offer the opportunity for change.

Not every American gets to vote. In San Quentin, a straw poll was held among prisoners in two of the cell blocks. Of the 176 ballots retrieved, a strong majority favored Biden. The men were given the opportunity to say why they voted the way they did, and why they wanted to vote at all. The Trump supporters liked the economic growth the president had created, along with his trade deals and his intention to build a wall on the southern border. "I want to vote because it is necessary that all voices be heard and to counter ethnic cleansing by way of prison," wrote Alex Ross, fifty-four, who had already served twenty-six years. Most of the men had never voted before they were incarcerated, but 98 percent said they would vote now if they had the chance. "The next president's job is going to be the hardest seat to fill because so many things are left broken," Rodney "Pit" Baylis, sixty, wrote. "To fill this seat everyone needs to help him. The Republicans and Democrats have to come together as one to fix this country."

My wife and I voted early, in a drop-off location in Travis County, where 97 percent of eligible voters were registered. It was a new way of voting—swift, efficient, and rather exhilarating. Austin is a deeply blue city, and Trump signs were rare. There was no doubt how the city was going to vote. But something was happening all over Texas. Nearly 17 million Texans were registered to vote in the state, a record, and 1.8 million of them were new voters. By October 30, more than 9 million Texans had already voted—more than the total vote in 2016. Moreover, Texas led the nation in voters under thirty, an increase of more than 600 percent over the last presidential election. Texas has long had the reputation of being a non-voting state, but even before November 3 it was clear that was no longer true. Whatever the outcome, the roots of democracy had sunk a little deeper in the obdurate soil of Texas.

The vote came amid a crescendo of bad news. The week before November 3, the country added half a million new Covid cases, reaching record highs in half the states. The stock market had its worst week since the swan dive in March, capping two straight months of losses. Eight million Americans had fallen into poverty since May. At least five members of Vice President Pence's staff were infected with Covid, as the virus continued to roam the halls of the White House. More than 130 Secret Service officers were quarantined or infected.

In Texas, as in many Republican states, there were naked attempts to suppress the vote. Governor Abbott restricted the number of drop-off sites to one per county, including in Harris County, which has over four million people. The attorney general, Ken Paxton, sued to block the enforcement of a mask requirement at the polls, endangering the voters as well as the poll workers, who tend to be older and more vulnerable. The governor readied a thousand National Guard troops in major cities in anticipation of violence. On the national scene, a "non-scalable" fence was erected around the White House. Store owners in cities around the country boarded up their windows, like beach communities in the face of an oncoming hurricane.

Voting is a simple act, but it is also an act of faith, a pledge of allegiance to the future of the country. All across America, people waited peacefully in long lines to vote—despite the disease, despite attempts to discredit or invalidate their vote, despite postal delays, despite threats of Russian or Iranian meddling, despite warnings from the White House that the president would not go quietly if he lost. They voted as if their country depended on it.

Epilogue

AFTER THE NEW YEAR, Matt Pottinger flew back to Washington to finish out his last weeks at the White House. As soon as he arrived, late Sunday evening, January 3, he began to hear about President Trump's threatening call to Brad Raffensperger, Georgia's secretary of state. After the ballots had been tabulated, and then manually recounted, it was determined that Joe Biden had won the state by 11,779 votes. According to the tape Raffensperger made of the telephone call, Trump claimed "We won very substantially in Georgia." Among his claims were that "at least a couple hundred thousand" ballots had been forged; thousands of voters had been turned away from the polls; others voted who weren't registered; thousands more voted who didn't have a valid address; and thousands of possible Trump votes had been dumped, shredded, or burned. "The other thing, dead people," the president said. "So dead people voted, and I think the number is close to five thousand people." Altogether, when the president toted up all these wholly imagined crimes, he figured that there were 300,000 fake ballots.

Raffensperger, a Republican, responded, "We don't agree that you have won."

"The people of Georgia are angry," Trump warned him. "The people of the country are angry. And there's nothing wrong with saying that, you know, that you've recalculated." But Raffensperger stood firm as the president tightened the screws, airing weird allegations about absent poll workers and compromised voting machines.

"We believe that we do have an accurate election," the Georgian said.

"No, no you don't!" Trump said. "Not even close." He finally got to the bottom line: "All I want to do is this. I just want to find 11,780 votes, which is one more than we [need] because we won the state. . . . And I think you have to say that you're going to reexamine it, and you can reexamine it, but reexamine it with people that want to find answers."

"We have to stand by our numbers," Raffensperger said.

When Pottinger heard the tape, his instinct was to resign on the spot. He'd already threatened to leave on at least seven occasions; there were several old resignation letters still stuck in his desk. But the implicit threats—"people are angry"—and the suggestion that the secretary of state, on his own, could simply "recalculate" and find the votes Trump needed, might have been voiced by a mafia boss. The president was in his final weeks in office; as much as Pottinger wanted to resign and walk away, he realized that until the new administration took over, the country faced profound security threats, which he characterized as a "white-knuckle ride through a haunted house."

Four years had passed since Mike Flynn, the former Marine general, had invited Pottinger to meet the president-elect in Trump Tower, to advise him about foreign policy. The invitation came as a result of a memo Pottinger had written about U.S. relations with Asia. He rode a Citibike to the glassy skyscraper on Fifth Avenue. Secret Service had cut off elevator access to the Trump quarters, so Pottinger walked up the remaining stairs, feeling a little disoriented. He emerged in an opulent apartment, slathered in blinding gilt. Steve Bannon, Trump's political guru, was there, along with Flynn. Jared Kushner wandered in with K.T. McFarland, who would serve briefly as deputy national security adviser, the position Pottinger would eventually hold. There were several other people Pottinger didn't know, none of whom had anything to do with Asia. Finally, Trump entered, and sat down, still wearing an overcoat, and went straight into a conversation with Kushner about Mexico, which took up most of the meeting.

At one point, Trump observed, "I am the greatest single negotiator in the world."

Who's he talking to? Pottinger wondered. Is he talking to me? I'm the only one in the room he doesn't know. But he's not looking at me. Is he talking to himself? Pottinger was rattled by Trump's narcissism and unfocused chatter. The fact this man was going to be president left Pottinger "scared shitless," as did the prospect of working for him. And yet the country was in grave danger. Flynn, the designated national security adviser, wanted Pottinger on his team. What was the right course of action?

He talked it over with Yen. They were a mixed couple, politically— she a Democrat, he a nominal independent who had voted for both parties, although he usually voted in a Republican primary. He explained that the country was at an inflection point in history, where everything could unravel. In some small way, he might be able to stand in the way of that. She had been heartbroken by the outcome of the election, and she wasn't happy about Matt's working for Trump, but she could see that Matt was tormented. She also realized that, if he didn't accept the job, he would be insufferable for the next four years, continually reprimanding himself whenever a false step was taken in Asia by the very naïve White House. Clearly, Matt was going to be miserable to live with, whether he took the job or not.

At first, she told herself that Matt was the perfect person for the job but he would be serving the wrong president. Eventually, she decided she had that backward. He would be far more needed by the Trump administration, which was so thinly staffed by foreign policy experts. Finally, she figured that, at his core, Matt was a good Marine. It was pointless to stand in the way of something he felt he had to do, to serve his country.

Everyone expected Pottinger's tenure would be brief, six months, maybe eighteen at the outside. His boss, Flynn, lasted only three weeks in the turbulent Trump White House, resigning after it was learned that he had misled Vice President Pence and other top White House officials about his communications with the Russian ambassador. Then H. R. McMaster took over the post, lasting a little more than a year; John Bolton, a month or two more than that. At each juncture, Pottinger was ready to leave, but somehow he never actually did. When O'Brien came in, he promoted Pottinger to be his deputy, replacing Charles Kupperman, who had been the acting national security adviser for all of eight days. Whatever institutional memory there was in the agency was invested in a still very conflicted Matt Pottinger.

He made a list of three reasons to stay: to keep the U.S. out of another war; to help the country compete effectively against China; and to protect the institution of the National Security Council, which the president repeatedly threatened to disband. In each of those categories, he had largely succeeded.

After Trump's attempted shakedown of the Georgia secretary of state, Matt called Yen again. Her advice was to get out, now. Trump continued to assail the legitimacy of the election, aided by the horn section of Fox News and by Republican elected officials who had placed their careers and reputations in the president's grip. But Matt had promised his chief, Robert O'Brien, that he would stay through the transition to the Biden team, which he felt obligated to do.

Much of the country knew that January 6, 2021, would be a day of reckoning. The electoral votes would be officially counted in Congress and Joe Biden would be formally designated president-elect. In the quadrennial ritual, electors from each of the fifty states and the territories arrive at the Capitol and present their votes. Trump had fixed on that day as his last stand. He had been rallying his supporters for weeks, encouraging them to come to Washington to join the "big protest" and overturn the "rigged election." It would take place as the pandemic was cresting, and the paranoia and social disruption caused by the yearlong siege was seeking catharsis. "Be there. Will be wild!" Trump tweeted.

Pottinger was staying in a house on Capitol Hill near the Library of Congress. That day, on his way to work, as he entered the Capitol South subway station, about 7:30 in the morning, he ran into a group of Trump supporters coming up the escalator, wearing flags and regalia. This group looked harmless; they were mostly gray-haired, with MAGA hats and hand-lettered signs. Dozens of groups had registered to march, but as far as Pottinger knew, there had been no warnings of a planned assault on the Capitol. As he rode in to work, Pottinger thought that, so long as no Biden supporters or Black Lives Matter counter-protesters got into the fray, there was little likelihood of violence.

The intelligence community gave daily briefings of terror threats; the Department of Justice, the FBI, the Department of Homeland Security, the National Counterterrorism Center, and the CIA all participate, along with the NSC. The FBI's only warning was that the bureau expected demonstrations at the Capitol by people "exercising their First Amendment rights." This was despite the fact that, on January 5, the FBI's office in Norfolk, Virginia, explicitly warned that extremists were coming to Washington to protest Trump's lost election and what they saw as unlawful lockdowns because of the coronavirus. The internet was choked with conspiracy threats. "Be ready to fight," one of the messages said. "Congress needs to hear glass breaking, doors being kicked in, and blood from their BLM and Pantifa [sic] slave soldiers being spilled. Get violent. Stop calling this a march, or rally, or a protest. Go there ready for war. We get our President or we die." None of this got into the daily terrorism briefing. It was the most inexcusable intelligence failure since 9/11.

Seeing the Trump supporters awakened in Pottinger the memory of the morning, four years before, when Hillary Clinton was defeated. Yen had cried herself to sleep that night, but Matt was too keyed up to sleep. He finally dressed and went for a walk. They were living in Manhattan's Upper West Side; it was early morning, still dark, and Matt walked down to the Javits Center, where Clinton had been expected to give her victory speech. It was dark and deserted. Then he crossed over to the New York Hilton Midtown, where Trump's supporters had celebrated their wildly unexpected victory. It was now nearly dawn and the party was over. Pottinger passed an open Starbucks near Columbus Circle. There was a girl crying, whom he pegged as a Clinton supporter. Other people were sleeping with their heads on the counters, a scene of exhaustion and abject desolation. Then, reflected in the glass, Pottinger noticed a group of construction workers on their way to work. They had a swagger in their step; one of them sported a Trump hat. Pottinger thought: Those are people who've been ignored for years. This is their moment. Maybe there's something in our political system that has gotten so out of kilter that only Trump's election might remedy.

Now, four years later, as the Trump supporters emerged from the subway—most of them older, working-class people who believed the president's lies about the stolen election—Pottinger felt that the country had come full circle, and neither party had remedied the social blight of the working class, the loss of jobs to China, the opioid crisis that followed, and the endless, futile foreign wars. The country was even more divided now than it had been then.

He got off at Farragut West Station and walked down 17th Street to the White House. There were larger crowds now. He made eye contact with a couple of middle-aged women wearing red, white, and blue. One of them smiled at him, so Pottinger struck up a conversation. They had driven all night from Charlotte, North Carolina, to hear the president speak at the "Save America" rally at noon. Pottinger asked them why they voted for Trump. They responded enthusiastically. He can't be bought, they said; he pays attention to people who've been ignored; he speaks his mind and doesn't care about polls. "We'd basically be living in a world run by China if not for him," one of them summed up. Pottinger was charmed; they were so undisillusioned. As they were standing just outside the White House gate, the women realized Pottinger actually worked there, and one of them blurted out, "Do you love Trump?"

Pottinger was caught short. He understood why these women adored Trump, but his own feelings were tangled and not yet sorted out. "Well, he's done some very important things, and he's got his flaws," he said lightly, trying to be both diplomatic and truthful.

"Don't say that!" one of them said. Her name was Stephanie; she identified herself as a realtor who had lost her job after posting pro-Trump messages on social media. She wasn't wearing a mask; fewer than half of the Trump supporters were. Pottinger wore an N95.

On a whim, he offered to take the women on a tour of the White House that afternoon. He was only going to be there a few more days himself, but he still had the power to grant these women a once-in-a-lifetime opportunity to peek into the most renowned chamber of power on earth. He reminded them that they would need to be masked. Then he went back to his office and forgot about it.

SINCE THE ELECTION, the president's calendar had been largely clear. Except for a few rounds of golf, he had practically no appointments the entire month of November. His wrathful mood suffused the White House; the staff and close advisers kept their distance. He passed his days brooding and tweeting about the "stolen" election. On January 4, he traveled to Georgia, where two Republican senators, David Perdue and Kelly Loeffler, were facing a runoff the next day, with control of the Senate in the balance. Trump had been floating the idea that the vice president could single-handedly subvert the results of the presidential election by refusing to accept the electoral votes, although Pence's actual role in the electoral college was ceremonial. "I hope Mike Pence comes through for us," Trump said in Georgia. "He's a great guy. Of course, if he doesn't come through, I won't like him as much." He drew a target on his most loyal officer for the mob he was summoning into action.

January 6 was chilly and partly cloudy in Washington. As thousands of his supporters assembled, the president and his family gathered with a few key insiders in a white tent on the Ellipse, below the South Lawn of the White House. Trump stood in front of a large video screen, staring at the images of the gathering throng. Around him, the mood was giddy. His son Don Jr. filmed a video selfie as Laura Branigan's disco hit "Gloria" blared out. The president was stoic and forbiddingly still. He appeared to be concentrating his powers on the host of followers who had responded to the siren of his implacable will.

The crowd filled the Mall, reaching from the Ellipse all the way to the Washington Monument, recently reopened after years of repairs following an earthquake in 2011. "All of us here today do not want to see our election victory stolen by emboldened and radical left Democrats, which is what they're doing, and stolen by the fake news media," Trump said when he took the stage, backed by a bank of American flags, and behind that, the majestic White House. "We will never give up. We will never concede. . . . We're going to have to fight much harder and Mike Pence is going to have to come through for us. And if he doesn't, that will be a sad day for our country. . . . We're going to walk down to the Capitol and we're going to cheer on our brave senators and congressmen and women, and we're probably not going to be cheering so much for some of them. Because you'll never take back our country with weakness. You have to show strength."

POTTINGER WAS LEAVING a lunch at the Indian Embassy when he got the word from his deputy that the mayor of Washington, D.C., Muriel Bowser, had ordered a curfew for 6:00 p.m. He wondered if something had happened. When he got back to the White House, his staff were transfixed by the scenes on television. Pottinger saw the crowd pushing down the metal barricades and shoving reporters, but they hadn't yet reached the Capitol. The president's supporters stretched for blocks down Pennsylvania Avenue, a sea of MAGA hats. They were carrying American flags and Trump banners and QAnon signs. For many—perhaps most—of them, their goal was already accomplished: they had listened to the president and they were marching to the Capitol. What they would do when they arrived was not settled in their minds. One could still call them demonstrators or protesters, but a crowd so large is aware of its power; and inside the ranks were some who had trained for this. They wore tactical outfits and carried makeshift weapons and gear—crowbars, bullhorns, Kevlar helmets, flexicuffs, hidden guns—signaling their intent. The cops tried flash bangs and tear gas to contain them, but the mob responded with bear spray, pummeling the police with fists and flagpoles. They chased the officers up the Capitol steps, wrestling polycarbonate riot shields out of their hands and using them to break the windows. One cop was dragged down the steps and beaten with a pole holding an American flag.

At 2:24 p.m., the president tweeted, "Mike Pence didn't have the courage to do what should have been done." A few minutes later, he added, "Stay peaceful!" but by then the delirious mob was roaming through the halls, past statues of the founders and the heroes of American history. Murder was on the mind of many who were crying "Hang Mike Pence!" They broke through the doors to Speaker Nancy Pelosi's suite as her staff cowered under a table in the conference room. A gallows was erected near the reflecting pool. It was a scene that summoned images of the Visigoths bursting through the gates of Rome. Eighteen seconds after 2:42 p.m., the seismograph recently installed on the Washington Monument recorded what appeared to be an earthquake radiating from the Capitol.

Senator Patty Murray was in her office, preparing to respond to the objections that were about to be raised to count the electoral votes. She felt safe; she had always felt safe in the Capitol, except for 9/11. That day, through her window, she had seen smoke rising from the Pentagon. Police officers had evacuated the Capitol. It was terrifying, but there was a consoling sense of solidarity among the members back then. There was none of that now, as she looked out the window again and saw the mob outside. Suddenly she heard explosions, and then there were people racing through the hallways, some yelling "Kill the infidels!" the battle cry of al-Qaeda, transported into an American mob that was emulating its terrorist model. Murray was struck by how jubilant their voices were.

"We saw them," one of the rioters said, as they pounded on Murray's door. "They're in one of these rooms."

Murray's husband, Rob Murray, sat on the floor holding the door closed with his foot. Patty couldn't remember if she had locked it or not. She looked at Rob. "The terror I saw in his eyes was something I have not seen, and we have been married for almost forty-nine years."

Inside the House chamber, Representative Paul Gosar of Arizona and Senator Ted Cruz of Texas posed their objections to certifying the votes from Arizona, the first of the four states that the obstructionists hoped to block from being counted. The Congress then divided into their separate chambers to debate the issue.

Shortly after 3:00 p.m. Pottinger went into his office and turned on his television. He got a message informing him that the Pentagon had rejected the National Guard troops the mayor had asked for. He ran to the president's reception area outside the Oval Office to tell Meadows about the mayor's request. The office was full of dazed and frantic advisers. Nobody was in charge. For Pottinger, it was "an out-of-body experience, like combat." The chief of staff came out of the private dining room, where the president was watching the riot on TV, and met Pottinger in the Oval Office. "I told them ten times, get the damn troops over there!" Meadows said. "My information may have been out of date," Pottinger admitted.

He went back to his office. It was now vividly clear to him that this was his last day in the White House. He had never expected to last this long. He had a secret rule that he would always be ready to leave in twenty minutes, so there were practically no personal items in his office, no framed photos, nothing on the wall except a laminated world map, with the Pacific—rather than the Atlantic—in the center, which is how Pottinger views the world. Everything else had to be packed in special boxes and sent to the National Archives; it all belonged to history, not to him.

In the middle of all this chaos, with the fate of the country in the balance, his assistant told him that a woman named Stephanie had been waiting for him for about an hour in the West Wing lobby. Her companion had forgotten her identification and wasn't allowed to enter.

Stephanie was having a lively conversation with the receptionist when Pottinger arrived. She was beside herself with excitement at being in the White House but disturbed by the desecration taking place in the Capitol by Trump's supporters. "That's not why we're here," she told Pottinger.

Pottinger took her to the Roosevelt Room and showed her the portraits of Theodore and Franklin, along with the Nobel Peace Prize and the Medal of Honor that Teddy had won. He told Stephanie that, when Democrats are in office, they swap the portraits, putting FDR over the mantle and Teddy on the side wall. Then he opened the door and pointed across the hall. "That's the Oval Office," he said. There was a Secret Service agent standing in front of the door, indicating that the president was inside. Stephanie was awed to be so close to her hero. Pottinger was thinking: This is my last time to see any of this.

He remembered a colleague, long since gone from the administration, who told him that every time he came through the White House gates he felt excitement, he felt honored by the privilege of serving, but mainly he felt joy. Pottinger had never experienced that. He was always weighed down by the burdens of the office, knowing the peril that the country was facing more intimately than nearly everyone, knowing every minute of his service how much was at stake, and how slender was the line between order and chaos—as the Capitol police were discovering at that very moment. He wondered if the day would come when he could look back on his time in the White House and discover the joy it provided others. He walked Stephanie down the colonnade to the first floor of the residence, showing her portraits of the First Ladies; then they were told to clear out of the area. Pottinger's staff helped send her off.

At 3:30 he watched his friend Mike Gallagher, a Republican congressman, tell Jake Tapper on CNN that he was hunkered down in his office. The only weapons he and his staff had to defend themselves were a pole holding the Wisconsin flag and Gallagher's ornamental Marine Corps sword. "I've not seen anything like this since I deployed to Iraq in 2007 and 2008," Gallagher said. Pottinger had served with him there. Now the congressman, a Trump supporter, told the president: "Call it off. It's over. The election is over." By now, 140 police were injured and one was dead. A female rioter was shot to death as she tried to crawl over a transom into the legislative chamber. Three other Trump supporters died in the riot, one by heart attack, one by stroke, and one was crushed by the mob she was a part of. Two police officers would commit suicide in the weeks immediately following.

The riot would prove to be the final superspreader event of the Trump presidency. Dozens of cops would soon test positive. Several Democratic lawmakers did as well, possibly from being confined in an undisclosed location with House Republicans who refused to wear the masks they were offered. Who knows how many cases the rioters took back to their own communities.

Pottinger phoned O'Brien and told him he was resigning. O'Brien was also considering leaving, but they worried that, if both left, the national security council could collapse in the midst of an attempted coup. The danger of a foreign adversary taking advantage of the chaos was on their minds. O'Brien decided to stay on.

Pottinger spent the night in his office, packing, writing emails to his staff, and filing his final financial disclosure. It all took a lot longer than twenty minutes. He watched the coverage of the riot. Mayor Bowser gave a press conference at Washington, D.C., police headquarters, flanked by masked officials, and Pottinger was struck once again by the fact that this entire drama was being played out against the backdrop of Covid-19, now eerily normalized.

He passed the night watching the sham Senate debate about accepting the electoral votes from four states. When it finally drifted to its inevitable conclusion, the vice president returned to the House chamber and resumed the somber but now defiant act of certifying the victory of a new president. The debris from the mob was still on the floor; windows were broken; and papers and personal items had been stolen from the lawmakers' desks. Only a few hours earlier, the lawmakers had run for their lives, down narrow stairways and back corridors, with the taunting mob mere steps away. Had they not been saved by the Capitol Police, some lawmakers would probably be dead, others captured and handcuffed by the zip ties rioters carried for that purpose, and yet 8 Republican senators and 139 Republican House members voted against accepting the results of the election.

At 3:30 a.m., Senator Amy Klobuchar finally announced that the deliberations were finished: "The report we make is that Joe Biden and

Kamala Harris will be the president and the vice president." The socially distanced legislators stood and applauded, and the vice president read out the final results. "The whole number of electors appointed to vote for the president of the United States is 538," he said. "Within that whole number, a majority is 270. The votes for president of the United States are as follows: Joseph R. Biden Jr., of the State of Delaware, has received 306 votes. Donald J. Trump, of the State of Florida, has received 232 votes." Then he read out the same votes for the vice president, announcing his own defeat. Democracy was speaking.

Pottinger rolled up the world map on his wall and walked out of the White House for the last time, carrying a shopping bag with his few personal items. He did not feel joy. With each step away from the White House, he felt a growing sense of rage.

THE STUMBLES OF the vaccine rollout were expectable, given the failures that had characterized the response to the coronavirus from the start. There was no coherent national plan. The CDC issued guidelines on December 3, 2020, proposing that the first doses should go to healthcare workers and residents of long-term care facilities; that was termed Phase 1a. Next in line would be essential workers, such as firefighters, police, corrections officers, food and agricultural workers, teachers and daycare workers, postal workers, and bus drivers. In that same category were people aged seventy-five and older. Phase 1c would include people over sixty-five and those with underlying health conditions. The FDA granted emergency use for the Pfizer vaccine on December 11.

The first problem was the scarcity of the vaccine. The Trump administration had promised 300 million doses by the end of the year. The chief scientific officer of Operation Warp Speed, Moncef Slaoui, reduced that to 35 to 40 million. That would be enough for up to 20 million people to receive the two shots recommended to achieve immunity. Some vaccine candidates were slow to emerge from trials; there were manufacturing problems; some of the raw materials were hard to obtain. In any case, by the end of the year, only about 2 million Americans had actually been vaccinated.

The states made up their own rules. Some prioritized homeless or incarcerated people, or those with high-risk health problems, or law-enforcement officers—each category had obvious merit, but the point was to get as many people inoculated as quickly as possible.

Texas governor Abbott quickly extended the list of prospective candidates in 1b to anyone over sixty-five—a huge cohort. But where to find a shot? Like everyone I knew in my age group, I began calling around. According to a chart the state put out, our neighborhood pharmacy had received five hundred doses, but they were all gone by the time I called. The hospitals were still administering them to healthcare workers only. The Austin Public Health website said that it was reserved for healthcare workers and "essential workers," not for seniors. I had friends that received backdoor vaccinations from well-connected doctors. Walk-ins began showing up at hospitals or grocery store pharmacies hoping to receive a shot drawn from leftover vaccine in the bottom of the vial.

President-elect Biden said that he planned to release nearly all the reserve doses of vaccine in order to get people immunized as quickly as possible, counting on increased production to secure the second dose. A few days later, Secretary Azar said he was doing just that, calling for inoculations for everyone over sixty-five. Suddenly, it seemed that the number of doses would double all at once. Then, just as quickly, Azar admitted there was no reserve.

My piano teacher was the first to tell me he had gotten a vaccine appointment. It had to be done online, but by the time I had filled out the form, the slot I selected had already been taken. This happened again and again. The following night at 11:00 p.m. I got a text from an unrecognized number with a link. It led to Austin Public Health's site. Within three tries, I was able to secure a date for my first shot. After that, their website crashed.

It was a chilly January morning. I thought I was arriving early, but cars were already backed up and waiting to enter the parking lot of a vast community center. There were about a hundred people already in line, my contemporaries, all of us wearing two masks—one covering our mouth and nose; the other, the one that age has inscribed on our features. Some of the quick-thinkers had brought camp chairs and thermoses full of coffee. A cold breeze whipped through my sweatshirt. I flipped up my hoodie and plugged in my AirPods and listened to Cyrus Chestnut play "Blues for Nita."

Finally the doors opened and we began the slow trek into the building, hopscotching from one designated standing spot to another as we
made our way toward the Visiting Team Dressing Room and finally
into the gymnasium, where about twenty stations were set up. Igloo
ice chests, bright red, containing the precious vaccine, were wheeled in
from time to time. The Texas and American flags hung above the blue
bleachers. It was quiet and orderly inside, the only voice rising above the
quiet murmur was calling "Next! Next!"

I scarcely felt the shot.

The doctor who administered the injection warned me that "things
are really goosey," and he wasn't able to make an appointment for the
booster twenty-eight days later. "Get it wherever you can," he advised.
Then he looked at my health history. "It says you had a severe reaction to
a vaccine before." There were two waiting areas; one for thirty minutes
and one for fifteen, to accommodate anyone who might have an allergic
reaction.

I told him about my experience with the tetanus shot when I was a
child.

"Well, it was a long time ago," he said.

I waited for fifteen minutes, occupying myself by sending a thank-
you note to Barney Graham and Jason McLellan.

SUDDENLY, the virus began to change. All viruses do. SARS-CoV-2 had
been remarkably stable as it coursed through the world, being already
so well adapted to the human host. This stability allowed the development of vaccines finely targeted for vulnerable regions of the virus's
spike protein. In February 2020, a new variant emerging from Italy had
proved to be far more infectious than the original Wuhan virus. After
that, scientists were on guard, expecting an assault of new mutations.
At the CDC, Greg Armstrong helped public health offices around the
country to prepare to sequence new variants. But where were they? "For
ten months, it was crickets," Armstrong said.

Then, in September 2020, just as the first vaccine candidates were
undergoing Phase 3 trials, the Trickster showed that it was not going
to be easily defeated. An aggressive new variant began circulating in
southeast England, centered in Kent, along the highway from London

to Dover. On Halloween, England announced a monthlong lockdown, which was dramatically successful in curbing the spread of Covid-19 in other parts of the country, but not in the Kent corridor. There were already a number of distinct variants of the novel coronavirus, with a few genetic variations of little consequence. But the U.K. variant, initially labeled a Variant Under Investigation, contained twenty-three different mutations, including several on the spike protein; moreover, it was rapidly driving out competitors and becoming the predominant virus in the country, especially among younger people. On December 18, it was upgraded to a Variant of Concern.

So what made the U.K. variant so much more successful than the original virus? One possibility is pure chance. It could have been amplified through some superspreader event, like the variant that took root at the Biogen conference, or perhaps it got seeded in a school or a church and spread rapidly among a tightly knit population. But as researchers went back and studied previously collected serum samples, they realized neither of these hypotheses could account for the accelerated pace of the spread. "Some mathematicians modeled how the variant has spread, and they found it was between 40 and 70 percent more infectious," the CDC's John Brooks told me. The current hypothesis was that the Kent variant, now called B.1.1.7, had a mutation that switched an amino acid in the spike protein, allowing it to bind more tightly to the body's ACE2 receptors. "That means it takes less virus to infect you," Brooks said. "That tighter binding also means that it can replicate more efficiently." Once infected with the new variant, a person will be shedding more virus than someone infected with another variant. "It's a wicked cycle," Brooks observed. B.1.1.7 quickly spread to dozens of countries. Historically, novel viruses have declined in mortality as they spread more successfully, but the U.K. variant turned out to be significantly deadlier.

England entered lockdown once again. By the second week in January, one out of thirty people in London was infected. The worrisome mutation in the B.1.1.7 variant affects the area of the virus where the antibodies that neutralize the disease do their work. The new mRNA vaccines command the immune system to produce neutralizing antibodies which target the spike protein of the invading virus, but it was that same spike that B.1.1.7 partially altered. That set off alarms in the public health community, because such mutations could erode the effectiveness of the vaccines. Viruses are always looking for hidden opportunities that mutations create, much as hackers search out flaws in application codes.

A month after the new strain was uncovered in England, a similar lineage emerged in South Africa, called B.1.351, quickly becoming the dominant variant in that country and setting off on its own tour of the world. It had the same mutation as B.1.1.7 that allowed it to adhere more tightly to the ACE2 receptors, but it also carried an additional mutation that is far more concerning. The mutation is denominated E484K, meaning that a single amino acid, glutamic acid (code letter E) has been replaced by another, lysine (code letter K), at position 484 of the genetic sequence of the spike protein. In a lab experiment, the E484K mutation caused more than a tenfold drop in the efficacy of the vaccine. Scientists began calling it the Eek mutation.

Yet another dangerous mutation turned up in Brazil, called P.1. A forty-five-year-old healthcare worker in the northeastern part of the country, who had no comorbidities, got Covid in May 2020. She was sick for a week with diarrhea, headaches, and exhaustion, but she fully recovered. Then, in October, 153 days later, she fell ill again with Covid-19, and this time the disease was more severe.

"This made the hair on my neck stand up," Brooks said. Like the South African variant, the Brazilian one had the mutation that makes it more infectious, as well as the Eek mutation, which raised the unsettling possibility that the coronavirus was evolving into a deadlier version of the flu or the common cold, which are constantly changing, dodging the body's immune system.

Greg Armstrong told me of an experiment to determine how many mutations it would take to create what is known as an "immune escape" strain. "They grew it up in tissue culture from a generic SARS-CoV-2 in diluted convalescent sera," he said. "They were eventually able to grow one that had three mutations that conferred almost complete resistance" to the antibodies in the survivors' blood.

"So how do we fight these mutants?" Brooks asked. "The best way is to suppress replication, and that means stopping infections." The more replications that occur, the greater the number of mutations. Occasionally, a slight error in replicating the genetic code creates a variant that spreads more successfully, and when that happens, evolution takes over.

Stopping transmission blocks the opportunity for viral mutation; it's the only thing that does. And the only means we have of standing in the way of the virus is vaccination. "It's a race," Brooks said. "We've got to get people vaccinated before more of these mutations occur."

The WHO says that herd immunity is reached when 60 to 70 percent of the population have had the disease or have been vaccinated, although Dr. Fauci has upped the figure incrementally, saying that a more reliable figure may be between 85 and 90 percent. The increased transmissibility of the mutant variants makes the higher figures more likely.

On January 19, two preprint research papers were published. One had good news: the Pfizer vaccine was just as effective at blocking the B.1.1.7 variant as the virus that originated in Wuhan. The other paper contained findings that Brooks and others had been dreading: the South African variant, B.1.351, showed that it can escape the antibodies in the blood of previously infected persons. That suggested that therapies using mono-clonal antibodies—the treatment President Trump received—could fail. The authors of the study underscored the implications for the effectiveness of SARS-CoV-2 vaccines: "These data highlight the prospect of reinfection with antigenically distinct variants and may foreshadow reduced efficacy of current spike-based vaccines." Indeed, the Novavax vaccine, while robustly effective in trials, was significantly less so when tested against the South African variant. The same was true for Johnson & Johnson's one-shot Covid vaccine.

Scientists in Barney Graham's lab working with Moderna found that their vaccine blocked both the U.K. and South African variants, although it was somewhat less effective against the latter. New variants began appearing in California and New York. Drug makers began designing boosters they hoped would take the mutations into account.

In the Bronx Zoo, a four-year-old Malayan tiger named Nadia tested positive for Covid. She probably got infected by an asymptomatic zoo-keeper. A few days later, three more tigers and three African lions tested positive. The virus was detected in marine mammals in the Mediterra-nean, snow leopards in the Louisville Zoo, and gorillas in the San Diego Zoo Safari Park. Seventeen million minks were culled in Denmark to block the outbreak in more than two hundred fur farms. Occasionally pets—cats and dogs—turned up positive as well. More than a hundred domestic cats in Wuhan were tested, and 14 percent were positive. There was always the possibility that SARS-CoV-2 could find a permanent reservoir in another mammal, as the H1N1 influenza is thought to have made a home in pigs during the 1918 Spanish flu.

As Stéphane Bancel, the CEO of Moderna, said, "We are going to live with this virus, we think, forever."

IMAGINE A FOREIGN ADVERSARY invaded America and killed half a million people. How would the country respond? No doubt the most powerful military in the history of the world would annihilate the invader. Partisan differences would fall away as the American people joined as one to defend their countrymen. History would mark the loss of life, unmatched by any military conflict in our country except the Civil War; but perhaps it would also note that it was the moment when the United States returned to its senses and concentrated on making the world a safer place.

But our invader is not a human adversary; it is nature that we struggle against, and in the face of this conflict there is a curious passivity. We were poorly armed for this contest, due to decades of cutbacks in our healthcare system. After 9/11, we spent trillions on homeland security and counterterrorism. Our military preparedness was unparalleled. We were ready to go to war with any other nation, but we were missing the fact that our own country was at war with itself, and that our weakened, broken society was easy prey for the contagion that was inevitably going to come.

At dusk on January 19, 2021, Joe Biden joined Kamala Harris at the Lincoln Memorial. The Washington Monument lay reflected in a golden light in the pool in front of them; and behind the obelisk was the brightly lit Capitol, pale and beautiful. This is the axis of the American republic, a touchstone of our history, the most sacred spot of our democracy. The next day, exactly a year from the day that the coronavirus officially arrived in America, Biden and Harris would be inaugurated on the steps of the same Capitol that was still cleaning up the debris from the siege.

"To heal, we must remember," Biden said. "It's important to do that as a nation." In the long siege of the coronavirus, the absence of a sense of collective loss was a failure few remarked, but it was costly to the spirit. Each death was a solitary event; every family grieved alone, until now. The words of solace that might have allowed the nation to grieve together were unsaid, until now. There had been no pause for reflection. Instead, there was confusion, blame, distrust, and division. The dead had been forgotten, until now.

Four hundred lamps lined the reflecting pool, each representing one thousand Americans who had already perished in the plague. More would come; 23,000 had died the previous week, and 1.5 million new cases had been reported. It would not end soon. But as the lamps came on in the gathering darkness, the nation began to remember.

Acknowledgments and Notes on Sources

This book comes at what must be near the end of a long and meaningful career, and I hope the reader will tolerate a brief valedictory. Journalism has given me a passport to visit other people's lives. The stories they share are incalculably precious, all the more so for being subject to erasure from the human experience by death or fading memories. A journalist's job is to gather them and weave them into a meaningful narrative, which awards them a kind of immortality.

Often, in movies or television, the press is depicted as a mob, arrogant and pitiless. My own experience is that reporting is a lonely and humble task. I picture myself with a backpack slung over my shoulder, awkwardly taking notes on a yellow legal pad, balancing a recorder in my hand, while following half a step behind a source who may not want to talk to me at all. I am still anxious when making the first calls on a story, realizing that I know so little, asking blundering questions of people who may be the world's greatest expert on this or that. It is also part of the job to delve into intensely personal matters, to probe the fresh wounds of people still grieving, or to interrogate liars, criminals, and sociopaths. Those experiences are balanced by the joy of penetrating a layer of truth that has been hidden until those words were uttered, and noted, and recorded, then written into the first draft of history.

———

When my editors at *The New Yorker*, David Remnick and Daniel Zalewski, first spoke to me about a major article on the pandemic, which this book grew out of, I considered that Covid-19 has deeply affected nearly every part of American society, including politics, race, science, the economy, and the culture at large. How could such a sprawling story be told? I chose to concentrate on notable institutions that define different sectors of our society and hope to find within them remarkable but representative individuals who could carry the reader into their world. In this, I was unbelievably fortunate.

I think of journalism as having two axes; one, which we can call the horizontal, consists of speaking to as many people as will speak to you. In the process of researching this book, I interviewed more than a hundred people. Casting a wide net allows the writer to draw from many sources and gain an overview; it also draws in contrasting narratives that provide a corrective to slanted perspectives. The horizontal axis creates a consensus about what has happened. The vertical axis is more about deep understanding. Some sources are simply more informed or more available, and to these I would return again and again.

At CDC, I want to sincerely thank John Brooks and Greg Armstrong for their guidance through the science and their patience with my endless queries. Robert Redfield was helpful in providing background information about the early days of the pandemic and offering his own perspective on the testing fiasco. Chin-Yih Ou was kind enough to describe laboratory procedures. Bruce Weniger and Stephen Redd were useful in describing the culture of CDC.

Barney Graham and Jason McLellan at NIAID are, I believe, real heroes in the effort to create a vaccine in record time. And of course Anthony Fauci has been a forthright and courageous leader of the public health community despite enormous political pressure exerted against him. Cliff Lane regaled me with stories about the history of NIAID and NIH.

Deborah Birx and Irum Zaidi provided insight into their spontaneous campaign to take the fight against the coronavirus to the individual states. Their role in this drama is uniquely valuable.

Stewart Simonson and David Heymann provided insights on the WHO. Philip Dormitzer, who helped out on my novel, spoke to me about vaccine development at Pfizer. Mark Ghaly, the secretary of California Health & Human Services, was helpful in describing the dilemma the state faced with quarantines and cruise ships. Lauren Ancel Meyers, a professor of Integrative Biology at the University of Texas, Austin, provided data on the early spread of SARS-CoV-2.

At the FDA, anonymous officials painstakingly took me through the chronology of the development of the test kit, and director Stephen Hahn responded to queries. At HHS, Robert Kadlec helped me through the decisions taken by that agency, and reviewed the Crimson Contagion exercise with me.

Howard Markel and Marty Cetron were wonderful fun to talk to. Their work on the 1918 pandemic, *Influenza Encyclopedia: The American Influenza Epidemic of 1918–1919,* is a highly original and useful document, which I commend to anyone interested in the history of that era.

I spoke to a number of U.S. senators about the impeachment hearings and the effect of the Covid contagion in their communities. I want to thank Lamar Alexander, Michael Bennet, Chris Coons, Amy Klobuchar, Mike Lee, Patty Murray, Marco Rubio, and Mark Warner for sharing their experiences. Governors Jay Inslee, Gretchen Whitmer, and Ned Lamont gave me many insights about their experiences in dealing with Covid and the Trump administration.

At the White House, Matt Pottinger may not have known what he was getting into when he first agreed to talk to me, but as a former reporter, he must have had an inkling. The skills he developed as a reporter himself turned out to be critically useful in uncovering developments in China that were apparently beyond the reach of U.S. intelligence. The Pottinger clan—Matt, Yen, and Paul—were ever so patient and candid in responding to my ceaseless questions. Peter Navarro and Olivia Troye were helpful in providing background about the Coronavirus Task Force.

I am sure Glenn Hubbard is a great teacher; he certainly was for me. He helped me frame the economic effects of Covid and provided a useful recording of his class at the Columbia School of Business. Steve Strongin and Jan Hatzius at Goldman Sachs were authoritative sources for the complex world of high finance. Heather Boushey helped frame my understanding of the economic effects of the pandemic. Raj Chetty taught me to see the economic consequences of the pandemic through the lens of his enlightening research. Lisa Cook showed me the historical consequences of a single tragic event—the Tulsa massacre—and how it still plays out in our own time.

Oskar Eustis was kind enough to allow me to share his story about his struggle with Covid. I long for the day we can work together again. Jordan Roth was a gracious guide to the darkened stages of Broadway.

Gianna Pomata was a serendipitous discovery for me. I wanted to talk to a medical historian, so I thought to look on the faculty of Johns Hopkins. I wrote her, not knowing she had retired, and she replied from Bologna. I profiled her in the July 20, 2020, issue of *The New Yorker* in a piece called "Crossroads." Her insights on the plague added much to my understanding of the effect of catastrophic diseases on society.

I decided to focus on Bellevue Hospital because my friend and former neighbor David Oshinsky had written a fascinating book about it, which led me to understand what a distinguished institution it is. David did me the favor of introducing me to Nate Link and Doug Bails, who were great informants, and they led me to Amit Uppal. Barron Lerner was still recovering from Covid when we first spoke, and he graciously recalled his experience. I came away from those interviews grateful for the dedication of those brilliant and compassionate doctors and the hospital they serve.

Ebony Hilton wrote a tweet about ethnic disparities in health outcomes that caught my eye, and I'm so glad it did. She introduced me to two worlds, her hospital and her hometown, Little Africa. I hope that her contribution to understanding the ethnic disparities in health outcomes will have real consequences in policy. Ebony's mother, Mary, was a delightful guide to her hometown and her remarkable family.

Deanne Criswell, New York City's emergency management commissioner, gave me a fascinating account of the preparations for a catastrophic pandemic. Oxiris Barbot, the former commissioner of health in the city, recounted the experience of the onset of the disease.

Photojournalist Al Drago and Reverend John Jenkins provided descriptions of the Rose Garden ceremony that proved to be a superspreader event. Jacob Lemieux took me through the intricacies of the Biogen study. Dimon Liu gave me a wonderful account of the Chinese New Year feast in her home. Johnny LaTouf made me long for the music to begin again at the Skylark Lounge. I also want to thank Emilia Sykes, an Ohio state representative with a master's degree in public health, for her thoughts on the politics of health. Matt McCarthy was an Army doctor and pandemic adviser in New York at the peak of the contagion. Qiming Wang, an engineer, told me about life in Wuhan during the shutdown.

For general scientific knowledge far outside my realm of understanding, I turned to Marc Lipsitch, a professor of epidemiology at the Harvard T.H. Chan School of Public Health; his colleague at the same institution, Tun-hou Lee, an emeritus professor of virology; Michael Osterholm, director of the Center for Infectious Disease Research and Policy at the University of Minnesota; and Tom Frieden, former head of CDC who now leads Resolve to Save Lives, an initiative aimed at preventing epidemics and cardiovascular disease. Each of these brilliant scientists helped me navigate some very tricky passages.

Some truths are only reached by swimming through a flood of tears—often, my own. I want to thank in particular Michael Miller, Melanie Cain Gallo, Corey and Jennifer Breen Feist, Chris Rogan, and Selene Meda-Schlamel for sharing stories that were wrenching and intensely personal, but which stood for so many other, similar experiences that will never be told.

The experience of writing this book, during the pandemic, has been different from my previous work in that nearly all the interviews were conducted by phone or Zoom. There's a loss of intimacy with my sources that I regret, but I hope we'll meet one day.

It's embarrassing to realize how many facts I can get wrong, despite my most earnest attempts at accuracy. Fortunately, fact checkers provide a net. Anyone who has been through the process at *The New Yorker* comes out chastened. While I was working on the article, also called "The Plague Year," in the January 4 & 11, 2021, issue of the magazine, Hélène Warner led a team of three additional checkers: Anna Boots, Dennis Zhou, and Zach Helfand. Checkers form an unappreciated diplomatic function, managing the anxiety of sources and the unconscious urges of the author who wishes facts to be true that aren't. For the book, Emily Gogolak, who was also trained in the rigorous *New Yorker* method, heroically undertook this delicate task.

I owe a particular debt to the expert readers who agreed to read all or portions of this book in manuscript: Ian Lipkin, Yanzhong Huang, Tun-hou Lee, Evan Osnos, and Mollie Saltskog provided useful insights and scrupulous corrections; Mollie graciously translated some material as well. The assistance of these distinguished readers is deeply meaningful to me. I have two other readers that I always turn to: Stephen Harrigan and my wife, Roberta, who have read nearly everything I've written and have always been my most trusted advisers.

When I first came to *The New Yorker* in 1992, I attended a party where I met many of the writers I had been reading since childhood. I thought at the time: I can grow old here. And I have. That relationship has been a source of pride and a deep well of friendship. Although separated from my colleagues during this time, I've had the benefit of their advice. At the beginning of this project, Josh Rothman pointed me toward several potential sources, who proved invaluable. I want to add my particu-lar thanks to Alex Barasch, who provided endless amounts of insight, along with difficult-to-track-down contacts for people I wanted to talk to. As always, I treasure my relationship with my editors. In the decades we've worked together, Daniel Zalewski has shaped and improved my craft. David Remnick has been a steady and inspiring leader, and he has trusted me with momentous stories, often at his suggestion.

I've had a parallel relationship with my publisher, Knopf, and my edi-tor, Ann Close. Our first book together, *In the New World,* a memoir of growing up in Dallas during the Kennedy assassination, was published in 1988. *The Plague Year* is our ninth book together. Over those years, I've benefitted from the assistance of the high level of professionalism that is a hallmark of Knopf. I am delighted to have the opportunity to thank that team once again: Paul Bogaards, Erinn Hartman, Todd Portnowitz, Julianne Clancy, Katherine Hourigan, Lydia Buechler, Kevin Bourke, Dan Novak, and Cassandra Pappas. Reagan Arthur is a dynamic and charming new leader for the Knopf enterprise. LuAnn Walther, head of Vintage, has been a great partner through many books.

My agent, Andrew Wylie, is a trusted ally, and I'm grateful for his advice and assistance, as well as that of James Pullen, in London.

Among the many awful legacies that Covid will leave, one blessing is that our understanding of viruses, and therefore our ability to treat and counter them, has been transformed. Much of that will be because of Barney Graham, Jason McLellan, John Brooks, Greg Armstrong, Ebony Hilton, Tony Fauci, Marty Cetron, Howard Markel, Lorna Breen, Barron Lerner, Tom Frieden, Amit Uppal, Nate Link, Doug Bails, Paul Pottinger, Deborah Birx, Irum Zaidi, and Yen Pottinger—to mention only those portrayed in this book. There has never been such an enormous, worldwide scientific effort so intently focused on a single disease. To them we all owe so much.

Notes

Quotations that are not attributed in the notes derive from interviews with the author.

PROLOGUE

3 **Video of the event:** Coleman Lowndes, "This photo triggered China's Cultural Revolution," *Vox*, Feb. 14, 2020. MacFarquhar, Roderick, and Michael Shoenhals, "Mao's Last Revolution," The Belknap Press of Harvard University Press, Cambridge, 2006, pp. 81-2.

4 **184,000 citizens:** Jung Chang and Jon Halliday, *Mao: The Unknown Story*, p. 539; Roderick Farquhar and Michael Shoenhals, *Mao's Last Revolution*, The Belknap Press of Harvard University Press, Cambridge, 2006, p. 214.
   Dr. Zhang Jixian: Xixing Li, Weina Cui, and Fuzhen Zhang, "Who Was the First Doctor to Report the COVID-19 Outbreak in Wuhan, China?" *Journal of Nuclear Medicine*, June 2020.
   "It is unlikely": "COVID-19 and China: A Chronology of Events (December 2019–January 2020," Congressional Research Service, updated May 13, 2020.
   authorities instructed: Debora MacKenzie, *COVID-19: The Pandemic that Never Should Have Happened and How to Stop the Next One*, New York: Hachette, 2020, p. 17.
   since November: Interview with Ian Lipkin, who was in China at the time. Retrospective modeling suggests the outbreak may have begun as early as mid-October. Jonathan Pekar, et al., "Timing the SARS-CoV-2 index case in Hubei Province," *Science*, March 18, 2021.
   a stream of patients: Kristin Huang, "Wuhan doctor 'muzzled for initially raising the alarm'; Posting of report on Sars-like virus by head of hospital's emergency department, which was shared by late whistle-blower, suggests officials missed opportunity to issue early warning," *South China Morning Post*, Mar. 12, 2020.
   10 of its 653 stalls: Dyani Lewis, "Can COVID spread from frozen wildlife? Scientists probe pandemic origins," *Nature*, Feb. 26, 2021.

5 **"pay attention":** "COVID-19 and China: A Chronology of Events," Congressional Research Service, May 13, 2020.

5 **hide the outbreak:** Yanzhong Huang, "The SARS Epidemic and its Aftermath in China: A Political Perspective," Institute of Medicine Forum on Microbial Threats; S. Knobler, A. Mahmoud, S. Lemon, et al., editors. *Learning from SARS: Preparing for the Next Disease Outbreak: Workshop Summary*, 2004.

Doctors in charge: Ibid.

first epidemic since HIV/AIDS: David P. Fidler, "SARS: Political Pathology of the First Post-Westphalian Pathogen," *Journal of Law, Medicine & Ethics*, 2003.

smuggled into ambulances: "China hid SARS patients—report," CNN, April 18, 2003.

thirty-two countries: "Cumulative Number of Reportable Probable Cases of SARS," from Nov. 1, 2002, to July 11, 2003, World Health Organization.

6 **He suspected:** Elsie Chen, with Chris Buckley and Steven Lee Meyers, "He Warned of Coronavirus. Here's What He Told Us Before He Died," *New York Times*, Feb. 7, 2020.

ordered hospitals to treat: "Covid-19 and China: A Chronology of Events," Congressional Research Service, May 13, 2020. "China Publishes Timeline on Covid-19 information sharing, int'l cooperation," *Xinhua*, April 6, 2020.

noticed the posts: Louise Watt, "Taiwan Says It Tried to Warn the World About Coronavirus," *Time*, May 19, 2020.

not to be SARS: www.who.int/docs/default-source/coronaviruse/transcripts/who-audio-emergencies-coronavirus-press-conference-20apr2020.pdf.

7 **strikingly low rate:** Yu-Jie Chen and Jerome A. Cohen, "Why Does the WHO Exclude Taiwan? Council on Foreign Relations, April 9, 2020.

Chinese technology companies: "The Origins of the COVID-19 Global Pandemic Including the roles of the Chinese Communist Party and the World Health Organization," House Foreign Affairs Committee Minority Staff Interim Report, June 12, 2020.

"damage stability": Kristin Huang, "Coronavirus: Wuhan doctor says officials muzzled her for sharing report on WeChat," *South China Morning Post*, March 11, 2020. Debora MacKenzie, *COVID-19*, op. cit., p. 17.

she was told: "COVID-19 and China," Congressional Research Service, May 13, 2020.

"If something happens": *Renwu* interview with Dr. Ai Fen. Translated by Mollie Saltskog.

"If I had known:" Lily Kuo, "Coronavirus: Wuhan doctor speaks out against the authorities," *Guardian*, Mar. 11, 2020.

"severely disturbed": Congressional Research Service, "COVID-19 and China," May 13, 2020.

His punishment: "The Origins of the COVID-19 Global Pandemic, Including the Roles of the Chinese Communist Party and the World Health Organization," House Foreign Affairs Committee Minority Staff Report, Sept. 21, 2020.

8 **"How can the bulletins":** Congressional Research Service: COVID-19 and China, May 13, 2020.

forced reporters into detention: Vivian Wang, "They Documented the Coronavirus Crises in Wuhan. Then They Vanished," *New York Times*, Feb. 14, 2020.

hospital authorities again: Jingqi Gong, "Whistleblower," *Renwu*, March 10, 2020.

highly inventive dissidents: Masha Borak, "Censored coronavirus news shows up again as emoji, Morse code and ancient Chinese," *Abacus*, March 12, 2020.

destroy existing stock: Zhuang Pinghui, "China confirms unauthorised labs were told to destroy early coronavirus samples," *South China Morning Post*, May 15, 2020.

"rectification": Congressional Research Service: COVID-19 and China, May 13, 2020.

8   **duplicity of local officials:** Edward Wong, Julian E. Barnes, and Zolan Kanno-Youngs, "Local Officials in China Hid Dangers From Beijing, U.S. Agencies Find," *New York Times*, Aug. 19, 2020, updated Sept. 17, 2020.

9   **demanded that researchers:** "China delayed releasing coronavirus info, frustrating WHO," Associated Press, June 1, 2020.

    by a couple of weeks: off the record interview with FDA authorities.

    revised to 3,869: "Wuhan Revises up Coronavirus Death Toll to 3,869 From 2,579," Bloomberg, April 16, 2020.

    3,500 urns: "Estimates Show Wuhan Death Toll Far Higher Than Official Figure," Radio Free Asia, Mar. 27, 2020; Christina Zhao, "Wuhan COVID-19 Death Toll May Be in Tens of Thousands, Data on Cremations and Shipments of Urns Suggest," *Newsweek*, Mar. 29, 2020.

    around 36,000: Mai He, Li Li, Louis P. Dehner, Lucia F. Dunn, "Cremation based estimates suggest significant under- and delayed reporting of COVID-19 epidemic data in Wuhan and China," *medRxiv,* June 16, 2020.

    including four other doctors: Alice Yan, "Fifth doctor from Wuhan hospital dies from Covid-19 after long battle," *South China Morning Post*, June 2, 2020.

    He left behind: Huang Chenkuang, "'Online wailing wall': How Chinese netizens continue to honor Li Wenliang, COVID-19 whistleblower," *SupChina*, March 31, 2020.

    "A healthy society": Han Zhang, "How the Coronavirus Has Tested China's System of Information Control," *The New Yorker*, Feb. 7, 2020.

10   **Not until then:** Debora MacKenzie, *COVID-19*, op cit., p. 17.

    about 650 million people: "IntelBrief: Coronavirus Continues to Spread Amid Growing Criticism of China," The Soufan Center, Feb. 20, 2020.

    nearly three billion trips: Karla Cripps and Serenitie Wang, "World's largest annual human migration now underway in China," CNN, Jan. 23, 2019.

    largest annual migration: "China Will Rack Up Three Billion Trips During World's Biggest Human Migration," Bloomberg, Jan. 20, 2020.

I. "IT'S GOING TO BE JUST FINE"

11   **One minute before midnight:** "Undiagnosed Pneumonia—China (Hubei): Request for Information," *ProMed*, Dec. 30, 2019, 23:59:00.

    learned of it almost: "COVID-19 and China: A Chronology of Events" (December 2019–January 2020), Congressional Research Service, May 13, 2020.

    "Whether or not it is SARS": "Undiagnosed Pneumonia—China (Hubei): Request for Information," *ProMed*, Dec. 30, 2019, 23:59:00.

    three family clusters: Interview with Robert Redfield.

12   **no clear evidence of human-to-human:** Julian Borger, "Caught in a superpower struggle: the inside story of the WHO's response to coronavirus," *The Guardian*, Apr. 18, 2020.

    no invitation: Interview with Matthew Pottinger.

    world's largest reporting system: Li Wang, Zhihao Wang, Qinglian Ma, Guixia Fang, and Jinxia Yang, "The development and reform of public health in China from 1949 to 2019," *BMC*, July 2, 2019.

    virus was already present: Sridhar V. Basavaraju, et al., "Serologic testing of U.S. blood donations to identify SARS-CoV-2-reactive antibodies: December 2019-January 2020," *Clinical Infectious Diseases*, Nov. 30, 2020.

    "I think we're too late": Interview with Robert Redfield.

14   **"It's one person":** Dan Mangan, "Trump dismissed coronavirus pandemic worry in January—now claims he long warned about it," CNBC, Mar. 17, 2020.

    "no doubt": Gerard Gallagher, *Infectious Disease News*, Jan. 11, 2017.

16   "Unfortunately, political will": *Global Health Security Index*, October 2019.

17   586,000 Americans: David E. Sanger, Eric Lipton, Eileen Sullivan, and Michael Crowley, "Before Virus Outbreak, a Cascade of Warnings Went Unheeded," *New York Times*, Mar. 19, 2020; interview with Robert Kadlec.
The Trump administration's own report: "Crimson Contagion 2019 Functional Exercise Key Findings," Coordinating draft.

2. THE TRICKSTER

20   The organization's mission broadened: *CDC Timeline*, Jan. 19, 2021.
lifespan of Americans: Dian Whitmore Schanzenbach, Ryan Nunn, and Lauren Bauer, "The Changing Landscape of American Life Expectancy," *The Hamilton Project*, June 2016.

22   "negative serial interval": Zhanwei Du, Xiaoke Xu, Uye Wu, Lin Wang, Benjamin J. Cowling, and Lauren Ancel Meyers, "The serial interval of COVID-19 from publicly reported confirmed cases," *medRxiv* preprint, March 20, 2020.

24   A German study: Valentina O. Puntmann, M. Ludovica Carej, and Imke Wieters, "Outcomes of Cardiovascular Magnetic Resonance Imaging in Patients Recently Recovered From Coronavirus Disease 2019 (COVID-19)," *JAMA*, July 27, 2020.

3. SPIKE

25   horse farms: Interview with Barney Graham.
not Covid-19: Stacy Kuebelbeck Paulsen, "Study finds no link between COVID-19, Guillain-Barré syndrome," *CIDRAP*, Dec. 14, 2020.

26   may have been misdiagnosed: Armond S. Goldman, et al., "What was the cause of Franklin Delano Roosevelt's Paralytic Illness?" *Journal of Medical Biography*, Nov. 1, 2003.
bankrolled by a lawyer: Brian Deer, "Revealed MMR research scandal," *The Sunday Times*, Feb. 22, 2021.
more than 100,000: "The Vaccine May Be The Cure For Our Economy, But Texas May Be An Obstacle," *Texas Standard*, Texas Public Radio, Jan. 12, 2021.
It used to infect: "Measles History," CDC, Nov. 5, 2020.
nearly 1,300 cases: www.cdc.gov/measles/cases-outbreaks.html.

27   more than 200,000: Michael Fitzpatrick, "The Cutter Incident: How America's First Polio Vaccine Led to a Growing Vaccine Crisis," *Journal of the Royal Society of Medicine*, March 2006.
the result of vaccination: Xiangdong Peng, Xiaojiang Hu, Miguel A. Salazar, "On reducing the risk of vaccine-associated paralytic poliomyelitis in the global transition from oral to inactivated poliovirus vaccine," *The Lancet*, Aug. 18, 2018.
until polio is fully eradicated: Interview with Gregory Armstrong.
Plandemic: Sheera Frenkel, Ben Decker, and Davey Alba, "How the 'Plandemic' Movie and Its Falsehoods Spread Widely Online," *New York Times*, May 20, 2020.

28   he found a match: Interview with Gary Noble.
273 men: Lawrence Wright, "Sweating out the swine flu scare," *New Times*, June 11, 1976.
"whole hog": Ibid.
vaccinate the entire country: Kat Eschner, "The Long Shadow of the 1976 Swine Flu Vaccine 'Fiasco'," *Smithsonian Magazine*, Feb. 6, 2017.

30   Forty-eight million: Michael Marshall and Debora MacKenzie, "Timeline: the secret history of swine flu," *New Scientist*, Oct. 29, 2009; Martin Furmanski, "Threatened pandemics and laboratory escapes: Self-fulfilling prophecies," *Bulletin of the Atomic Scientists*, Mar. 31, 2014.

31 **only just repealed:** Stacy Barchenger, "Tennessee's marriage recognition laws rarely used," *Tennessean*, May 3, 2015.

32 **vaccine enhanced disease:** Jon Cohen, "Structural Biology Triumph Offers Hope Against a Childhood Killer," *Science*, vol. 342, Nov. 1 2013.

4. "AN EVOLVING SITUATION"

38 **The Democrats targeted:** Norman Eisen, *A Case for the American People: The United States v. Donald J. Trump*, Crown, New York, 2020, p. 203.

39 **"We have the votes":** Nicholas Fandos, "McConnell Says He Will Proceed on Impeachment Trial Without Witness Deal," *New York Times*, Jan. 7, 2020.
"We have a constitutional duty": Lamar Alexander statement on impeachment.

40 **"This virus in China":** Interview with Lamar Alexander.
"In the morning": *Congressional Record*, January 24, 2020.

41 **"We are prepared":** Meeting notes supplied by Senator Patty Murray's office.
"isn't something the American people": Warren Fiske, "Fact-check: Did Fauci say coronavirus was 'nothing to worry about'?" *PolitiFact.com*, April 29, 2020.

42 **"Reactivating these machines":** Katz, Marshall & Banks, LLP, "Addendum to the Complaint of Prohibited Practice and Other Prohibited activity by the Department of Health and Human Services Submitted by Dr. Rick Bright," April 29, 2020.

43 **"No way to prevent it":** Ibid.
"Rick, I think": Aaron C. Davis, "In the early days of the pandemic, the U.S. government turned down an offer to manufacture millions of N95 masks in America," *Washington Post*, May 9, 2020.
"I remember how": Joe Biden, "FLASHBACK by Joe Biden: Trump is worst possible leader to deal with coronavirus outbreak," *USA Today*, Jan. 27, 2020.

45 **"biggest national security threat":** Bob Woodward, *Rage*, p. xiii.
half a million in January: Ibid., p. 276.

46 **"Is all the money dumb?":** Interview with Matthew Pottinger.
Mulvaney barred him: Interview with Peter Navarro.
also tested positive: Isaac Ghinai, et al., "First known person-to-person transmission of severe acute respiratory syndrome coronavirus 2 (SARS-CoV-2) in the USA," *The Lancet*, March 13, 2020.

47 **Three major U.S. carriers:** Michael Corkery and Annie Karni, "Trump Administration Restricts Entry Into U.S. From China," *New York Times*, updated Feb. 20, 2020.
direct and one-stop flights: Robert Farley, "The Facts on Trump's Travel Restrictions," *FactCheck.org*, March 6, 2020.
unlike Taiwan: David Leonhardt, "The Unique U.S. Failure to Control the Virus," *New York Times*, Aug. 6, 2020.
"against the advice": Robert Farley, "The Facts on Trump's Travel Restrictions," *FactCheck.org*, March 6, 2020.
"Just because actions": Marco Rubio, "My Statement on the President's Impeachment Trial," Jan. 31, 2020, medium.com.

5. "FLATTEN THE CURVE"

50 **"a large fraction":** Robert G. Webster and Elizabeth Jane Walker, "Influenza," *American Scientist*, March-April 2003.

51 **New York City was the first:** *Influenza Encyclopedia: The American Influenza Epidemic of 1918-1919*, University of Michigan Center for the History of Medicine and Michigan Publishing, University of Michigan Library.

52 **nearby Navy Yard:** Alfred W. Crosby, *Epidemic and Peace, 1918*, Westport, Connecticut: Greenwood Press, 1976, p. 71.

53 **40,000 to 50,000 orphans:** *Influenza Encyclopedia*, op. cit., p. 1.

54 **among the worst:** Ibid.

56 **in more than fifty years:** Transcript for CDC Media Telebriefing: Update on 2019 Novel Coronavirus (2019-nCoV), Jan. 31, 2020.
"The best way": Bill Chappell, "Coronavirus: CDC Puts Americans Who Left Wuhan Into 'Unprecedented' 14-Day Quarantine," NPR, Jan. 31, 2020.

6. "IT'S COMING TO YOU"

59 **"the fastest we've ever":** Rebecca Ballhaus and Stephanie Armour, "Health Chief's Early Missteps Set Back Coronavirus Response," *Wall Street Journal,* April 22, 2020. Azar denies the quote.

60 **German test:** Peter Whoriskey and Neena Satija, "Coronavirus: German company developed 1.4m tests in six weeks while US production stalled," *Independent*, Mar. 17, 2020.
Just as the test kits: Dina Temple-Raston, "CDC Report: Officials Knew Coronavirus Test Was Flawed But Released It Anyway," NPR, Nov. 6, 2020.
"This is either going to": Leonardo Santamaria and Laura Lannes, "Inside the Fall of the CDC." ProPublica, Oct. 15, 2020. The CDC would not make Lindstrom available for comment.

63 **insisted on sticking:** David Willman, "The CDC's failed race against Covid-19: A threat underestimated and a test overcomplicated," *Washington Post*, Dec. 26, 2020.
The CDC admitted: Stephanie Armour, Brianna Abbott, Thomas M. Burton, and Betsy McKay, "What Derailed America's Covid Testing: Three Lost Weeks," *Wall Street Journal*, Aug. 18, 2020.
fewer than 500: Julie Steenhuysen, Andrew Hay, and Brad Brooks, "Mixed messages, test delays hamper U.S. coronavirus response," Reuters, Feb. 27, 2020.
1.6 million per week: "Scoop: Lab for coronavirus test kits may have been contaminated," Axios, March 1, 2020.

64 **"filthy":** Interview with FDA officials. Sheila Kaplan, "C.D.C. Labs Were Contaminated, Delaying Coronavirus Testing, Officials Say," *New York Times*, May 7, 2020.
"When Dr. Stenzel": FDA: "Regulatory history of CDC's molecular diagnostic test for SARS-CoV-2," draft, Dec. 1, 2020.

66 **Biogen:** Sarah Kaplan and Chris Mooney, "Genetic data show how a single super-spreading event sent coronavirus across Massachusetts and the nation," *Washington Post*, Aug. 25, 2020; Emma Brown, "A look inside coronavirus preparations at a major U.S. hospital," *Washington Post*, March 9, 2020; "Second Presumptive Positive Case Identified by Massachusetts State Laboratory," Massachusetts Department of Health, March 5, 2020.
Of the 175 attendees: Hanna Krueger, "Biogen conference in Boston likely linked to as many as 300,000 COVID-19 cases worldwide, researchers say," *Boston Globe*, Dec. 10, 2020.
CDC constraints: Emma Brown, "A look inside coronavirus preparations at a major U.S. hospital," *Washington Post*, March 9, 2020.

67 **"While superspreading events":** Jacob E. Lemieux, Katherine J. Siddle, Bennet M. Shaw, et al., "Phylogenetic analysis of SARS-CoV-2 in Boston highlights the impact of superspreading events," *Science*, Feb. 5, 2021.

68 **"go rogue":** Matt Richtel, "Frightened Doctors Face Off With Hospitals Over Rules on Protective Gear," *New York Times*, March 31, 2020.
"We're in for a disaster": "Covid War," CNN, March 28, 2021.
A Chinese report: The Novel Coronavirus Pneumonia Emergency Response Epidemiology Team, "The Epidemiological Characteristics of an Outbreak of 2019 Novel Coronaviruses Diseases (COVID-19)–China, 2020," Feb. 14, 2021.

69   **PEPFAR:** Vivian Salama, Pamela Brown, Kristen Holmes, and Kate Bennett, "How Dr. Deborah Birx's political skills made her the most powerful person on the coronavirus task force," *CNN,* July 17, 2020.
effective and data-driven: "Audit of the Department of State's Coordination and Oversight of the U.S. President's Emergency Plan for AIDS Relief," Office of the Inspector General, U.S. State Department, Feb. 2020.
she found $200 million: Interview with Matthew Pottinger.
70   **end of her career:** Full interview with Deborah Birx on *60 Minutes,* Jan. 24, 2021.
152 of the 186: Seoyun Choe, Hee-Sung Kim, and Sunmi Lee, "Exploration of Superspreading Events in 2015 MERS-CoV Outbreak in Korea by Branching Process Models," *International Journal of Environmental Research and Public Health,* Aug. 24, 2020.
3 percent of the patients: "Small number of 'superspreaders' caused most Ebola infections, drove West Africa epidemic," *Infectious Disease News,* Feb. 22, 2017.
71   **"eccentric genius":** Richard L. Riley, "What Nobody Needs to Know About Airborne Infection," *American Journal of Respiratory and Critical Care Medicine,* 163(1), p. 7.
On the roof: Karen Kruse Thomas, "The Experiment That Proved Airborne Disease Transmission," *Hub,* July 22, 2020.
Grand Princess: "Grand Princess Updates," April 7, 2020.
a single infected passenger: Smriti Mallapaty, "What the cruise-ship outbreaks reveal about COVID-19," *Nature,* March 26, 2020; Expert Taskforce for the COVID-19 Cruise Ship Outbreak, "Epidemiology of COVID-19 Outbreak on Cruise Ship Quarantined at Yokohama, Japan, February 2020," *Emerging Infectious Diseases,* Nov. 2020.
through aerosol droplets: Parham Azimi, et al., "Mechanistic Transmission Modeling of COVID-19 on the Diamond Princess Cruise Ship Demonstrates the Importance of Aerosol Transmission," *medRxiv,* July 15, 2020.
72   **put at 19.2 percent:** Interview with Martin Cetron.
it reached 60 percent: Uki Goñi, "Cruise ship stranded off Uruguay says 60% onboard have Covid-19," *The Guardian,* April 7, 2020.
"go home": Leonardo Santamaria and Laura Lannes, "Inside the Fall of the CDC," ProPublica, Oct. 15, 2020.
fifty-seven-year-old woman: Rob Barry, Joel Eastwood, and Paul Overberg, "Coronavirus Hit the U.S. Long Before We Knew," *Wall Street Journal,* Oct. 8, 2020.
Those passengers who: Mario Koran, *The Guardian,* March 14, 2020.
73   **a healthcare worker:** "CDC, Washington State Report First COVID-19 Death," CDC media statement, Feb. 29, 2020.

7. "NOTHING CAN STOP WHAT'S COMING"

75   **thirty-eight states:** Rob Barry, Joel Eastwood, and Paul Overberg, "Coronavirus Hit the U.S. Long Before We Knew," *Wall Street Journal,* Oct. 8, 2020.
"full of cobwebs": Joseph Goldstein and Andrea Salcedo, "For 4 Days, the Hospital Thought He Had Just Pneumonia. It Was Coronavirus," *New York Times,* Mar. 11, 2020.
"I think this patient": Priscilla DeGregory, "Hospital failed to protect nurse from NY's coronavirus 'patient zero': suit," *New York Post,* May 31, 2020.
"Am I going to die?": Christian Nolan, "Lawrence Garbuz, New York's First Known COVID-19 Case, Reveals What He Learned About Attorney Well-Being From the Virus," *New York State Bar Journal,* Aug. 11, 2020.
76   **ninety people:** Joseph Goldstein and Andrea Salcedo, "For 4 Days, the Hospital Thought He Had Just Pneumonia. It Was Coronavirus," *New York Times,* March 10, 2020.

76   synagogue was shut down: Sarah Maslin Nir, "Coronavirus in N.Y.: Inside New Rochelle's 'Containment Area'," *New York Times*, March 12, 2020.

out of eleven cases: "2014-2016 Ebola Outbreak in West Africa," CDC, Dec. 27, 2017.

"STOP THE FLIGHTS!": Gabriel Schoenfeld, "Trump tweeted heartlessly about Ebola in 2014. He's ill-equipped to handle the 2019 outbreak," *USA Today*, July 28, 2019.

3,200 direct flights: John Kelly and Pierre Thomas, "Disaster in motion: Where flights from coronavirus-ravaged countries landed in US," ABC News, April 7, 2020.

Sixty percent of flights: John Kelly and Steven Cioffi, "Coronvirus News: How international travel left NY vulnerable," WABC, April 6, 2020.

100,000 cases: "WHO Director-General's opening remarks at the media briefing on COVID-19," World Health Organization, March 11, 2020.

77   "We are coordinated": Cuomo press briefing, Mar. 2, 2020.

"if you don't see a problem": Interview with Marc Lipsitch.

more than 50,000: "Scenario exploration for SARS-CoV-2 infections," paper by Rebecca Kahn and Marc Lipsitch provided to author.

Starting in January: Interview with Deanne Criswell.

78   "a little perturbed": Joe Sexton and Joaquin Sappien, "Two Coasts. One Virus. How New York Suffered Nearly 10 Times the Number of Deaths as California," ProPublica, May 16, 2020.

"Ultimately, we expect": Transcript for the CDC Telebriefing Update on COVID-19, CDC, Feb. 26, 2020.

"incredibly quickly": CDC press briefing, Feb. 28, 2020.

79   Three law-enforcement officials: Gus Burns, "Third Michigan law enforcement death attributed to the coronavirus," Mlive, March 26, 2020.

Orleans Parish: Gordon Russell, "Orleans Parish has highest per-capita coronavirus death rate of American counties—by far," *The Times-Picayune/The Advocate*, March 26, 2020.

"My uncle": Steve Benen, "Trump thinks he may have 'a natural ability' to address viral outbreaks," MSNBC, March 9, 2020.

80   devout Catholic: Kristen Holmes, Nick Valencia, and Curt Devine, "CDC woes bring Director Redfield's troubled past as an AIDS researcher to light, CNN, June 5, 2020.

"God's judgment": Laurie Garrett, "Meet Trump's New, Homophobic Public Health Quack," *Foreign Policy*, March 23, 2018.

"a terrific, dedicated": Eric Lipton, Abby Goodnough, Michael D. Shear, Megan Twohey, Apoorva Mandavilli, Sheri Fink, and Mark Walker, "The C.D.C. Waited 'Its Entire Existence for This Moment.' What Went Wrong?" *New York Times*, Aug. 14, 2020.

81   "Anybody that wants a test": www.whitehouse.gov/briefings-statements/remarks-president-trump-tour-centers-disease-control-prevention-atlanta-ga/.

82   "You hear any bad things": David A. Fahrenthold, Anne Gearan, and Michelle Ye Hee Lee, "Trump defiant on testing and handshakes even as third Mar-a-Lago case emerges," *Washington Post*, March 13, 2020.

"I could just feel": Joe Hagan, "'Dishonesty . . . Is Always an Indicator of Weakness': Tucker Carlson on How He Brought His Cornavirus Message to Mar-a-Lago." *Vanity Fair*, March 17, 2020.

"Nothing can stop": Timothy Bella, "Trump tweets a meme of himself fiddling, drawing a comparison to Roman emperor Nero," *Washington Post*, Mar. 9, 2020.

"Every message": Joe Sexton and Joaquin Sappien, "Two Coasts. One Virus. How New York Suffered Nearly 10 Times the Number of Deaths as California," ProPublica, May 16, 2020.

83 **"Greater than 99 percent":** William K. Rashbaur, J. David Goodman, Jeffery C. Mays, and Joseph Goldstein, "He Saw 'No Proof' Closures Would Curb the Virus. Now He Has De Blasio's Trust," *New York Times*, May 14, 2020.

"If you're under fifty": David Freedlander, "When New York Needed Him Most, Bill de Blasio Had His Worst Week As Mayor," *New York* magazine, March 26, 2020.

84 **abnormalities in 78:** Valentina O. Puntmann, M. Ludovica Carej, and Imke Wieters, "Outcomes of Cardiovascular Magnetic Resonance Imaging in Patients Recently Recovered From Coronavirus Disease 2019 (COVID-19)," *JAMA*, July 27, 2020.

heart transplants: Jennifer Couzin-Frankel, "As evidence builds that COVID-19 can damage the heart, doctors are racing to understand it," *Science*, Sept. 15, 2020.

8. THE DOOM LOOP

85 **3,656 new cases:** Interview with Matt Pottinger.

"The center of gravity": Ibid.

"We need to take steps": Ibid.

86 **"Better safe than sorry":** Ibid.

87 **"Forget about ballgames":** Quotes in this passage come from interviews with Matt Pottinger, Olivia Troye, off the record interviews, and contemporaneous notes.

6.64 percent: Andrea Remuzzi and Giuseppe Remuzzi, "COVID-19 and Italy: what next?" *The Lancet*, Mar. 13, 2020.

88 **"This is going to bankrupt":** Woodward, *Rage*, op. cit., p. 277; and interview with Matt Pottinger.

"Oh, oh, I got": David Lipson, "Donald Trump's address was meant to lay out US plans to tackle coronavirus. Instead it sparked confusion," ABC News, March 13, 2020.

"We are marshaling": www.whitehouse.gov/briefings-statements/remarks-presi dent-trump-address-nation/

90 **"When Keynes saw":** R. Glenn Hubbard, "Ideas Are Shaping Responses to the Pandemic and a Business Path Forward," lecture in the course "Highlights of Modern Political Economy," Columbia Business School, Aug. 17, 2020. This section also relies on interviews with Hubbard.

Jimmy Wales: Katherine Mangu-Warad, "Wikipedia and Beyond," *Reason*, June 2007.

93 **"We went from":** Interview with Chris Coons.

"If we told Alaska": Kevin Hassett's remarks come from a recording of Glenn Hubbard's class, "Ideas Are Shaping Responses to the Pandemic and a Business Path Forward," lecture in the course "Highlights of Modern Political Economy," Columbia Business School, Aug. 17, 2020.

9. "LET IT BE MARCH"

96 **70 to 80 percent:** Interview with Dr. Douglas Bails.

a hundred translators: David Oshinsky, *Bellevue: Three Centuries of Medicine and Mayhem at America's Most Storied Hospital*, New York: Doubleday, 2016, p. 1.

97 **1.4 million:** Denise Grady, "Ebola Cases Could Reach 1.4 Million Within Four Months, C.D.C. Estimates," *New York Times*, Sept. 23, 2014.

28,616 reported cases: "2014-2016 Ebola Outbreak in West Africa," CDC report, undated.

99 **"Under the direction":** Michael Paulson, "Broadway, Symbol of New York Resilience, Shuts Down Amid Virus Threat," (photo) *New York Times*, Mar. 12, 2020.

100 **$1.8 billion:** "2018-2019 Broadway End-of-Season Statistics," The Broadway League, May 28, 2020.

10. "IT'S LIKE A WIND"

103 **just eclipsed China:** "Italy Coronavirus Deaths Rise by 919, Highest Daily Tally Since Start of Outbreak," Reuters, March 27, 2020.

104 **biological warfare:** Philip Ziegler, *The Black Death*, HarperCollins edition, 1971; p. 15.

105 **Medieval mortality figures:** Robert S. Gottfried, *The Black Death: Natural and Human Disaster in Medieval Europe*, New York: The Free Press, 1983, pp. 45-6.

seventy-five million people: Kevin Shau, "Petrarch, Boccaccio, and the Black Death," *Medium*, Sept. 2, 2019.

"layer by layer": Marchione di Coppo Stefani, "The Florentine Chronicle," www2 .iath.virginia.edu/osheim/marchione.html.

106 **triple conjunction:** Barbara W. Tuchman, *A Distant Mirror: The Calamitous 14th Century*, New York: Knopf, 1978; p. 103.

107 **nobody was left alive:** Ibid., p. 93.

latrines were immune: Ziegler, *The Black Death*, op cit., p. 74.

"The advice of doctors": Boccaccio, *The Decameron*, translated by Wayne A. Rebhorn," ebook, p. 65.

11. BELLEVUE

109 **"I'm a New York City":** Chandelis Duster and Paul LeBlanc, "New York governor dismisses possibility of shelter in place order after mayor urged New Yorkers to prepare for it," CNN, March 17, 2020.

"If you are in": Sayna Jacobs, Devlin Barrett, and Ben Guarino, "New York governor orders shutdown of all nonessential businesses," *Washington Post*, March 20, 2020.

110 **"I hate to say this":** Ibid.

more AIDS patients: David Oshinsky, *Bellevue*, op. cit., p. 9.

111 **only thirty-two tests:** Interview with Dr. Matt McCarthy.

115 **using their phones:** Richard Levitan, "The Infection That's Silently Killing Coronavirus Patients," *New York Times,* April 20, 2020.

116 **eight hundred people a day:** Interview with Deanne Criswell.

storing bodies: Katie Shepherd, "As New York morgues ran out of space, a funeral home filled U-Haul trucks with dozens of bodies, police say," *Washington Post*, April 30, 2020.

12. THE NO PLAN PLAN

117 **"tremendous control":** Danile Dale, "Fact check: Trump falsely claims US has 'tremendous control' of the coronavirus," CNN, March 15, 2020.

"We're marshalling": Jonathan Martin, "Trump to Governors on Ventilators: 'Try Getting It Yourselves,'" *New York Times*, March 16, 2020.

118 **"That would be equivalent":** Interview with Jay Inslee.

"You're actively setting us up": Interview with Olivia Troye; response to query from Larry Hogan.

for their next shift: Interview with Gretchen Whitmer.

"The federal government": Quint Forgey, "'We're not a shipping clerk': Trump tells governors to step up efforts to get medical supplies," *Politico*, March 19, 2020.

119 **never replenished:** Ben Elgin and John Tozzi, "Hospital Workers Make Masks From Office Supplies Amid U.S. Shortage," Bloomberg, March 17, 2020.

least popular governors: *Morning Consult,* undated.

120 **"If you were hoping":** "Governor Cuomo Shuts Down NYC Due To Coronavirus," YouTube, March 16, 2020.

121   "This could be catastrophic": Larry Hogan, "Fighting alone," *Washington Post*, July 16, 2020.
       "redirected": Joel Rose, "A 'War' For Medical Supplies: States Say FEMA Wins By Poaching Orders," NPR, April 15, 2020.
       "We took seriously": Ibid.
       paid $2 million: Ibid.
       disguised his plans: Frank Main, "Pritzker arranging secret flights from China to bring millions of masks and gloves to Illinois," *Chicago Sun-Times*, April 14, 2020.
122   "I hate the idea": *NewsHour*, April 6, 2020.
       "We weren't going to let": Larry Hogan, "Fighting alone," *Washington Post*, July 16, 2020.
       "Vendors with whom": Chad Livengood, "Whitmer: Feds told vendors not to send medical supplies to Michigan," *Crain's Detroit Business*, March 27, 2020.
       "Don't call the woman": Ibid.
       "It's a struggle": Don Lemon interviewing Jared Polis, CNN, April 4, 2020.
123   South Florida firefighters: "Feds confiscate 1 million masks meant for Miami firefighters, rescue officials say," Associated Press, April 24, 2020.
       An order of thermometers: Noam N. Levey, "Hospitals say feds are seizing masks and other coronavirus supplies without a word," *Los Angeles Times*, April 7, 2020.
       "I spent hours": Michael Grunwald, "How the Smallest State Engineered a Big Covid Comeback," *Politico*, July 8, 2020.
       "You've suggested": "I want them to be appreciative: Trump to governors," ABC News, March 27, 2020.
124   "We *were* the team": Jane Mayer, "A Young Kennedy, In Kushnerland, Turned Whistleblower," *The New Yorker*, Sept. 21, 2020.
       "VIP Update": Jack Elsom, "Whistleblower claims Jared Kushner's 'frat-party' PPE task force hampered coronavirus response," *MailOnline*, May 6, 2020; Peter Baker, Maggie Haberman, Zolan Kanno-Youngs, and Noah Weiland, "Kushner Puts Himself in Middle of White House's Chaotic Coronavirus Response," *New York Times*, April 2, 2020; Yasmeen Abutaleb and Ashley Parker, "Kushner coronavirus effort said to be hampered by inexperienced volunteers," *Washington Post*, May 5, 2020.
       "We would call factories": *Totally Under Control*, documentary, directed by Alex Gibney, Ophelia Harutyunyan, and Suzanne Hillinger, Jigsaw Productions, Oct. 2020.
       Yaron Oren-Pines: Rosalind Adams and Ken Bensinger, "After One Tweet to President Trump, This Man Got $69 Million From New York For Ventilators," *BuzzFeed*, Apr. 29, 2020.
       $55.5 million: Mark Maremont, "FEMA Cancels $55.5 Million Contract With Panthera," *Wall Street Journal*, May 12, 2020.
125   "These volunteers": Yasmeen Abutaleb and Ashley Parker, "Kushner coronavirus effort said to be hampered by inexperienced volunteers," *Washington Post*, May 5, 2020.
       yearlong contract: Aaron C. Davis, "In the early days of the pandemic, the U.S. government turned down an offer to manufacture millions of N95 masks in America," *Washington Post*, May 9, 2020.
       "I saw him as the key": Andrew Cuomo, *American Crisis*, p. 122.
126   "cheat death": Daniel Bates, "'Gift from God' coronavirus 'cure' touted by Donald Trump is promoted by a FAKE Stanford University 'researcher' who is actually a cryptocurrency-hustling Long Island lawyer whose bogus science paper was removed by Google," *MailOnline*, March 23, 2020.
127   "My hobby": Nick Robins-Early, "The Strange Origins of Trump's Hydroxychloroquine Obsession," *The Huffington Post*, May 13, 2020.
       "We know how to cure": Scott Sayare, "He Was a Science Star. Then He Promoted a Questionable Cure for Covid-19," *New York Times*, May 12, 2020.

127   "hundred-percent cure rate": *Tucker Carlson Tonight,* March 18, 2020.
      "It's been around": Anna Edney, "Trump Touts Drug that FDA Says Isn't Approved for Virus," Bloomberg, March 19, 2020.
      "a game changer": Libby Cathey, "Timeline: Tracking Trump alongside scientific developments on hydroxychloroquine," ABC News, Aug. 8, 2020.
      three hundred times: Kayla Gogarty and Alex Walker, "A comprehensive guide to Fox's promotion of hydroxychloroquine and chloroquine," *Media Matters,* April 16, 2020.
      "We have to be careful": "One-on-One with Dr. Fauci," *The Ingraham Angle,* March 17, 2020.

128   "I used to have koi": Libby Cathey, "Timeline: Tracking Trump alongside scientific developments on hydroxychloroquine," ABC News, Aug. 8, 2020.
      "serious cardiac adverse events": "Coronavirus (COVID-19) Update: FDA Revokes Emergency Use Authorization for Chloroquine and Hydroxychloroquine," FDA News Release, June 15, 2020.
      twice as likely: Libby Cathey, "Timeline: Tracking Trump alongside scientific developments on hydroxychloroquine," ABC News, Aug. 8, 2020.
      "It certainly didn't hurt": Katie Thomas, "F. D.A. Revokes Emergency Approval of Malaria Drugs Promoted by Trump," *New York Times,* June 15, 2020.
      "opened up and raring": John Wagner and Brady Dennis, "Trump wants U.S. economy 'opened up and raring to go' by Easter," *Washington Post,* March 24, 2020.
      overall is 2 percent: Interview with Matthew Pottinger.

129   a quarter of the staff: Ellen Barry, " 'Total Pandemonium': What Went Wrong at a Veterans' Home Where 76 Died," *New York Times,* June 24, 2020.
      "walking [the patients]": Mark W. Pearlstein, "The COVID-19 Outbreak at the Soldiers' Home in Holyoke: An Independent Investigation Conducted for the Governor of Massachusetts," June 23, 2020, unpublished.

130   "They're not thinking": Interview with Michael Miller.

13. LITTLE AFRICA

136   For every 10,000: Richard A. Oppel Jr., Robert Gebeloff, K. K. Rebecca Lai, Will Wright, and Mitch Smith, "The Fullest Look at the Racial Inequity of Coronavirus," *New York Times,* July 5, 2020.
      three times greater: David Leonhardt, "The Unique U.S. Failure to Control the Virus," *New York Times,* Aug. 6, 2020.

14. THE MISSION OF WALL STREET

138   continued robust growth: Jan Hatzius, Daan Struyven, and Ronnie Walker, "A Break in the Clouds," *Goldman Sachs Economic Research,* Nov. 20, 2019.

144   about $375,000: Raj Chetty, et al., "The Economic Impacts of COVID-19: Evidence from a New Public Database Built Using Private Sector Data," unpublished, Oct. 2020.
      hundreds of investigations: Ryan Tracy, "Evidence of PPP Fraud Mounts, Officials Say," *Wall Street Journal,* Nov. 8, 2020.
      more than $850,000: Aaron Gregg, "The Trump administration bailed out prominent anti-vaccine groups during a pandemic," *Washington Post,* Jan. 18, 2021.

145   "lost Einsteins": Alex Bell, Raj Chetty, Xavier Jaravel, Neviana Petkova, and John Van Reenen, "Who Becomes an Inventor in America? The Importance of Exposure to Innovation," The Equality of Opportunity Project.

147   20,000 confirmed cases: Taylor DesOrmeau, "Michigan becomes 3d state to eclipse 20,000 coronavirus cases, *Mlive,* Apr. 8, 2020.

15. THE MAN WITHOUT A MASK

150   **when masks were worn:** "Considerations for Wearing Masks," CDC, updated Dec. 18, 2020.

two long bus rides: Xiaopeng Liu, Sisen Zhang, "COVID-19: Face masks and Human-to-human transmission," letter to the editor, *Influenza*, March 29, 2020.

failed to detect: Nancy H. L. Leung, et al., "Respiratory virus shedding in exhaled breath and efficacy of face masks," *Nature Medicine*, April 2020.

"It turns out": Interview with Matthew Pottinger.

"This is voluntary": Associated Press, April 3, 2020.

"If you're going to cough": Daniel Lippman, "The Purell presidency: Trump aides learn the prsident's real red line," *Politico*, July 7, 2019.

151   **"a psychological problem":** Sophia Tesfaye, "Newly released Howard Stern Show tapes feature Trump admitting to psychological problems," *Salon*, Sept. 25, 2017.

he avoided his son: Daniel Lippman, "The Purell presidency: Trump aides learn the prsident's real red line," *Politico*, July 7, 2019.

"I had a man": www.whitehouse.gov/briefings-statements/remarks-president -trump-vice-president-pence-members-coronavirus-task-force-press-conference/.

"politically correct": John T. Bennett, " 'You want to be politically correct': Trump asks reporter to take mask off then mocks him when he says no," *Independent*, May 26, 2020.

mask-making factory: Greg Sargent, "New questions arise about Trump's event at Honeywell mask factory," *Washington Post*, May 6, 2020.

"bail out": J. Edward Moreno, "Trump nods at reputation as germaphobe during coronavirus briefing: 'I try to bail out as much as possible' after sneezes," *The Hill*, Feb. 26, 2020.

not just Republicans: "Republicans, Democrats Move Even Further Apart in Coronavirus Concerns," Pew Research Center, June 25, 2020.

"send the wrong message": Will Weissert and Jonathan Lemire, "Face masks make a political statement in era of coronavirus," Associated Press, May 7, 2020.

152   **to show their disapproval:** Michael C. Bender, "Trump Talks Juneteenth, John Bolton, Economy in WSJ Interview," *Wall Street Journal*, June 19, 2020.

"deadly stuff": Woodward, *Rage*, op. cit., pp. xix-xx.

actively discouraged their use: "Media Statement: the role and need of masks during COVID-19 outbreak," World Health Organization, Mar. 6, 2020. Also, see the statement: "We don't generally recommend the wearing of masks in public by otherwise well individuals, because it has not been up to now associated with any particular benefit," "FULL TRANSCRIPT: WHO Press Briefing COVID-19," Mar. 30, 2020.

"If it's not fitted": Jeremy Reynolds, "Are homemade face masks effective in protection against COVID-19?" *Pittsburgh Post-Gazette*, April 24, 2020.

"Right now in the United States": "Dr. Anthony Fauci Talks with Dr. Jon Lapook about COVID-19," *60 Minutes Overtime*, March 8, 2020.

153   **"[wear] cloth face coverings":** Lea Hamner, et al., "High SARS-CoV-2 Attack Rate Following Exposure at a Choir Practice—Skagit County, Washington, March 2020," *Morbidity and Mortality Weekly Report*, May 15, 2020.

guidance be dropped: Leonardo Santamaria and Laura Lannes, "Inside the Fall of the CD," ProPublica, Oct. 15, 2020.

"There will be people": Ibid.

fewer than a thousand: Shan Soe-Lin and Robert Hecht, "Guidance against wearing masks for the coronavirus is wrong—you should cover your face," *Boston Globe*, March 19, 2020.

154   **172 observational studies:** Derek K. Chu, et al., "Physical distancing, face masks, and eye protection to prevent person-to-person transmission of SARS-CoV-2 COVID-19: a systematic review and meta-analysis," *The Lancet*, June 1, 2020.
mask-wearing counties: Miriam E. Van Dyke, et al. "Trends in County-Level COVID-19 Incidence in Counties With and Without a Mask Mandate—Kansas, June 1-August 23, 2020." *Morbidity and Mortality Weekly Report*, Nov. 27, 2020.
Wu Lien-teh: "From the Black Death to Covid-19: The evolution of medical masks as disease control," Agence France-Presse, May 18, 2020.
"the growth rate": Jan Hatzius, Daan Struyven, and Isabella Rosenberg, "Face Masks and GDP," *Goldman Sachs Economics Research*, June 29, 2020.

155   **"Nobody knew":** Aaron Blake, "Trump keeps saying 'nobody' could have fore-seen cornoavirus. We keep finding out about new warning signs," *Washington Post*, March 19, 2020.

157   **53,000 American soldiers:** Carol R. Byerly, "War Losses (USA)," *International Encyclopedia of the First World War*.
average life expectancy: Michael T. Osterholm and Mark Olshaker, "Chronicle of a Pandemic Foretold," *Foreign Affairs*, July / August 2020.
worst natural disaster: Ibid.
nearly twelve years: Andrew Noymer and Michel Garenne, "The 1918 Influenza Epidemic's Effects on Sex Differentials in Mortality in the United States," *Population and Development Review*, Sept. 10, 2009.

158   **one in five:** Rachel Siegel and Andrew Van Dam, "3.8 million Americans sought jobless benefits last week, extending pandemic's grip on the national workforce," *Washington Post*, April 30, 2020.
Over one million: Amy Woodyatt, Jessie Yeung, and Adam Renton, "April 30 coronavirus news, CNN, April 30, 2020.

159   **"In recent days":** Mike Pence, "There Isn't a Coronavirus 'Second Wave,'" *Wall Street Journal*, June 16, 2020.
oldest state building: Patricia Leigh Brown, "Prison Makes Way for Future, but Preserves Past," *New York Times*, Jan. 18, 2008.

160   **not be tested:** Roy W. Wesley, Inspector General, "COVID-19 Review Series, Part Three: California Correctional Health Care Services and the California Department of Corrections and Rehabilitation Caused a Public Health Disaster at San Quentin State Prison When They Transferred Medically Vulnerable Incarcerated Persons From the California Institution for Men Without Taking Proper Safeguards," Feb. 1, 2021.
largest coronavirus outbreaks: Zoe Schiffer and Nicole Wetsman, "'They're Trying to Kill Us,'" *The Verge*, Aug. 28, 2020.
188 percent of capacity: Juan Moreno Haines, "'Man Down:' Left in the Hole at San Quentin During a Coronavirus Crisis," *Solitary Watch*, July 7, 2020.
"prisoners are reluctant": Juan Moreno Haines, "In the Middle of a Pandemic, Prisoners at San Quentin Are Punished for Being Sick," *The Appeal*, June 23, 2020.
In Kansas . . . general population: Beth Schwartzapfel, Katie Park, and Andrew Demillo, "1 in 5 Prisoners in the U.S. Has Had COVID-19," *The Marshall Project*, Dec. 18, 2020.

161   **"the entrance into":** Diane M.T. North, "California and the 1918-1920 Influenza Pandemic," *Boom California*, June 18, 2020.
"This assessment": Roy W. Wesley, Inspector General, "COVID-19 Review Series, Part Three: California Correctional Health Care Services and the California Department of Corrections and Rehabilitation Caused a Public Health Disaster at San Quentin State Prison When They Transferred Medically Vulnerable Incarcerated Persons From the California Institution for Men Without Taking Proper Safeguards," Feb. 1, 2021.

16. WAVES

162 **A third of the population of Egypt:** McNeill, *Plagues and Peoples* (paperback), p. 165.
six million people: Ziegler, *The Black Death*, New York: HarperCollins, 2009, p. 25.

163 **scores died:** Becky Little, "The First Time the Plague Broke Out in the US, Officials Tried to Deny It," *History*, March 23, 2020.
As many as two thousand: Julia Filip, "Avoiding the Black Plague Today," *The Atlantic*, April 11, 2014.
"a human tragedy": Mario Draghi, "Draghi: we face a war against cornavirus and must mobilise accordingly," *Financial Times*, March 25, 2020.

164 **reading Cicero's letters:** Francisco Petrarca, *Petrarch's Letters to Classical Authors*, Mario Emilio Cosenza, translator, University of Chicago Press, 1910.

165 **The Plague of Athens:** Katherine Kelaidis, "What the Great Plague of Athens Can Teach Us Now," *The Atlantic,* March 23, 2020.
disparities of wealth: Emmanuel Saez and Gabriel Zucman, "Exploding wealth inequality in the United States," *Equitable Growth*, Oct. 20, 2014.

17. I CAN'T BREATHE

168 **"a big teddy bear":** Angelina Chapin, "If I Would Have Been Here, George Floyd Would Be Alive," *The Cut*, June 2, 2020.
the pandemic put him out: "George Floyd: What happened in the final moments of his life," BBC, July 16, 2020.

169 **J. Alexander Kueng:** Kim Barker, "The Black Officer Who Detained George Floyd Had Pledged to Fix the Police," *New York Times*, June 27, 2020.
Thomas Lane: Sachin Jangra, "Who Is Thomas Lane?" *The Courier Daily*, June 12, 2020.
"stiffened up": *State of Minnesota vs. Derek Michael Chauvin*, Statement of Probable Cause, May 29, 2020.
largest concentration of Hmong: Minnesota Historical Society.
Mrs. Minnesota: "Kellie Chauvin, Wife of Police Officer Derek Chauvin, Seeks Name Change in Divorce," *International Business Times News*, June 3, 2020.
had a mixed record: Pilar Melendez, "Minneapolis Man: Cop Who Kneeled on George Floyd 'Tried to Kill Me' in 2008," *Daily Beast*, May 29, 2020.

170 **over half of all the Black males:** Dan Olson, "Racial Disparities—An Overview," Minnesota Public Radio, Nov. 2001.
seven times higher: Richard A. Oppel Jr., and Lazaro Gamio, "Minneapolis Police Use Force Against Black People at 7 Times the Rate of Whites," *New York Times*, June 23, 2020.

171 **five times as likely:** Tracy Jan, "Minneapolis had progressive policies, but its economy still left black families behind," *Washington Post,* June 30, 2020.
"The biggest predictor": "The Secret Shame," *brightbeam*, Jan. 2020.

172 **"excited delirium":** Andy Mannix, "Patients sedated by ketamine were enrolled in Hennepin Healthcare study," *Minneapolis Star Tribune*, June 23, 2018.
The police encouraged: Ibid.
enrolled in clinical trials: Ike Swetlitz, "African-Americans are disproportionately enrolled in studies that don't require informed consent," *STAT*, Oct. 1, 2018.
African Americans account for: Joe Carlson, "COVID widens racial gap in Minnesota's healthcare system," *Minneapolis Star Tribune*, Sept. 14, 2020.
first white officer: Catherine Kim, "What we know about the officers involved in George Floyd's death," *Vox*, May 31, 2020.

173 **"very fine people":** "In Context: Donald Trump's 'very fine people on both sides' remarks," *Politifact*, Aug. 15, 2017.

174 **"Our profession is hurting"**: Manny Fernandez, Richard Pérez-Peña, and Jonah Engel Bromwich, "Five Dallas Officers Were Killed as Payback, Police Chief Says," *New York Times*, July 8, 2016.

"We're hiring": "Dallas police chief to protesters: We're hiring," KCRA3, July 12, 2016.

overreaction by the Dallas police: "After Action Report: George Floyd Protest, May 29, 2020 Thru June 1, 2020," Aug. 14, 2020.

175 **"I am telling the truth"**: Diane Solis, "40 years after the murder of Santos Rodriguez, scars remain for family, neighbors and Dallas," *Dallas Morning News*, July 21, 2013.

her father, a police officer: Tristan Hallman and Steve Thompson, "New Dallas police chief's life was shaped by tragedy, self-discipline and Detroit's struggles," *Dallas Morning News*, July 22, 2017.

"We were responsible then": "When Police Chief Reneé Hall stood at the grave of Santos Rodriguez, she made a quiet statement that all of us should hear," *Dallas Morning News* editorial, July 29, 2020.

18. TULSA

178 **"I did something good"**: Michael C. Bender, "Trump Talks Juneteenth, John Bolton, Economy in WSJ Interview," *Wall Street Journal*, June 19, 2020.

179 **stepped on Page's foot**: Doug Stanglin, "Fact check: Devastating 1921 Tulsa Race Massacre wasn't worst U.S. riot, isn't ignored in books," *USA Today*, June 17, 2020.

"a hell of a night": Michael C. Bender, "Trump Talks Juneteenth, John Bolton, Economy in WSJ Interview," *Wall Street Journal*, June 19, 2020.

TikTok pranksters: Taylor Lorenz, Kellen Browning, and Sheera Frenkel, "TikTok Teens and K-pop Stans Say They Sank Trump Rally," *New York Times*, June 21, 2020.

180 **"We've tested now"**: "Speech: Trump Holds a Political Rally in Tulsa, Oklahoma," *Factbase*, June 20, 2020.

182 **"Accounts of the Tulsa riot"**: Lisa D. Cook, "Violence and Economic Activity: Evidence from African American Patents, 1870 to 1940," Michigan State University, June 2012.

The peak year: Interview with Lisa D. Cook.

19. THELMA AND LOUISE

183 **"So, supposedly we hit the body"**: "President Trump asks about using ultraviolet light and injecting disinfectants to treat coronavirus," CNBC, April 23, 2020; "White House task force briefing," April 23, 2020.

184 **"safe return"**: "Pediatricians, Educators and Superintendents Urge a Safe Return to Schools This Fall," press release, American Academy of Pediatrics, July 10, 2020.

"herd immunity": "Fewer than 1 in 10 Americans have antibodies to coronavirus, study finds," Stanford Medicine press release, Sept. 28, 2020.

Sweden would experience: Christie Aschwanden: "The false promise of herd immunity for COVID-19," *Nature*, Oct. 21, 2020. Sweden had 58.12 deaths from Covid per 100,000 versus 5.23 for Norway.

"His voice is really": Geoff Brumfiel and Tamara Keith, "President Trump's New COVID-19 Adviser Is Making Public Health Experts Nervous," NPR, Sept. 4, 2020.

185 **Pence declined**: Yasmeen Abutaleb, Philip Rucker, Josh Dawsey, and Robert Costa, "Trump's den of dissent: Inside the White House task force as coronavirus surges," *Washington Post*, Oct. 19, 2020.

186   "Little lady": Much of this section is derived from interviews with Deborah Birx and Irum Zaidi.

   hundred-dollar fine: Dan Boyd and Dan McKay, "Gov: Mask mandate will be enforced," *Albuquerque Journal*, July 1, 2020.

   "She gave me a tutorial": www.whitehouse.gov/briefings-statements/remarks-presi dent-trump-meeting-governor-ducey-arizona/.

187   "absolutely the oldest": "COVID-19 UPDATE: Gov. Justice hosts Dr. Deborah Birx, White House Coronavirus Response Coordinator, to discuss West Virginia virus response," press release, Office of the Governor Jim Justice., Aug. 19, 2020.

   sat on Birx's report: Chris Polansky, "Local Officials Across Oklahoma 'Blindsided,' 'Shocked' by White House Report Not Shared by Governor," Tulsa Public Radio, Aug. 21, 2020

   40 percent of adults: "Adult Obesity Facts," CDC, June 29, 2020.

   half have cardiovascular: "Cardiovascular diseases affect nearly half of American adults, statistics show," *American Heart Association News*, Jan. 31, 2019.

   one in thirteen: "Most Recent National Asthma Data," CDC, Oct. 26, 2020.

   94 percent: "Weekly Updates by Select Demographic and Geographic Characteris tics," CDC National Center for Health Statistics, Mar. 31, 2021.

188   "We were in your grocery": Jack Dura, "White House virus response leader tours Bismarck, sees 'least use' of masks in COVID-19 fight," *Bismarck Tribune*, Oct. 26, 2020.

   "It starts with the community": Meredith Deliso, "Dr. Deborah Birx calls out North Dakota for poor mask use during pandemic," ABC News, Oct. 27, 2020.

20. THE HEDGEHOG AND THE FOX

189   "We had this interesting relationship": Michael Barbaro, host, *The Daily*, Jan. 26, 2021.

190   "unflappable bullet": Natalie Angier, "Scientist at Work: Anthony S. Fauci; Con summate Politician on the AIDS Front," *New York Times*, Feb. 15, 1994.

   power-walking: Nsikan Akpan and Victoria Jaggard, "Fauci: No scientific evidence the coronavirus was made in a Chinese lab," *National Geographic*, May 4, 2020.

   "being with my wife": "First Person: Anthony S. Fauci," *The Scientist*, May 4, 2003.

   the president pushed him: Jim Acosta and Brian Stelter, "White House hasn't approved requests for TV interviews with Fauci, official says," CNN Business, July 3, 2020.

191   "by Fauci & the Democrats": Alex Leary and Sarah E. Needleman, "Trump Retweets Attacks Against Fauci on Coronavirus," *Wall Street Journal*, July 28, 2020.

   "a nice man": Yasmeen Abutaleb, Josh Dawsey, and Laurie McGinley, "Fauci is side lined by the White House as he steps up blunt talk on pandemic," *Washington Post*, July 11, 2020.

   "He's got this high approval": Morgan Phillips, "Trump says his 'personality' is giv ing him a low coronavirus approval rating," Fox News, July 28, 2020.

   67 percent: Yasmeen Abutaleb, Josh Dawsey, and Laurie McGinley, "Fauci is side lined by the White House as he steps up blunt talk on pandemic," *Washington Post*, July 11, 2020.

192   "I mean the importance": "Coronavirus Pandemic Expert and Holy Cross Alumnus Dr. Anthony Fauci '62: A Man for and with Others," *Holy Cross in the News*, March 18, 2020.

   "One day during lunch break": Donald N. S. Unger, " 'I saw people who were in pain'," *Holy Cross Magazine*, Summer 2002.

   "Could you come translate": "Dr. Christine Grady Oral History 1997," National Institutes of Health.

193   "Curiously, they were all gay": The American Association of Immunologists Oral
History Project, "Anthony S. Fauci, M.D.," Dec. 9, 2015. Interview conducted by
Brien Williams.
"I call you murderers": Larry Kramer, "An Open Letter to Dr. Anthony Fauci," *San
Francisco Examiner*, June 26, 1988.
"No one had ever": Brent Lang, "Dr. Anthony Fauci on His 'Dear, Deep Friendship'
With Larry Kramer," *Variety*, May 28, 2020.

194   "What they were saying": "Anthony S. Fauci, M.D.," interviewed by Brien Williams, PhD., The American Association of Immunologists Oral History Project,
Dec. 9, 2015.
"Here I am": Ibid.
"With AIDS in those days": Michael Specter, "How Anthony Fauci Became Ameri-
ca's Doctor," *The New Yorker*, April 10, 2020.
"dear, deep friendship": Brent Lang, "Dr. Anthony Fauci on His 'Dear, Deep Friend-
ship' With Larry Kramer," *Variety*, May 28, 2020.
"I was on a C-SPAN": Natalie Angier, "Scientist at Work: Anthony S. Fauci; Con-
summate Politician on the AIDS Front," *New York Times*, Feb. 15, 1994.
"I love you, Tony": Brent Lang, "Dr. Anthony Fauci on His 'Dear, Deep Friendship'
With Larry Kramer," *Variety*, May 28, 2020.

196   "This is a war": Andy Chow, "Amy Acton Steps Down as DeWine's Chief Health
Adviser," WYSO, Aug. 6, 2020.
"medical dictator": Griff Witte, "Ohio's Amy Acton inspires admiration, and a
blacklash, with tough coronavirus response," *Washington Post*, May 18, 2020.
twenty-seven top health officials: Jackie Borchardt and Jessie Balmert, "First came
the pandemic, then came the politics: Why Amy Acton quit," *The Columbus Dispatch*,
June 15, 2020.

197   puff of white powder: Michael Barbaro, host, *The Daily*, Jan. 26, 2021.
"I might have to write": Michael Klinski, "Mount Trumpmore? It's the president's
'dream,' Rep. Kristi Noem says," *Sioux Falls Argus Leader*, updated Aug. 9, 2020.
"Now here's what I do": Alana Abramson, "I Can Be More Presidential Than Any
President," *Time*, July 26, 2017.

198   55,595 new infections: "Trump Hosts July 4 Event at White House as U.S. Coronavirus Cases Soar," *New York Times*, July 4, 2020.
"We are not even": Will Feuer, "CDC says U.S. has 'way too much virus' to control
pandemic as cases surge across country," CNBC, June 29, 2020.

21. DARK SHADOWS

200   "Biden says he's going": "Donald Trump Laura Ingraham Interview Transcript
August 31: Says People 'in the Dark Shadows' Controlling Biden," *Rev Transcripts*,
Sept. 1, 2020.
seventeen-year-old Trump supporter: John Fritz, Kevin Johnson, and David Jackson, "Trump defends Kyle Rittenhouse on eve of visit to Kenosha," *USA Today*, Aug.
31, 2020.

201   widest margin: Alec Tyson and Shiva Maniam, "Behind Trump's victory: Divisions
by race, gender, education," Pew Research Center, Nov. 9, 2016.

202   "unbreakable lead": Nate Silver, "The Comey Letter Probably Cost Clinton The
Election," *FiveThirtyEight*, May 3, 2016.
opioid epidemic: Dean Reynolds, "Overdoses now leading cause of death of Americans under 50," CBS News, June 6, 2017; Adam Dean and Simeon Kimmel, "Free
trade and opioid overdose death in the United States," *SSM Population Health*, Aug. 8,
2019.

203 **likely to vote for Trump:** James S. Goodwin, et al. "Association of Chronic Opioid Use with Presidential Voting Patterns in US Counties in 2016," *JAMA Network*, June 1, 2018; Wasfy, Jason H., Charles Stewart III, and Vijeta Bhambhani. "County community health associations of net voting shift in the 2016 U.S. presidential election," *PLOS ONE*, Oct. 2, 2017; Julianna Pacheco and Jason Fletcher, "Incorporating Health into Studies of Political Behavior: Evidence for Turnout and Partisanship," *PubMed*, July 12, 2018.

likely to vote Republican: Julianna Pacheco and Jason Fletcher, "Incorporating Health into Studies of Political Behavior: Evidence for Turnout and Partisanship," *PubMed*, July 12, 2018.

higher mortality rates: Shannon M. Monnat, "Deaths of Despair and Support for Trump in the 2016 Presidential Election," Research Brief, Department of Agricultural Economics, Sociology, and Education, University of Pennsylvania, Dec. 4, 2016.

"If you carry guns": Michael Caputo, Facebook, Sept. 13, 2020.

Vladmir Putin's image: Peter W. Stevenson, "Which Trump associates have been caught up in the Russia investigation? A running list," *Washington Post*, June 16, 2017.

204 **"defeat despair":** Dan Diamond, "'Helping the president': HHS official sought to rebrand coronavirus campaign," *Politico*, Oct. 29, 2020.

"publicly endorsed Obama": Yasmeen Abutaleb, "Trump's $250 million coronavirus ad campaign had 'partisan' edge, down to the celebrities chosen to participate," *Washington Post*, Oct. 30, 2020.

205 **"reckless when drunk":** Zusha Elinson, Erin Ailworth, and Rachael Levy, "In Michigan Plot to Kidnap Governor, Informants Were Key," *Wall Street Journal*, Oct. 18, 2020.

"sick of being robbed": "Video appears to show Whitmer kidnapping plot suspects training," CNN, Oct. 19, 2020; Paul Egan and Tresa Baldas, "New and shocking details revealed at hearing for Gov. Whitmer kidnap plot," *Detroit Free Press*, Oct. 13, 2020.

Red Dawn: Hannah Knowles, "Wolverine watchmen, extremist group implicated in Michigan kidnapping plot, trained for 'civil war'," *Washington Post*, Oct. 9, 2020.

206 **called themselves "watchmen":** Andrew Feather, "What we know about the Wolverine Watchmen," WWMT, Oct. 9, 2020.

shut down the gyms: David Eggert and Ed White, "AG says Michigan governor, family were moved as plotters tracked," Associated Press, Oct. 9, 2020.

Breakin' 2: Electric Boogaloo: Alex Woodward, "Why far-right protesters are wearing Hawaiian shirts," *Independent*, June 17, 2020.

207 **Although the plotters:** "Most suspects share a bond: Troubled pasts," *Detroit Free Press*, Oct. 11, 2020; LifeZette staff, "Report: Michigan Militia Members Charged in 'Whitmer Kidnapping Plot' Possibly Aligned with Antifa," *Newstex Blogs*, Oct. 12, 2020; Kim Bellware, Alex Horton, Devlin Barrett, and Matt Zapotosky, "Accused leader of plot to kidnap Michigan governor was struggling financially, living in basement storage space," *Washington Post*, Oct. 9, 2020.

"Snatch and grab": *United States of America v. Adam Fox, Barry Croft, Ty Garbin, Kaleb Franks, Daniel Harris, and Grandon Caserta,* Case No. 1:20-mj-416, Oct. 6, 2020.

208 **"Words matter":** "Transcript of Gov. Gretchen Whitmer addressing Michigan after charges of kidnapping plot," WWMT, Oct. 8, 2020.

"a threat against our governor": Kelly House, Paula Gardner, and Riley Beggin, "'Liberate Michigan': Months of angry rhetoric precede Whitmer kidnap plot," *Bridge Michigan*, Oct. 8, 2020.

22. THE ROSE GARDEN CLUSTER

210 **"The flag . . . is still flying"**: "Judge Barrett Gives Remarks on Nomination, Pays Homage to Justices Ginsburg and Scalia," C-SPAN, Sept. 26, 2020.

"I don't want to move": Henry J. Gomez and Kadia Goba, "When Did Trump Test Negative For COVID-19? Officials Won't Say," *BuzzFeed News,* Oct. 6, 2020.

211 **had not been contacted**: Apoorva Mandavilli and Tracey Tully, "White House Is Not Tracing Contacts for 'Super-Spreader' Rose Garden Event," *New York Times,* Oct. 5, 2020.

"Nobody from the White House": Brian Stelter, "New York Times reporter infected with Covid-19 says White House is not doing contact tracing," CNN, Oct. 5, 2020.

"disregarding gathering limits": "Gov. Wolf Issues Statement on Trump Rallies in PA," press release, Sept. 25, 2020.

212 **"Possibly I did"**: "Donald Trump NBC Town Hall Transcript October 15," *Rev Transcripts,* Oct. 15, 2020.

"highest ratings": John Koblin, "In TV Ratings, Trump vs. Biden Was No Match for Trump vs. Clinton," *New York Times,* Sept. 30, 2020.

Mexico was paying: "Speech: Donald Trump Holds a Campaign Rally in Duluth, Minnesota," *Factbase,* Sept. 30, 2020.

No one told: Sarah Ellison and Josh Dawsey, "Hope Hicks returned to the White House to pull Trump across the finish line. Then coronavirus hit," *Washington Post,* Oct. 9, 2020.

1 in 25: James Gallagher, "Covid: What is the risk to Donald Trump's health?" BBC, Oct. 2, 2020.

dropped into the 80s: Noah Weiland, Maggie Haberman, Mark Mazzetti, and Annie Karni, "Trump Was Sicker Than Acknowledged With Covid-19," *New York Times,* Feb. 11, 2021.

supplemental oxygen: Jacqueline Howard, "Trump's Covid-19 so far has caused high fever and drops in oxygen, doctors say," CNN, Oct. 4, 2020.

213 **"Trump is in great danger"**: Clara O'Rourke, "No evidence showing doctors endangered Trump," *PolitiFact.com,* Oct. 7, 2020.

"Recovering from an illness": "First Lady Melania Trump: 'My personal experience with COVID-19," U.S. State Department reprint, Oct. 14, 2020.

214 **"I could be one of the diers"**: Olivia Nuzzi, "The Entire Presidency Is a Superspreading Event," *New York Magazine,* Oct. 9, 2020.

"He went to the hospital": "Donald Trump Virtual Town Hall Transcript," *Rev Transcripts,* May 3, 2020.

"Am I going out": Gabriel Sherman, "'This is Sprialing Out of Control': Allies Panic About Trump's Hospital Stay as White House Deflects," *Vanity Fair,* Oct. 3, 2020.

"I'm not good for medical": Marlow Stern, "The Time Donald Trump Turned Away in Disgust While a Man Was Bleeding to Death in Front of Him," *Daily Beast,* Sept. 28, 2017.

23. THE SEARCH FOR PATIENT ZERO

216 **Patient Zero**: Josephine Ma, "Coronavirus: China's first confirmed Covid-19 case traced back to November 17," *South China Morning Post,* March 13, 2020.

"It now turns out": Jonathan Latham and Allison Wilson: "A Proposed Origin for SARS-CoV-2 and the COVID-19 Pandemic," jonathanlatham.net/, jamiemetzl.com/.

217 **"China created this pandemic"**: Jake Tapper interview with Peter Navarro, CNN, June 21, 2020.

"enormous evidence": Jack Brewster, "Pompeo: 'Enormous Evidence' Linking Wuhan Lab To Covid Outbreak," *Forbes,* May 4, 2020.

217 **"I lost the race"**: Peter Navarro, *San Diego Confidential: A Candidate's Odyssey*, San Diego: QT Press, 1998, pp. 231-7.

"Trump Democrat": Peter Navarro, "My journey to Trumpland," CNN, Aug. 28, 2016.

218 **Kushner phoned Navarro:** Sarah Ellison, "The Inside Story of the Kushner-Bannon Civil War," *Vanity Fair*, April 14, 2017.

25 percent tax: Alan Rappeport and Ana Swanson, "President Trump has embraced a deal that his top trade adviser lobbied against," *New York Times*, Dec. 26, 2019.

"engaged in classified research": Statement by John Ullyot, NSC spokesman.

"The disease was acute": Li Xu, "The Analysis of Six Patients with Severe Pneumonia Caused by Unknown Viruses," Master's Thesis, School of Clinical Medicine, Kun Ming Medical University, May 2013. Translated by *Independent Science News*, embedded in Jonathan Latham and Allison Wilson, "A Proposed Origin for SARS-CoV-2 and the COVID-19 Pandemic," jonathanlatham.net/.

219 **led by Shi Zhengli:** Jane Qiu, "How China's 'Bat Woman' Hunted Down Viruses from SARS to New Coronavirus," *Scientific American*, June 1, 2020.

in the distant past: "Middle East respiratory syndrome coronavirus (MERS-CoV)," World Health Organization, March 11, 2019.

incidental victims: L.-F Wang and B. T. Easton, "Bats, Civets, and the Emergence of SARS," in J. E. Childs, J. S. Mackenzie, and J. A. Richt, eds., *Wildlife and Emerging Zoonotic Diseases,* Berlin: Springer, 2007, p. 334.

220 **pangolin scales:** "Pangolins: Hong Kong finds 'record' haul of scale in shipping container," BBC News, Feb. 1, 2019.

"These animals were sent": Kangpeng Xiao, "Isolation and Characterization of 2019-mCoV-like Coronavirus from Malayan Pangolins," *bioRxiv* preprint, Feb. 20, 2020.

found in the sewage: Milton Leitenberg, "Did the SARS-CoV-2 virus arise from a bat coronavirus research program in a Chinese laboratory? Very possibly," *Bulletin of the Atomic Scientists*, June 4, 2020.

gene samples that precisely matched: David Cyranoski, "Bat cave solves mystery of deadly SARS virus—and suggests new outbreak could occur," *Nature*, Dec. 1, 2017.

Chinese traditional medicine: Debora MacKenzie, *COVID-19*, op. cit., p. 102.

no naturally occurring bat virus: Antoni G. Wrobel, et al., "SARS-CoV-2 and bat RaTG13 spike glycoprotein structures inform on virus evolution and furin-cleavage effects," *Nature Structural & Molecular Biology*, July 9, 2020.

221 **96 percent of its genome:** Shi-Hui Sun, et al., "A Mouse Model of SARS-CoV-2 Infection and Pathogenesis," *Cell Host & Microbe,* July 8, 2020.

common ancestor: Jon Cohen, "Trump 'owes us an apology.' Chinese scientist at the center of COVID-19 origin theories speaks out," *Science*, July 24, 2020.

The NIH: Nicholson Baker, "The Lab-Leak Hypothesis," *New York* magazine, Jan. 4, 2021.

collected about 15,000: Nurith Aizenman, "Why The U.S. Government Stopped Funding A Research Project On Bats And Coronaviruses," NPR, April 29, 2020.

"alive and well": Betsy McKay and Phred Dvorak, "A Deadly Coronavirus Was Inevitable. Why Was No One Ready?" *Wall Street Journal*, Aug. 13, 2020.

a thousand-fold: Antoni G. Wrobel, et al., "SARS-CoV-2 and bat RaTG13 spike glycoprotein structures inform on virus evolution and furin-cleavage effects," *Nature Structural & Molecular Biology*, July 9, 2020.

"appears to be missing": Shing Hei Zhan, Benjamin E. Deverman, and Yujia Alina Chan, "SARS-CoV-2 is well adapted for humans. What does this mean for re-emergence?" *biRxiv* preprint, May 2, 2020.

221   **a poor candidate:** Antoni G. Wrobel et al., "SARS-CoV-2 and bat RaTG13 spike gly-coprotein structures inform on virus evolution and furin-cleavage effects," *Nature Structural & Molecular Biology*, July 9, 2020.
intermediate animal host: Kristian G. Andersen, Andrew Rambaut, W. Ian Lipkin, Edward C. Holmes, and Robert F. Garry, "The proximal origin of SARS-CoV-2," *Nature Medicine*, March 17, 2020.

222   **pathogens do escape:** Martin Furmanski, "Threatened pandemics and laboratory escapes: Self-fulfilling prophecies," *Bulletin of the Atomic Scientists*, March 31, 2014.
"It takes only one": Milton Leitenberg, "Did the SARS-CoV-2 virus arise from a bat coronavirus research program in a Chinese laboratory? Very possibly," *Bulletin of the Atomic Scientists*, June 4, 2020.
just moved: Sanjay Gupta, "Covid War," CNN, March 28, 2021.
Dr. Redfield believes: Ibid.
Shi has downplayed: Jane Qiu, "How China's 'Bat Woman' Hunted Down Viruses from SARS to New Coronavirus," *Scientific American*, June 1, 2020.

223   **In 2011, two virologists:** Robert Roos, "Experts call for alternatives to 'gain-of-func-tion' flu studies," *CIDRAP News*, May 22, 2014.
fiery debate: Marc Lipsitch, "Why Do Exceptionally Dangerous Gain-of-Function Experiments in Influenza?" *Influenza Virus*, Aug. 28, 2018.
"virus infectivity experiments": George Arbuthnott, Jonathan Calvert, and Philip Sherwell, "Revealed: Seven year coronavirus trail from mine deaths to a Wuhan lab," *The Sunday Times*, July 4, 2020.
"a serious shortage": Josh Rogin, "State Department cables warned of safety issues at Wuhan lab studying bat coronaviruses," *Washington Post*, April 14, 2020.

224   **"That really took":** Jane Qiu, "How China's 'Bat Woman' Hunted Down Viruses from SARS to New Coronavirus," *Scientific American*, June 1, 2020.
humanized mice: Josh Rogin, "In 2018, Diplomats Warned of Risky Cornoavirus Experiments in a Wuhan Lab. No One Listened," *Politico*, March 8, 2021.
"high degree of confidence": Jeff Mason, "Trump confident that coronavirus may have originated in Chinese lab," Reuters, April 30, 2020.
"President Trump's claim": Jon Cohen, "Trump 'owes us an apology.' Chinese sci-entist at the center of COVID-19 origin theories speaks out," *Science*, July 24, 2020.
U.S. intelligence community: Office of the Director of National Intelligence, "Intel-ligence Community Statement on Origins of COVID-19," April 30, 2020.
"Nature created this virus": Zachary Brennan, "NIH director: 'No way of knowing' if coronavirus escaped from Wuhan lab," *Politico*, May 27, 2020.

225   **"The CREID network":** "NIAID Establishes Centers for Research in Emerging Infectious Diseases," NIAID press release, Aug. 27, 2020.
"Science must stay open": Simone McCarthy, "WHO team heading to China as politics weigh on search for Covid-19 origin," *South China Morning Post*, July 8, 2020.
China forbade: Selam Gebrekidan, Matt Apuzzo, Amy Qin, and Javier C. Hernán-dez, "In Hunt for Virus Source, W.H.O. Let China Take Charge," *New York Times*, Nov. 2, 2020.
There was no mention: "WHO-convened Global Study of the Origins of SARS-CoV-2," World Health Organization, Nov. 5, 2020.
Not until January 2021: Robert Hart, "China Finally Green Lights WHO Investiga-tion Into Coronavirus Origins As Daily Covid-19 Cases Spike To Five-Month High," *Forbes*, Jan. 11, 2021.
"Sometimes emotions": Jeremy Page and Drew Hinshaw, "China Refuses to Give WHO Raw Data on Early Covid-19 Cases," *Wall Street Journal*, Feb. 12, 2021.
spreading in Wuhan in November: Betsy McKay, "Covid-19 Was Spreading in China Before First Confirmed Cases, Fresh Evidence Suggests," *Wall Street Journal*, Feb. 19, 2021.

226 **can remain infectious:** Dyani Lewis, "Can COVID spread from frozen wildlife? Scientists probe pandemic origins," *Nature*, Feb. 26, 2021.

packaging of frozen cod: Peipei Liu, et al., "Cold-chain transportation in the frozen food industry may have caused a recurrence of COVID-19 cases in destination: Successful isolation of SARS-CoV-2 virus from imported frozen cod package surface," *Biosafety and Health*, Dec. 2020.

"reasonable hypothesis": Dyani Lewis, "Can COVID spread from frozen wildlife? Scientists probe pandemic origins," *Nature*, Feb. 26, 2021.

"It was my take": Javier C. Hernández and James Gorman, "On W.H.O. Trip, China Refused to Hand Over Important Data," *New York Times*, Feb. 12, 2021.

"not off the table": Betsy McKay, "Covid-19 Virus Studies Yield New Clues on Pandemic's Origin," *Wall Street Journal*, March 1, 2021.

China had withheld: Stephanie Nebehay and John Miller, "Data withheld from WHO team probing COVID-19 origins in China: Tedros," Reuters, March 30, 2021.

several bats taken: Supaporn Wacharapluesadee, Chee Wah Tan, et al., "Evidence for SARS-CoV-2 related coronaviruses circulating in bats and pangolins in Southeast Asia," *Nature Communications*, Feb. 9, 2021.

wildlife farms: Michaeleen Doucleff, "WHO Points to Wildlife Farms in Southern China as Likely Source of Pandemic," NPR, March 25, 2021.

24. SURVIVORS

227 **"My husband":** Shanshan Wang, "Widow of Wuhan whistleblower doctor Li Wenliang gives birth to their son," CNN, June 12, 2020.

His social media page: Yvette Tan, " 'Wailing Wall' for China's Whistleblowing doctor," BBC, June 22, 2020; Huang Chenkuang, " 'Online wailing wall': How Chinese netizens continue to honor Li Wenliang, COVID-19, whistleblower," *SupChina*, March 31, 2020; Emily Feng, "Dear Dr. Li: Chinese Netizens Confess To The Late Coronavirus Whistleblower," NPR, Feb. 7, 2021.

228 **"Dr. Li did":** "Remarks by Deputy National Security Advisor Matt Pottinger to the Miller Center at the University of Virginia," *Foreign Policy*, May 4, 2020.

still detaining activists: "China: Free Journalists, Activists," Human Rights Watch, Dec. 26, 2020.

229 **Blacks were incarcerated:** Richard A. Oppel Jr. and Richard Fausset, "Klobuchar Ramped Up Prosecutions, Except in Cases Against Police, *New York Times*, Feb. 26, 2020.

about three thousand: Christina Jewett, Robert Lewis, and Melissa Bailey, "More Than 2,900 Healthcare Workers Died This Year—And the Government Barely Kept Track," *Kaiser Health News*, Dec. 23, 2020.

Nurses are the most likely: "3373 US healthcare worker deaths," *The Guardian* and *Kaiser Health News*.

230 **"little or no effect":** "WHO: Remdesivir Has "Little or No Effect" as Hospital COVID-19 Treatment," *Clinical IMICs*, Oct. 19, 2020.

234 **"My grandmother lived":** Aamer Madhani, "Birx tells grandmother's story in social distancing plea," Associated Press, March 25, 2020.

"an absolute necessity": Lena H. Sun and Josh Dawsey, "Top Trump adviser bluntly contradicts president on covid-19 threat, urging all-out response," *Washington Post*, Nov. 2, 2020.

235 **shrank by 3.5 percent:** Rachel Siegel, Andrew Van Dam, and Erica Werner, "2020 was the worst year for economic growth since World War II," *Washington Post*, Jan. 28, 2021.

Perhaps a third: Matthew Haag, "One-Third of New York's Small Businesses May Be Gone Forever," *New York Times*, updated Dec. 24, 2020.

235   **More than half:** Rodney A. Brooks, "More than half of Black-owned businesses may not survive COVID-19," *National Geographic,* July 17, 2020.

"**We are crushing**": Alex Samuels, "Dan Patrick says 'there are more things than living and that's saving this economy,' " *The Texas Tribune,* April 21, 2020.

237   "**bradykinin hypothesis**": Thomas Smith, "A Supercomputer Analyzed Covid-19— and an Interesting New Theory Has Emerged," *Medium.com,* Sept. 1, 2020.

25. SURRENDER

240   **West Virginia:** Laura Strickler and Lisa Cavazuti, " 'We crushed it,' How did West Virginia become a national leader in Covid vaccination?" NBC News, Jan. 31, 2021.

"**This should be the model**": Tucker Doherty, Victoria Guida, Bianca Quilantan, and Gabrielle Wanneh, "Which States had the best pandemic response?" *Politico,* Oct. 14, 2020.

241   **death rate per 100,000:** Johns Hopkins University of Medicine, Coronavirus Resource Center.

life expectancy: Sabrina Tavrnise and Abby Goodnough, "A Grim Measure of Covid's Toll: Life Expectancy Drops Sharply in U.S.," *New York Times,* Feb. 18, 2021.

lowest death rate: Mike Baker, "Seattle's Virus Success Shows What Could Have Been," *New York Times,* March 11, 2021.

had more cases: Neil A. (Tony) Holtzman, "Invited commentary: The Covid-19 pandemic in the United States," *International Journal for Equity in Health,* Jan. 4, 2021.

35 percent of Covid: Mary Van Beusekom, "US leads 19 nations in COVID-19, all-cause death rates," Center for Infectious Disease Research and Policy, Oct. 12, 2020.

242   **Lowy Institute:** "Covid Performance Index," Lowy Institute.

deadliest year: Erin Banco, "Virus drove record U.S. death rate, C.D.C. finds," *Politico,* March 20, 2021.

In Denmark: Jacob Poushter and J. J. Moncus, "How people in 14 countries view the state of the world in 2020," Pew Research Center, Sept. 23, 2020.

"**a voluntary thing**": Steve Holland and Alexandra Alper, "Trump advises voluntary mask use against coronvirus but won't wear one himself," Reuters, April 3, 2020.

244   "**getting hit very, very hard**": Ibid.

"**Covid, Covid**": Jocelyn Grzeszczak, "As U.S. Cases Hit New Daily High, Trump Jokes Media Reports on COVID will Stop on Nov. 4," *Newsweek,* Oct. 24, 2020.

up 46 percent: Giulia McDonnell, Nieto del Rio, Simon Romero, and Mike Baker, "Hospitals Are Reeling Under a 46 Percent Spike in Covid-19 Patients," *New York Times,* Oct. 27, 2020.

245   "**If I can get better**": "Donald Trump Rally Speech Transcript Tampa FL," *Rev Transcripts,* Oct. 29, 2020.

Covid cases often followed: Nadia Kounang, "Many counties that hosted Trump rallies had a significant increase in Covid-19 cases," CNN, Oct. 29, 2020.

"**So much pain**": "Joe Biden Drive-In Campaign Rally in Tampa," C-SPAN, Oct. 29, 2020.

"**a whole lot of hurt**": Josh Dawsey and Yasmeen Abutaleb, " 'A whole lot of hurt': Fauci warns of a Covid-19 surge, offers blunt assessment of Trump's response," *Washington Post,* Oct. 31, 2020.

246   "**The effects of this pandemic**": Bill Zeeble, "Collin College Doesn't Post A COVID-19 Dashboard. Faculty, Students Ask Why," KERA, Nov. 11, 2020.

249   "**They made Pullman**": Tucker Carlson, "Why Donald Trump supporters love him so much," *Tucker Carlson Tonight,* Nov. 2, 2020.

makeshift monument: Kayla Molczan, "Overdose Memorial Honors Those Lost To Addictions," WISR, Dec. 18, 2017.

249 **highest levels ever:** "Overdose Deaths Accelerating During COVID-19," CDC press release, Dec. 17, 2020.

"So, given all of that": Tucker Carlson, "Why Donald Trump supporters love him so much," *Tucker Carlson Tonight,* Nov. 2, 2020.

250 **"I want to vote":** Juan Moreno Haines and Kevin Deroi Sawyer, "We can't vote in San Quentin prison. So we held a mock election," *The Guardian,* Oct. 28, 2020.

Nearly 17 million: Nicole Cobler, "Texas sets voter registration record after adding 1.8 million voters since 2016 election," *Austin American-Statesman,* Oct. 13, 2020.

more than 9 million: Alex Samuels, Matthew Watkins, and Mandi Cai, "More than 9 million Texans have cast ballots so far, surpassing the state's total votes cast in 2016," *The Texas Tribune,* Oct. 30, 2020.

more than 600 percent: Fares Sabawi and Paul Venema, "The youth vote in Texas is up more than 600% from last presidential election," KSAT, Oct. 27, 2020.

two straight months: Anneken Tappe, "Stocks just wrapped up their worst week since March," CNN, Oct. 30, 2020.

Eight million Americans: Jason DeParle, "With Aid Spent, Poverty Traps Millions More," *New York Times,* Oct. 16, 2020.

251 **130 Secret Service:** Carol D. Leonnig and Josh Dawsey, "More than 130 Secret Service Officers are said to be infected with cornavirus or quarantining in wake of Trump's campaign travel," *Washington Post,* Nov. 13, 2020.

naked attempts to suppress: Avery Travis, "Gov. Abbott says National Guard will 'play no role whatsoever' in election process," KXAN, Oct. 29, 2020.

"non-scalable": Dom DiFurio, Jeremy Hallock, and Maria Halkias, "Downtown Dallas businesses prepping for potential Election Day unrest," *Dallas Morning News,* Nov. 2, 2020.

EPILOGUE

252 **"We won very substantially":** Amy Gardner and Paulina Firozi, "Here's the full transcript and audio of the call between Trump and Raffensperger," *Washington Post,* Jan. 5, 2021.

256 **"Be ready to fight":** Devlin Barrett and Matt Zapotosky, "FBI report warned of 'war' at Capitol, contradicting claims there was no indication of looming violence," *Washington Post,* Jan. 12, 2021.

258 **"He's a great guy":** Maegan Vazquez, Ryan Nobles, and Nikki Carvajal, "Trump says he hopes Pence 'comes through' while he rallies for Georgia senators," CNN, Jan. 4, 2021.

"All of us here today": Aaron Blake, "What Trump said before his supporters stormed the Capitol, annotated," *Washington Post,* Jan. 11, 2021.

an earthquake: Interview with Matt Pottinger.

259 **"Kill the infidels!":** "Sen. Patty Murray recounts her narrow escape from a violent mob inside the U.S. Capitol," *PBS NewsHour,* Feb. 12, 2021.

261 **only weapons:** Mike Gallagher, "Republican congressman: To keep safe during Capitol attack, we barricaded my office door," *USA Today,* Jan. 14, 2021.

"I've not seen anything like this": "GOP lawmaker on Capitol riot: Trump needs to call it off," CNN, January 6, 2021.

262 **Dozens of cops:** Nadia Kounang and Whitney Wild, "38 Capitol Police officers test positive for Covid-19 after Capitol riot," CNN, Jan. 24, 2021.

263 **300 million:** Christopher Rowland, Lena H. Sun, Isaac Stanley-Becker, and Carolyn Y. Johnson, "Trump's Operation Warp Speed promised a flood of Covid vaccines. Instead, states are expecting a trickle," *Washington Post,* Dec. 5, 2020.

35 to 40 million: Katie Thomas and Jesse Drucker, "When Will You Be Able to Get a Coronavirus Vaccine?" *Washington Post,* Sept. 17, 2020.

264 **no reserve:** Isaac Stanley-Becker and Lena H. Sun, "Vaccine reserve was exhausted when Trump administration vowed to release it, dashing hopes of expanded access." *Washington Post*, Jan. 15, 2021.

265 **aggressive new variant:** Public Health England, "Investigation of novel SARS-CoV-2 variant," technical briefing, Dec. 2020.

266 **significantly more deadly:** Peter Horby, et al., "NERVTAG note on B.1.1.7 severity," SAGE meeting paper, Jan. 21, 2021.
one out of thirty: Jill Lawless, "Johnson under fire as UK again faces onslaught of COVID-19," Associated Press, Jan. 10, 2021.

267 **another dangerous mutation:** Carolina Kymie Vasques Nonaka, et al., "Genomic evidence of a SARS-CoV-2 reinfection case with E484K spike mutation in Brazil." Preprint; posted Jan. 6, 2021.

268 **effective at blocking:** Alexander Muik, et al., "Neutralization of SARS-CoV-2 lineage B.1.1.7 pseudovirus by BNT162b2 vaccine-elicited human sera." *bioRxiv* preprint, Jan. 19, 2021.
"These data highlight": Kurt Wibmer, et al., "SARS-CoV-2 501Y.V2 escapes neutralization by South African COVID-19 donor plasma." *bioRxiv* preprint, Jan. 19, 2021.
Novavax: Katie Thomas, Carl Zimmer, and Sharon LaFraniere, "Novavax's Vaccine Works Well—Except on Variant First Found in South Africa," *New York Times*, Jan. 28, 2021.
Johnson & Johnson's one-shot: Carl Zimmer, Noah Weiland, and Sharon LaFraniere, "Johnson & Johnson's Vaccine Offers Strong Protection but Fuels Concern About Variants," *New York Times*, Jan. 29, 2021.
effectively blocked: Kai Wu, et al., "mRNA-1273 vaccine induces neutralizing antibodies against spike mutants from global SARS-CoV-2 variants," *bioRxiv* preprint, Jan. 25, 2021.
began designing boosters: Carolyn Y. Johnson, Laurie McGinley, and Joel Achenbach, "New coronavirus variants accelerate race to make sure vaccines keep up, *Washington Post*, Jan. 25, 2021.
In the Bronx Zoo: "Update: Bronx Zoo Tigers and Lions Recovering from COVID-19," *WCS Newsroom*, April 22, 2020.
marine mammals: Tania Audino, et al., "SARS-CoV-2, a threat to marine mammals? A study from Italian seawaters," *bioRxiv*, March 29, 2021.
hundred domestic cats: Sarah Boseley, "Origin story: what do we know about where coronavirus came from?" *The Guardian*, Dec. 12, 2020.

269 **"live with this virus":** Zack Guzman, "Moderna CEO offers a bleak assessment of Covid-19," Yahoo! Jan. 25, 2021.

270 **1.5 million new cases:** "U.S. sets COVID-19 death record for third week hospitalizations fall," Reuters, Jan. 19, 2021.

Index

LAWRENCE WRIGHT is a staff writer for *The New Yorker*, a playwright, a screenwriter, and the author of ten books of nonfiction, including *The Looming Tower, Going Clear*, and *God Save Texas*. His second novel, *The End of October*, was a *New York Times* best seller. Wright's books have received many honors, including a Pulitzer Prize for *The Looming Tower*. He is the keyboard player in the blues collective WhoDo. He and his wife are longtime residents of Austin, Texas.

A NOTE ON THE TYPE

This book was set in Monotype Dante, a typeface designed by Giovanni Mardersteig (1892–1977). Conceived as a private type for the Officina Bodoni in Verona, Italy, Dante was originally cut for hand composition by Charles Malin, the famous Parisian punch cutter, between 1946 and 1952. The Monotype Corporation's version of Dante followed in 1957. Although modeled on the Aldine type used for Pietro Cardinal Bembo's treatise *De Aetna* in 1495, Dante is a thoroughly modern interpretation of the venerable face.

Composed by North Market Street Graphics,
Lancaster, Pennsylvania

Printed and bound by Friesens,
Altona, Manitoba, Canada

Designed by Cassandra J. Pappas